Guided Reflection: Advancing Practice

Guided Reflection: Advancing Practice

Christopher Johns

With contributions from Aileen Joiner, Alexia Stenning, Yvonne Latchford, Bella Madden, Jane Groom, & Dawn Freshwater.

Blackwell
Science

© 2002 by Blackwell Science Ltd, a Blackwell Publishing company

Editorial offices:
Blackwell Science Ltd, 9600 Garsington Road, Oxford OX4 2DQ, UK
    Tel: +44 (0) 1865 776868
Blackwell Publishing Inc., 350 Main Street, Malden, MA 02148-5020, USA
    Tel: +1 781 388 8250
Blackwell Science Asia Pty, 550 Swanston Street, Carlton, Victoria 3053, Australia
    Tel: +61 (0)3 8359 1011

First published 2002
4   2007

ISBN 978-0-632-05975-1

Library of Congress Cataloging-in-Publication Data is available

A catalogue record for this title is available from the British Library

Set in 10/12.5 Sabon
by DP Photosetting, Aylesbury, Bucks
Printed and bound in India by Replika Press Pvt. Ltd

The publisher's policy is to use permanent paper from mills that operate a sustainable forestry policy, and which has been manufactured from pulp processed using acid-free and elementary chlorine-free practices. Furthermore, the publisher ensures that the text paper and cover board used have met acceptable environmental accreditation standards.

For further information on Blackwell Publishing, visit our website:
www.blackwellpublishing.com

Contents

List of Contributors

Dawn Freshwater PhD BA (Hons) RNT RGN DipPsych
Head of Academic Research Centre in Practice (Mental Health and Primary Care), Institute of Health and Community Studies, Bournemouth University and North Dorset Trusts

Jane Groom RN BA (Hons)
Staff nurse, Accident & Emergency Department, Kettering General Hospital NHS Trust

Christopher Johns RN PhD
Reader in Advanced Nursing Practice, University of Luton

Aileen Joiner RMN BA
Staff nurse, Department of Mental Health & Elderly, Milton Keynes General Hospital NHS Trust

Yvonne Latchford RN HV BA (Hons)
Health visitor, Bedfordshire & Luton Community Trust

Bella Madden RN RM BA (Hons) MSc
Senior lecturer, Faculty of Health & Social Studies, University of Luton

Alexia Stenning RN MSc
Clinical leadership, Bedford Hospital NHS Trust

Preface
Freedom to Practise

' "If one has not seen what is, how can one go beyond it?" Unfortunately, academic practice shows little or no understanding of "seeing what is" in the context of genuine self-inquiry.'
Anderson (1996) (quoted words within quotation by Krishnamurti)

This book is a process of genuine self-inquiry as a way of working with health care practitioners in developmental programmes and formal research. Words like genuine, rather like truth, are notoriously difficult to use within a post-modern world-view. By the end of the book the reader will decide whether this is so. My work is to help the reader reach such decisions. Reflective practice is well established within health care disciplines such as nursing, health visiting and midwifery, and it is from these disciplines I have constructed narratives. Like a soft dawn, reflective practice shines a light across the darkened landscape of health care practice. Caught in the glare many practitioners will scurry to their dark caves of habitual practice. Others, intrigued by new vistas will grasp the opportunity of reflection as an opportunity to realise desirable practice. This must be the quest of all practitioners, to know and realise self as caring within everyday practice. Through the narratives of nurses, health visitors and midwives this book explores the way practitioners do make a difference and the way this difference is nurtured and developed through guided reflection as co-developmental and collaborative research process. Practitioners must be committed to what they do and accept responsibility for ensuring they are most effective, always challenging habitual ways of viewing and responding to practice situations with the mindset to develop self and practice. By placing self at the core of the learning process of self-inquiry, then commitment and responsibility are foremost in the developmental lens.

The book is presented in three parts. Part 1 prepares the reader to read the narratives with a tuned eye, tuned to challenge the theoretical ideas for their ability to adequately structure meaning through the narrative. Part 2 is a collection of narratives that exemplify guided reflection. However, each narrative stands alone and can be read purely as a story that illuminates clinical practice. Part 3 tidies up the loose ends and moves the reader into new dimensions.

In the three chapters that make up Part 1, I unfold and explore the various influences that have guided my thinking about the nature of guided reflection as a co-developmental and collaborative research process working with practitioners to enable them to realise desirable and effective practice. While I draw on an extensive literature to frame my development of guided reflection, the primary source of knowing has been reflection on my own practice of guiding reflection over the past 11 years. In this sense, the chapters are partially written as a personal narrative of my own journey of realisation. I have inserted three pieces of text written by Bella Madden, whom I guided through her masters' dissertation, that illuminate the way she moulded the philosophical influences of guided reflection to her own style and, in doing so, expand the philosophical background of guided reflection.

Guided reflection is driven by practical concerns. To realise desirable practice, the practitioner first needs to know what desirable practice is. Only then can the contradictions between what is desirable and actual practice be framed and action contemplated for resolution. In doing so, the practitioner needs to understand those factors that constrain realising desirable practice and become adept at changing the conditions of practice so desirable work can be realised. Guided reflection is the weaving of two strands of *being* and *becoming*. *Being* is the reflection of the practitioner's clinical practice as known through reflection – the stories written in a reflective journal or shared in guided reflection. *Becoming* is the reflection of the practitioner's journey from where she is at now to where she wants to be, as known by looking back through the unfolding series of reflected-on experiences to perceive self as transformed or not. The perception is given form by drawing on appropriate markers. Guided reflection unfolds and weaves the practitioner's unique pattern of being and becoming in narrative form.

This idea of knowing as being was inspired by Doug Boyd (1974). He wrote, in relation to his experience with Rolling Thunder, a Western Shoshone Native American medicine man:

> 'Rolling Thunder ... said that truth cannot be expressed verbally, that it can only be experienced: "You have to live it and be part of it and then you might get to know it." My first step was to learn what Rolling Thunder meant by understanding. Understanding is not the sort of thing my modern, establishment education had me believing it was. Understanding, to what Rolling Thunder calls the establishment mind, is simply a rather low-level dance and shuffle, a kind of churning process by which a number of ideas and concepts are juggled around with the newcomer idea until they all somehow fit together. This fitting provides a feeling of knowing which gratifies the mind. A person simply feels the satisfaction of having all his assumptions fit together, and he says, "I know." To Rolling Thunder, knowing is being.' (p. 71)

In this spirit, the reader is encouraged to read this work as a living experience, relating to the narratives on a personal level rather than as an intellectual observer.

Part 2 is a collection of narratives that illuminate the process of guided reflection and its impact on realising self in practice. It is the skill of the narrator to turn the apparent mundane, the ordinary into something extraordinary, in ways that grip the reader's attention. Each narrative offers a deep insight into everyday practice and invites the reader to relate to the narrative in terms of her own experiences. In this way the narratives intend to be both challenging and informative, and provide a powerful learning milieu.

Part 3 has two chapters. In chapter 11 I reflect on the narratives, drawing out on a deeper level the significance of the narratives. Whilst the narratives are deeply subjective, their contextual nature provides insight into cultural and organisational norms. In chapter 12 Dawn Freshwater critically gazes across the landscape of the book within a view of her own journey and towards a fusion of horizons. Dawn and I agree that narrative is a word that is already threatened with multiple under-standings, some well grounded and others less so. Dawn has a background as a psychotherapist, and as part of her everyday therapeutic work, works with the per-son's life narrative, a depth exploration and revealing of self in its quest to move towards self-realisation. My approach might be viewed as a journey along the sur-face following the signs to the deeper self, whereas Dawn's approach might be viewed as a journey towards the surface from reading the deep signs within. We both concur on the need for an integrated approach to caring as narrative, the inte-gration of mind/body/soul as strands of the human consciousness. In this way we pay attention to complementary ideas within nursing, moving towards an integra-tion of ideas rather than the fragmentation and isolation of much-claimed nursing scholarly work.

Dawn's contribution is titled 'Guided reflection in the context of post-modern practice'. Her post modern gaze may initially feel like an assault upon the intellect. Some of the ideas may be difficult to grasp written in its post-modern style. Yet her contribution offers a challenge to embrace these ideas because guided reflection and its narrative form inevitably get drawn into this genre. Her gaze opens new vistas for the narrative explorer to tread. It suggests that the potential influences to guide our conception of self-inquiry and transformation are vast indeed depending which way you turn your head or follow your heart. But we must not lose sight of the essential nature of this work. It is not primarily an intellectual pursuit. Rather it is an honest endeavour to become better at what we seek to do. For nurses and health care practitioners generally that must mean becoming most effective in our caring and healing practices. It is both our destiny and responsibility if we chose to walk this path. Guided reflection can help us realise ourselves. If it is riddled with contradiction as a developmental and research process that is only a reflection of life itself. As reflective practitioners we learn through experience. We can never era-dicate contradiction because as we understand one contradiction another emerges. Dawn's vision helps to point out issues that are problematic, at least for her, and demand a closer look, just like practice itself. As Tony Ghaye says, in reviewing this book for Blackwell Science: 'I think this chapter has made me appreciate, again, how I must learn to tolerate, work with and understand difference. It's not the kind of final chapter I was expecting.' Tony continues by drawing out some contentious issues from Dawn's contribution – highlighting yet further perspectives. The post-modern turn may challenge our taken-for-granted ways and partial views of being in the world, yet it can feel detached like a cold blade dissecting a living body. In doing so it can lose sight of the (he)art of the work. Tony finishes his review by saying 'Enough. Thank you Dawn for making me think. I loved the idea of writing a text that has to be responded to, in some way, rather than "just read".'

Thank you Tony. In this spirit we invite you to dialogue with this book.

References

Anderson, A. (1996) Introduction. In *Total freedom: The essential Krishnamurti* (ed. J. Krishmurti), pp. xi–xiv. Harper Collins, San Francisco.
Boyd, D. (1974) *Rolling Thunder*. Delta, New York.

Acknowledgements

My thanks to all the contributors to this book for engaging with me in guided reflection. Their efforts made the book possible. My thanks to all at Blackwell Publishing, notably Beth Knight, for helping me turn the rough draft into a fine production, and to Professor Tony Ghaye for his critical and encouraging reviews.

My heartfelt thanks to Valerie Young, my colleague at the University of Luton, for helping me to see the feminine in narrative through the work of Virginia Woolf, and to Roddy McKenzie, for gifting me Ben Okri's 'A way of being free'.

Part 1

Introduction

Chapter 1

Revealing the Nature of Reflection

Guided reflection is a process of self-inquiry to enable the practitioner to realise desirable and effective practice within a reflexive spiral of being and becoming. Such work is of immense value to the practitioner simply as a developmental process. When written as a narrative, it also becomes of immense value to inform other practitioners, especially with regard to situations which are indeterminate and have no easy answers (Schön 1987).

Guided reflection fuses teaching and research as one activity. Being in guided reflection groups is reminiscent of the 'campfire' approach to storytelling, reflecting on our own wisdom as practitioners, giving voice to our personal knowing, ideas and opinions, learning to dialogue, and working our stories into the caring-healing tradition of nursing and health care. In this sense reflective teaching balances an increasing trend towards open learning and virtual teaching. I endeavour to work with students in small communities of inquiry where mutual challenge and support are the norm, where wheels are not re-invented, and where supervision time can be maximised. It's also more fun than being alone. At the core of any reflective curriculum is the practitioner's everyday practice that can be grasped in all its whole complexity and unravelled for its meanings through the reflective lens. Contradiction between beliefs, theory and actual practice is the essential learning opportunity of guided reflection; to be understood and worked towards resolution, thus enabling the practitioner to work towards realising desirable practice as a lived reality.

In a new Masters of Clinical Leadership programme at the University of Luton, students commence their dissertation on day 1, extending as a core activity through the two years course duration, researching self being and becoming a clinical leader. As they move through the course they integrate the theoretical modules into their practice (within the dissertation form). Journeying through the course is like moving through a fair, sampling the side shows and applying what is relevant into the journey.

Beginnings

In 1989 I commenced a guided reflection relationship with Gill. My role was senior nurse at Burford Community Hospital. I appointed Gill as an associate nurse on the understanding that she entered into guided reflection as a study to monitor the impact of guided reflection to enable her to become an effective practitioner. Over 18 months Gill and I experienced 25 guided reflection sessions. We contracted to meet at two-weekly intervals for one hour. In practice this slipped to three weeks due to the exigencies of everyday practice. Our relationship terminated when she left on maternity leave.

At this time, the new undergraduate programme at Oxford Polytechnic (now Oxford Brookes University, UK) required students to reflect as evidence of meeting learning objectives to complete their learning contracts (Davies & Sharp 2000). My role as a lecturer-practitioner required me to both supervise the students' practice and deliver the theoretical component of the module. What an opportunity to link theory and practice through the milieu of reflection. To adequately fulfil this role I needed to be a reflective practitioner to guide the students and my colleagues to learn through reflection.

Working with Gill in guided reflection also enabled me to fulfil my role as a clinical leader in enabling and supporting her and subsequently other practitioners to become effective in their roles and work towards constructing a mutually supportive relationship that is considered necessary to support primary nursing and therapeutic work with patients and families. In this way guided reflection is a *mutual process* of becoming effective in our respective roles.

Like me, Gill was new to Burford. She had previously worked in an acute care setting where the philosophy for practice was very different from Burford's holistic philosophy (Johns 2000). Gill acknowledged that shifting from a medical model mentality to a holistic attitude was very challenging. She was also new to the responsibility of primary nursing roles whereby she accepted responsibility for the decisions and actions she made in contrast to the diffuse responsibility she was accustomed to. The need to support Gill was very apparent. Guided reflection offered this support in context of her lived experience, enabling her to reflect on her way of being rather than taking a theoretical approach about how she should work with patients and colleagues. By reflecting on experience, Gill was helped to see the contradictions between the way she thought, felt and acted about her practice, and the holistic values she aspired to her in her practice. She could feel these contradictions and fathom the reasons she acted in contradictory ways with her new values. She could then explore new ways of acting to realise her values as a lived reality. In doing so she broke free from previous norms that governed the way she viewed practice. She could also reflect on affirming experiences, things that went well, enabling her to get positive feedback and boost her confidence and self-esteem.

As Gill disclosed her experiences I listened carefully to what she was saying, clarifying what she had said and asking questions to help her reflect deeper on what was significant within the experience. During each session I took extensive verbatim notes of the dialogue between us. I word-processed the notes within 24 hours and returned the notes to Gill for her agreement that they adequately represented what took place between us. We used the notes to pick up issues from session to session to ensure the developmental continuity through the sessions. In this way, Gill was encouraged to apply insights gained from one session into practice and then subsequently to reflect on the impact of doing this. At the same time I drew Gill's attention to published papers that contained research findings and theoretical ideas that she might find relevant to the practice issues we were exploring. We explored and found meaning in the beliefs and values of holistic practice that we espoused in terms of everyday practice. We came to understand those embodied forces within practice that constrained Gill's ability to realise desirable practice.

Guided reflection emerged as a deeply interpersonal and transpersonal process. It spread beyond our relationship to infiltrate all aspects of practice as a consequence of the issues it raised. Periodically, we could look back and review Gill's reflexive development through the guided reflection sessions. Similarly we could reflect on the guided reflection process and its efficacy as a means towards its ends. At the end of our relationship, I used a phenomenological 'attitude' to construct a narrative by analysing the learning themes of Gill's practice that were significant for her becoming an effective practitioner.

My work with Gill began an intense eight year PhD project (1989–1997). The methodology for this study was 'guided reflection', or what I then called a 'critical reflexive phenomenology' (Johns 1998a). The result was an understanding of the nature of effective practice and the dynamics of guided reflection to enable practitioners to realise it.

Influences on guided reflection methodology

When I commenced the study with Gill, no theory of guided reflection directed the research process. As the research unfolded, I accessed and critiqued literature from diverse sources that informed my developing ideas of guided reflection. However, this literature was kept at a distance to avoid falling into an epistemological trap of having to justify guided reflection in terms of some extant theory, particularly a literature that views reflection in terms of cause–effect relationships and outcomes. Typical of this literature is Burton's (2000) view:

> 'It will be argued that reflective theory and practice has not yet been adequately tested and there is a pressing need for evidence to demonstrate irrefutably the effectiveness of reflection on nursing practice, particularly with respect to patient outcomes.' (p. 1009)

I have no pressing need to contribute to this argument. Developing appropriate ways to monitor effective practice was a focus for the research, not simply in terms of patient outcomes, but more significantly the process of working with patients. Of course, this should be the acid test of all developmental programmes. Yet to what extent has any nursing educational programme been tested for its impact on patient outcomes? Words like *irrefutably* reveal the facile thinking behind such a comment, reflecting the legacy of mechanistic ways of thinking that have resulted in a neglect of developing and researching ways of being and relating between nurses, patients and families. From the holistic perspective of practice at Burford hospital, such ways of being and relating *are* nursing. I have always been struck by Florence Nightingale's words that 'We have to put a person in the best possible place so that nature can work on them'. If this is so, then understanding this *place* is the true focus for nursing research. The practitioner reflects on creating an environment (place) whereby she can be available to work with the patient and family to meet their health needs. My view is that narrative adequately demonstrates the efficacy of guided reflection to enable practitioners to become effective practitioners and reveal the quality of the relationship between the process of guided reflection and practitioner development.

Methodological influences

In constructing my ideas about guided reflection I have been and continue to be influenced by the work of many writers (see Fig. 1.1). I have attempted to weave these influences within a patterned whole and it is this pattern I will try and set out in its complexity. My understanding of this pattern continues to evolve through reflection with practitioners on the nature of guided reflection. Without doubt, my understanding of the nature of these influences is tentative because of their deep philosophical nature and the inevitable partiality of interpretation. However, I must emphasise that the major influence has been my own reflexive understanding of guided reflection. The various ideas of others have been challenges to look at my own work as it evolves. Hence, I have always sought to understand and assimilate such ideas into my own work as appropriate.

Critical social theory	Hermeneutics	Phenomenology
• Fay • Habermas	• Gadamer • Heidegger	• Giorgi
Evolutionary consciousness • Wilber • Newman	Guided reflection: A co-developmental and collaborative research process	**Literature** • Woolf • Okri
Dialogue • Krishnamurti • Bohm		**Ancient & spiritual wisdom** • Rinpoche • Blackwolf
Empowerment theory • Freire • Kieffer	**Reflective and supervision theory** • Schön • Mezirow	**Feminist** • Belenky *et al.* • Cixous

Fig. 1.1 Some personal influences on my view of guided reflection methodology (Hermeneutic cycle/Kosmos/Gestalt).

The nature of experience

Put simply, *experience* is the way an individual perceives self and others within the context of a particular event or series of events. Such a view is deeply subjective. How can such knowing be known? Wilber (1998, 2000) offers the 'Four quadrants' as a model to integrate partial views of knowing self within experience (Fig. 1.2). Wilber identifies two pathways, the left hand path which represents the 'subjective' self and the right hand path which represents the 'objective' self.

	Subjective (left hand path)	Objective (right hand path)
Individual	Upper left 'I'	Upper right *Behavioural fit*
Collective	*Cultural fit* Lower left	*Functional fit* Lower right

Fig. 1.2 The four quadrants as a model to integrate partial views of knowing self within experience.

Upper left – the individual subjective view

I could ask you to tell me about or reflect upon your particular experience. Reflection is concerned with revealing the subjective world of 'I' by reading the surface signs to reveal the deeper nature of self, a self that may be hidden. Reflection would prompt you to reveal to yourself the way you were thinking, feeling and responding within the experience. Cope (2001) describes these as the head, heart and hand dimensions. Of course your perception of the event is not observable and therefore I am reliant on the truthfulness of your reflection. However, you may unwittingly distort your reflection due to subconscious factors. It follows that such qualities as authenticity, sincerity, integrity and commitment are essential for reflection (Wilber 2000). As I shall expand later, people distort reflection for reasons which are in themselves an important focus for reflection.

Upper right – the individual objective view

However, if I was to observe you within the particular experience I may pick up signs that give me specific information about your behaviour and lead me to draw certain conclusions based on research findings. This is an objective perspective which may or may not correlate with your reflection of the event. As a guide I might encourage and guide you to explore issues emerging from your reflection in a more objective light.

Lower left – the collective subjective view

As you reflect on 'I' within the particular experience, you would also begin to reveal normal patterns of relationships that structure your everyday world or what Wilber (2000) describes as *the shared cultural worldspace necessary for the communication of any meaning at all* (p. 143). You do not live in isolation from others but share a world that is largely pre-governed by cultural norms that strongly, albeit unwittingly, shape the way you think, feel and respond within situations. Reflection gives you access to understand these patterns of relationships and ways they have influenced you within experience.

Lower right – the collective objective view

Besides helping you reveal and understand cultural patterns, reflection also helps you view or place your experience in terms of social systems that shape everyday practice. For example, working in a hospital is a complex social system which is part of the National Health Service in the UK. From this perspective your responses within situations can be viewed in terms of functional fit within the organising system. Reflection will help you reveal and understand the way things fit together and whether the system is adequate as an organising structure.

To summarise, Wilber's four quadrants offer an organising structure to view self in ways that integrate diverse world views. The model guides us to place the 'I' in context of the other three quadrants; a self in context of inter-subjective cultural meanings, within existing social systems and contradictions between interior thoughts and feelings and observable practice. It is the peeling back of layers to reveal the integral core of the experience. Each moment of experience has these inseparable aspects that are, in Wilber's (2000) words, 'intimately correlated with, dependent upon, but not reducible to, the others' (p. 145). Wilber urges caution, that because these quadrants are all intimately related, the subjective path has tended to be aggressively reduced into the objective path. Guided reflection offers a path for integrating the four quadrants from the direction of the subjective 'I'.

In chapter 3 I shall explore the way each quadrant has its own truth claims and shall challenge the prevailing dominance of the 'objective' quadrant's truth claims.

Defining reflection

Wilber's work is grounded in an integrated model of evolutionary consciousness that seeks to integrate partial and seemingly contradictory world views of the nature of consciousness. This 'fits' with a view of guided reflection as a process of transforming self, and here we could say consciousness, as necessary to realise desirable practice.

The subjective 'I' is accessed through reflection and dialogue. Reading the literature, theories of reflection tend to portray reflection as an educational or emancipatory technology, as an elaborate cognitive activity to access and learn through experience. In practice, I have *generally* found that when practitioners *commence* guided reflection, they tend to share experiences that are imbued with strong negative feelings towards themselves or towards those others who they see as causing these feelings. Like cream, the negative feeling rises to the surface of consciousness from the vast weight of experience that resides in the subconscious and which has never been consciously paid attention to precisely because it was uneventful. Over time, say six months of four-weekly guided reflection, the practitioner tends to shift the focus of reflection from negative feelings, characterised by such feelings and emotions as guilt, outrage, distress, frustration, anger, resentment, to reflect on affirming self. However, what is reflected on is just the tip of the iceberg, as much of experience is simply taken for granted within habitual ways of responding to the world. There is a view that reflection may take place on a subliminal level because people do seem to naturally learn through experience. For example, how do people become 'experts'? Dreyfus and Dreyfus (1986), in their model of skill acquisition adopted by Patricia Benner (1984) in her work on expert practice, suggest that people do move along a continuum from novice to expert without the opportunity for overt reflective opportunities. What is characteristic about the move to expertise is the shift from reliance on linear models of decision making to intuition based on prior experience. I assume that overt reflection speeds this learning process.

With experience the reflective practitioner can reflect on self within the most mundane aspects of work because nothing is taken for granted but always viewed with an open and curious mind. In other words, reflection is a way of paying attention to self both within the unfolding moment and after the event. It is a holistic process that draws on all the senses to know self, rather than merely a cognitive process.

When Gill and I commenced working together we reflected from a naive or intuitive sense. The advantage of this approach was that it did not impose a framework within which to fit Gill's stories. This was significant as I came to realise that people tell their stories in their own ways. I describe reflection as a window through which the practitioner can view and focus self within the context of her own lived experience in ways that enable her to confront, understand and work towards resolving the contradictions within her practice between what is desirable and actual practice. Through the conflict of contradiction, the commitment to realise desirable work, and understanding why things are as they are, the practitioner can become empowered to take more appropriate action in future situations within a reflexive spiral of being and becoming. The practitioner may require guidance to realise the potential of reflection.

The emphasis on *being* acknowledges the existential moment of the unfolding moment, whilst the emphasis on *becoming* acknowledges the transformative nature of reflection. Reflexivity is the looking back and seeing self as a changed person through the series of unfolding experiences that have been reflected on and learnt through. Many practitioners do not have a clear vision of desirable practice although they easily sense contradiction as an affront to their beliefs. By exploring contradiction, the practitioner is challenged to articulate and confront her beliefs for their meaning in practice and congruence within a wider community health care community. For example, consider the way Yvonne (in Chapter 8) explored her practice beliefs and framed these within a critique of Government policy and contemporary nursing literature on the role of the health visitor in child protection.

Structured reflection

'While we cannot learn or be taught to think, we do have to learn how to think well, especially how to acquire the general habit of reflecting.' (Dewey 1933 p. 35)

If I asked you to reflect on experience you may be uncertain as to what this meant. In response a number of 'models' have been constructed with the intention of guiding this process (Gibbs 1988, Boud *et al.* 1985, Boyd & Fales 1983 and Mezirow 1981, to name a few). In my own work I analysed my own patterns of dialogue with practitioners to construct the model of structured reflection (MSR) (Johns 2000) to guide the practitioner to access the breadth and depth of experience for learning to take place.

Over time I have continually tested the adequacy of the MSR to guide practitioners, and in response have reflexively developed the model – culminating in the 13th edition (see Fig. 1.3). Using the reflective cues prompts the practitioner to deconstruct her experiences in ways that hopefully will lead to understanding and insights that can be applied to new experiences.

- Bring the mind home
- Write a description of an experience that seems significant in some way
- What issues seem significant to pay attention to?
- How was I feeling and what made me feel that way?
- What was I trying to achieve?
- Did I respond effectively and in tune with my values?
- What were the consequences of my actions on the patient, others and myself?
- How were others feeling?
- What made them feel that way?
- What factors influenced the way I was feeling, thinking or responding?
- What knowledge did or might have informed me?
- To what extent did I act for the best?
- How does this situation connect with previous experiences?
- How might I respond more effectively given this situation again?
- What would be the consequences of alternative actions for the patient, others and myself?
- How do I *now* feel about this experience?
- Am I now more able to support myself and others better as a consequence?
- Am I more available to work with patients/ families and staff to help them meet their needs?

Fig. 1.3   Model for structured reflection, 13th edition (adapted from Johns 2000).

Commentary on the MSR

Bring the mind home

In the 12th edition I divided the MSR into two parts: 'looking in' and 'looking out'. 'Looking in' was the posture or mind-set necessary to enhance the reflective process concerned with finding the place of stillness free from distraction. I wanted to emphasise that reflection was a holistic approach and not merely a cognitive model and that people may need to set special time aside to reflect as they might to meditate. In the 13th edition I have summarised the cues of 'looking in' as 'bring the mind home'.

Reflection is a way of contemplating self, an opportunity to bring the self together, a self that may be fragmented within the turmoil of everyday existence. As Rinpoche (1992) notes:

'We are fragmented into so many different aspects. We don't know who we really are, or what aspects of ourselves we should identify with or believe in. So many contradictory voices, dictates, and feelings fight for control over our inner lives that we find ourselves scattered everywhere, in all directions, leaving nobody at home. Reflection then helps to bring the mind home. (p. 59) . . . yet, how hard it can be to turn our attention within! How easily we allow our old habits and set patterns to dominate us! Even though they bring us suffering, we accept them with almost fatalistic resignation, for we are so used to giving in to them.' (p. 31)

Reflection is a state of mind, like a quiet eddy in a fast moving stream, a place to pause in order to consider the fast moving stream and the way self swims within it. The space of guided reflection can be viewed as a space of stillness that enables the practitioner to reconstitute the wholeness of experience, a place to bring the heart home, what the Objiway Native Americans call Ain-dah-ing:

'The gifts waiting for you are many. In the silent space between the [heart] beats, you discover intuitions. Here is where knowledge freely flows. Peace abides in the place of nothing. And insights occur while being quiet. Ain-dah-ing is the place where your heart rests, where you heart connects to the drum of life. Here is where you learn to be capable and self-sufficient. In the home within your heart you will thrive.' (Blackwolf and Gina Jones 1995, p. 53)

Such words help balance the image of reflection as a cognitive activity. The ancient wisdom keepers know the secrets of the universe and consciousness, whilst the theorists grasp for explanation. Reflection is where the Buddhist and quantum theorist collide in the way they talk of the whole and the relationships between things. Bentz and Shapiro (1998) have drawn together Buddhist thinking with Western thinking in their 'mindful inquiry in social research' that resonates with my own thinking. The word 'mindful' could easily replace 'reflective'.

It may be difficult cognitively for the practitioner to focus on self, especially if the self is well defended from looking in, fearful of what might be unearthed. As such the practitioner and guide may benefit from contemplative practices such as meditation to help her tune into 'who I am' and become more sensitive to self and the ways she responds to issues. Of course, this sets up certain expectations that the guide is able to help prepare the practitioner for this work. Spending a few minutes 'quiet time' before a session relaxing and focusing self will also help establish guided reflection as a special place for reflection, creating a sense of connection between practitioner and guide. It will also help the guide to be more aware of her own concerns and the need to suspend these for effective dialogue and co-creating meaning.

Description

The cue 'Write a description of an experience that seems significant in some way' encourages the practitioner to write about an experience. There is no one method of doing this. In reality, people tell their stories as best they can. Over time they will develop a certain style that suits them. I write a reflective account or story after each shift I work at the hospice as a bank nurse. Consider the way I commenced my last reflective account:

'Saturday 18th August

I love this time of the morning – 06.45 – the day is soft, the rising sun tinges the sparse cloud cover gold. Few cars on the road. I can centre myself and find such a stillness that I find so helpful in preparing to work at the hospice. It is as if I am going to a sacred place. At report Diana does not commence with a few words for reflection to honour the sacredness of our work. However Leslie, who is on the morning shift, moves into this space to say a few words after Diana has finished. Leslie is a keeper of tradition. She chooses a poem which is very moving.

I am working with Sue [the team leader] in the 'red team' this morning. Our patients are June and Sue. Walking into Sue's room she seems peaceful. She lays there, her skin yellow from the jaundice. Her body is very toxic now. Curtains are pulled. I say hello Sue – she opens her eyes yet she is barely responsive but she knows me. She closes her eyes again as I take her hand and focus on sending her my deep compassion. She is hot. I can feel the heat around her head and body. I use therapeutic touch to move the heat out of her body, visualising a cool blue waterfall. The heat shifts. About her liver area I feel the tumour bulk. It is massive. I try and flood it with light but it is very dense. I can take some heat away from the surface.'

Storytelling enables the practitioner to articulate the way they intuitively responded within often complex situations, 'drawing on their own private data base, immediate and persuasive, which informs them of the truth value of any particular concept' (Spence 1982, p. 212).

The cue 'What issues seem significant to pay attention to?' challenges me to sift the description for significant moments. What seems significant in my description? Perhaps the morning ritual? Perhaps my response using therapeutic touch? Perhaps how I felt seeing Sue close to death? My sense of compassion? This cue gives description a focus for reflection.

Surfacing feelings

The cue 'How was I feeling and what made me feel that way?' acknowledges that reflection is often triggered by strong feelings. Boud *et al.* (1985) highlight the way feelings influence the way things are perceived, and hence the significance of paying attention to feelings within relation to taking action. They note:

'Of particular importance within description is the observation of the feeling evoked during the experience. On occasions our emotional reactions can override our rationality to such an extent that we react unawarely and with blurred perceptions.' (p. 28)

I don't agree that feelings blur perceptions. Perception is always within the context of feelings. Hence practitioners' accounts are always influenced by their feelings within their experiences and by their subsequent feelings on reflection. Boud *et al.* suggest that it is necessary to remove obstructive or negative feelings as only positive feelings are conducive to learning. However, I feel they place too much emphasis on rationality as the basis for learning when clearly feelings are so influential. The expression of such feelings is always cathartic. The issue is not so much removing them but accepting them as valid and harnessing this energy for taking positive action. However, feelings can also be positive and reflection the opportunity to affirm self.

One meaningful way to access reflection is to commence by expressing any feelings, as it is these feelings that draw the practitioner's attention to the particular experience. This can be done by writing the strong feeling in the middle of the journal page:

'I am angry'
'I feel guilty'
'I feel satisfied'

Then to ask 'Why do I feel this way? With regard to negative feelings, the work of Pennebaker (1990) and De Salvo (1999) indicate that the therapeutic impact of writing hinges around making connections between feelings and events. This is a significant insight to support the idea that guided reflection is a healing modality.

Stories can be very long and complex. One part of a story can unfold to lead into further stories. Sometimes stories are told that unfold over weeks. The way practitioners tell their stories cannot be prescribed although using reflective cues and writing them in a journal does seem to help practitioners tell their stories more coherently. I let the practitioner tell her story until she pauses. It is best to allow the pause rather than rushing to fill the space the silence opens up. My primary response is usually two-fold. Firstly, to ask why they are sharing this particular experience? What is significant within it? I listen with the intent to unearth significance. Yet it is always better to ask the practitioner what is significant rather than say first what you, the guide, feel is significant, especially if the story is long and complex.

Secondly, if the story has been very emotional or I suspect emotions ripple below the storyline, then I will be cathartic – 'I can sense this is tough for you?' 'I feel your anger', etc., pulling the emotion up onto the surface where it can be explored. With some space between the practitioner and her emotion we can view it with a measure of detachment and even disdain. What is this thing? Where does it come from? What is its nature? What can we do with it? My mind set is to enable the practitioner to dissipate the energy, converting the energy into 'positive' energy necessary for taking appropriate action. This is not to deny or dismiss the emotion as 'negative', but to honour and accept the negative emotion as valid.

Often the practitioner will feel a failure because they feel the way they do. Often feelings are not expressed, perhaps because there has been no culture for expressing feelings. This presents a huge paradox for the practitioner. 'I need to express my feelings but I cannot because it would show I am not coping and therefore a failure.' It is as if nurses construct a stereotype of an ideal nurse and then judge themselves harshly. Jourard (1971) noted that failure to meet ideal self inevitably leads to self-alienation where the self is not available to use in therapeutic ways. As such, feelings may be hidden within the story. Being cathartic pricks a tension bubble. It also enables the guide to reflect within the moment on the way they feel about the emotion. Does the guide feel comfortable working with strong feelings? Does the guide identify with the feeling or the situation around the feeling? If so, better to say something like 'I can feel this myself'. Working in this way with the practitioner is intense and intimate. I once described it as 'this space between us a river of tears'(Johns 2000). Drawing out this energy is important because it may be difficult for the practitioner to talk through the situation otherwise.

Achieving and responding

The cue 'what was I trying to achieve?' challenges the practitioner to consider what she was aiming to achieve and intends to encourage her to become more purposeful and sensitive to her actions. In the description above, I was trying to help Sue find stillness and realise that she was not alone as she prepared for her death.

The cue 'Did I respond effectively and in tune with my values?' challenges the practitioner to surface contradiction between what is desirable and actual practice. Many practitioners may struggle to express their values because nursing is defined from a more functional perspective. Yet values and beliefs give meaning to practice and nurture a sense of commitment, responsibility and compassion. Knowing what is 'desirable' is central to understanding the nature of contradiction. As such, the cue challenges the practitioner to consider such questions as:

- What are your values?
- What do they mean in practice?
- Are they appropriate values to hold?
- Are your values shared with your colleagues?

The cues 'How were others feeling' and 'What made them feel that way?' enable the practitioner to be sensitive and empathic to others within the situation and to suspend their own feelings in order to recognise and understand the feelings of others.

The cue 'What factors influenced the way I was feeling, thinking or responding?' challenges the practitioner to acknowledge and understand those factors which constrain her ability to realise desirable practice, and to consider ways these influences can be shifted to realise desirable practice. I have explicated common influencing factors into an 'influences grid' (Fig. 1.4) as a check list to guide the practitioner

Expectations from self about how I should act? Conforming to normal practice?	Negative attitude towards the patient/family?	Expectations from others to act in certain ways? Need to be valued by others?
Information/theory/research to act in a certain way?	What factors influenced my actions?	Doing what was felt to be right?
Emotional entanglement/over-identification? Strong feelings?		Misplaced concern? Loyalty to staff versus loyalty to patient/family?
Limited skills/discomfort to act in other ways? Lack of confidence?	Time/priorities?	Anxious about ensuing conflict? Fear of sanction?

Fig. 1.4 Grid for considering 'what factors influenced my action?' (adapted from Johns 2000).

in exploring these influences. Exploring these influences challenges the practitioner to position herself squarely within Wilber's cultural and organisational quadrants (see Fig. 1.2).

The cue 'What knowledge did or might have informed me?' draws the practitioner's attention to access and critique relevant extant theory for its usefulness to inform practice. In this way theory is juxtaposed with and assimilated within personal knowing. I term this 'theoretical framing' and discuss its nature in greater depth under 'Framing perspectives' later in this chapter.

Ethical mapping

The response to the cue 'To what extent did I act for the best?' can be structured through 'ethical mapping' (Fig. 1.5). The map focuses the practitioner to pay attention to multiple and competing perspectives about the particular situation, including her own. In this sense the practitioner positions herself 'in-between' (Parker 1997, p. 22).

Patient's/family's position	Who had authority to make the decision/act within the situation?	The doctor's position
If there is a conflict of perspectives/values – how might these be resolved?	The situation/dilemma	What ethical principles inform this situation?
The nurse's position	Consider the power relationships/factors that determined the way the decision/action was actually taken	The organisation's position

Fig. 1.5   Ethical mapping (Johns 1998b, 2000).

Parker notes that 'a number of temporalities will intersect to create an uneasy space' (p. 22). This space 'in-between' is tense with potential and actual conflict about an unpredictable future. Where is each person coming from, what are their interests and agendas? Why are they responding as they do? The practitioner in mediating this space needs to be reflective of her own perspective and its influence in mediating the other perspectives. From this perspective no one perspective is privileged, confronting authority claims for a dominant perspective. Mediation is given an objective edge by a claim on ethical principles to reflect on ethical decision making and consequent action. The map guides the practitioner to view these competing perspectives from diverse ethical perspectives and to review the interface between ethical principles and the ethics of the situation (Cooper 1991).

Mediation reveals any conflict of interest and prompts consideration of ways in which any conflict might be resolved for the best. The map draws the practitioner's attention to explore issues around authority and autonomy to make decisions and finally to examine the way the decision was actually taken in terms of power. The analysis of power ways of relating enables the practitioner to review herself in these terms and to consider ways of countering power in order for the best decision to be made. Mapping enables multiple discourse although some are less influential. However, as Rudge (1997) notes, citing Buchbinder (1994, p. 30):

> 'Just as discourses reflect dominant positions, and prescribe "what is said and to whom; and with regard to who is to be heard and thus empowered by being given a voice, and who is to be silenced and hence disempowered", they do allow the possibility of alternative or *resistant* discourses.' (p. 83)

From this perspective ethical mapping has the potential to facilitate discourse and shift taken-for-granted or hegemonic practices.

Ethical mapping intends to help practitioners 'see' the various contextual factors within any ethical decision. At each point within this 'map', the supervisor challenges the practitioner to understand and balance the dynamics towards making the 'right' decision within the particular circumstance.

Trail through the map (Fig. 1.5)

(1) Consider each perspective in turn commencing with the nurse's own perspectives.
(2) Consider which ethical principles apply in terms of the best (ethically correct) decision.
(3) Consider what conflict exists between perspectives/values and how these might be resolved.
(4) Consider who had the authority for making the decision/taking action?
(5) Consider the power relationships/factors that determined the way the decision/action was actually taken.

Past experience

The cue 'How does this situation connect with previous experiences?' enables the practitioner to reflect on the way past experience influences present actions, notably habitual patterns of behaviour that are contradictory with desirable practice.

The cue 'How might I respond more effectively given this situation again?' enables the practitioner to explore other ways of responding and the consequences of these ways of responding. This is lateral thinking aimed at enabling the practitioner to challenge the way she habitually sees and responds to situations. The cue encourages her to be creative and imaginative and consequently to develop her repertoire of available and effective responses. New ideas are planted like seeds to germinate within subsequent situations. New ways of responding can be watered by rehearsal.

The cue 'How do I *now* feel about this experience?' enables the practitioner to harness together the bits of energy dissipated within the reflective space and focus this energy to take positive action. The cue 'Am I now more able to support myself and others better as a consequence' enables the practitioner to reflect on their support systems within practice. The cue often exposes impoverished support systems, and challenges the practitioner to develop more effective systems. The cue 'Am I more available to work with patients, families and colleagues to help them meet their needs?' prompts the practitioner to review the way reflection on the experience has enabled their growth of effective practice, using the being available template to frame effective practice (see the section 'Framing effective practice' in Chapter 3).

Guarding against a prescriptive legacy

I must emphasise that the MSR *is not a prescription for reflection*. Nursing, in particular, has a culture of fitting experience to models rather than using models creatively to perceive the nature of experience (Johns & Graham 1996). As Emden (1991) suggested, adhering to a model (she used the model devised by Boud *et al.* 1985) may be unhelpful because it encouraged her to fit experience into arbitrary stages rather than using the model creatively. This is a legacy of the way many practitioners are socialised into a received knowledge of practice. From this view the model authoritatively defines the nature of reality although always from a partial view. From a reflective perspective, the value of any model is the extent to which it helps the practitioner see something in its wholeness rather than impose a rigid world view. A paradox of the MSR is that the cues might be perceived as fragmenting the holistic essence of experience, and yet practitioners often perceive experience as fragmentary. Rather than fragmenting experience, by using the MSR the guide can enable the practitioner to bring together the fragments of experience into a meaningful whole. Although there is a logical flow through the cues they are not intended to be sequential.

Whilst I advocate the use of the MSR, I also encourage the practitioner to choose a model that works best for them. Using a model is important because it gives reflection shape and rigour and hence helps to counter criticism that reflection lacks rationality. It is still a sign of our times that we have to try and justify our subjective processes.

The struggle of keeping a reflective journal

By initially using the cues in an overt way, the practitioner integrates reflection within her consciousness until reflection becomes a natural process. Rather like choosing a pair of shoes, try various styles until one seems to fit. Whilst using the MSR may seem straightforward, many practitioners struggle with the idea of using a model of reflection and keeping a reflective diary. Nina was a community nurse respondent within my PhD study. Donna was her guide. In their twelfth session (which took place after 10 months of commencing the guided reflection relationship) Nina still struggled using the MSR:

> Nina: 'I've tried to use the MSR for this experience from last session, but something else has happened. I wrote about that too but didn't use the model. I'm not quite sure about a couple of things. I seem to repeat myself. I shall see if you think it is a reflection or just a description. I'm concerned I'm not using it properly. My biggest problem is paperwork. I find it difficult,

like care plans. What I find difficult is everything that is paper – there's a trend now that we have to write things down.'

Donna: 'Hang on a moment. What are you saying? You mean the diary – you don't find it useful?'

Nina: 'I don't know – it's helping me to think and therefore it is useful. Where I am finding it difficult is going through each section [of the MSR] knowing what to put where. I think I could get as much from just discussing it, not writing it down. The other experience I shared I just wrote down how I felt. I let it flow. I didn't use the model.'

Nina resisted the model because it involved writing things down. She had a barrier with any sort of paperwork which she felt interfered with being with the patient. As it was, the description of the experience she read was muddled. Yet, the corner had been turned. In their next session Nina shared an experience using the MSR which led to a much deeper exploration of the experience. She told how the structure had 'redefined my thinking'.

Donna was acting to reassure Nina when in fact she needed to guide Nina much earlier in the research process to become reflective. This can be done by using the MSR cues as a check list at the end of the session or during a pause in the dialogue when either the guide or practitioner feel uncertain about continuing the dialogue.

Nina's comments reflect the way many practitioners try and fit experience into a model whether it is a model of reflection or a nursing model, rather than use the model creatively as a way of seeing and making sense of experience.

Karen was an associate nurse at Burford who I worked with in guided reflection over 18 months as part of my PhD study. In our session 7 Karen felt that the expectation of keeping a diary was oppressive:

> *Chris:* 'Did you look forward to our supervision today?'
> *Karen:* 'No, it felt like added pressure. I have to prepare for the session. I feel like a little schoolgirl who hasn't done her homework!'
> *Chris:* 'That does sound almost oppressive.'
> *Karen:* 'It has been this time and I haven't been able to keep up with the diary.'
> *Chris:* 'You are saying that makes you feel that supervision is for my benefit not yours?'
> *Karen affirmed:* 'Yes, like this is CJ's research. Why do I spend time writing a diary?'
> *Chris:* 'Is that how you really feel?'
> *Karen softened:* 'Not always . . . just at the moment.'
> *Intuitively Chris asked:* 'Because of your personal life?'
> *Karen affirmed:* 'Yes . . . I do see the benefits of reflection but when I've got more time.'
> *Chris:* 'Is it useful to get these feelings into the open?'
> *Karen:* 'I feel guilty, because it's something I agreed to take on, agreed to participate in and now I'm not regretting it but it's taking a lot out of me at the moment. I was looking forward to that but what with other pressures I'm just shattered.'
> *Chris:* 'I get the feeling you don't want to disappoint me but that you are?'
> *Karen:* 'I'm disappointed that I am not helping you with the research project as much as I could do.'

Karen experienced a sense of guilt in failing to keep a diary as agreed. She had a mind-set that she was keeping a diary for my benefit rather than for hers. Writing had become a burdensome task, made worse by the expectation that she should keep a diary. She hadn't been able to share these feelings with me because she hadn't wanted to disappoint me and because she felt guilty. This perception is much less a problem for practitioners who are the primary researchers. They have to take responsibility for the work. With Karen, as with Caitlin and Tessa (Chapters 5 and 6), the responsibility for the research was mine, no matter how hard I challenged them with responsibility.

In session 8 I picked up the feelings from the last session:

Chris: 'What was good about the session?'
Karen: 'I felt I really got to the bottom of things rather than skimming over the top. I felt I really got to grips with it... I have been using the diary since I've been back [from her honeymoon]. I've written about two incidents. The last session has helped me so much to see the benefit of all this.'

Karen had derived great benefit from being confronted with her resistant attitude. It had also been an extremely productive session in terms of the experiences she had shared. It had been a breakthrough session in terms of finding meaning within guided reflection. She had found a sense of commitment and purpose in her work that enabled her to see a purpose in keeping a diary. I had noticed with other practitioners that the 6th or 7th sessions were often the sessions when practitioners came of age as reflective practitioners. The dynamics of guided reflection need always to be surfaced and resistance worked through whilst reinforcing that reflection is the practitioner's primary responsibility. A host of factors emerge that impinge on her diary keeping – lack of time, commitment, expectations of others, personal–work divide, habit, tiredness, coping patterns, stressful events, social forces, responsibility, etc. Yet at times, the practitioner's head is turned and distracted. The guide needs to read the signs and surface the issues.

The oral tradition of nursing (Street 1992) and the prescriptive nature of nursing models undoubtedly mitigate against writing reflective journals. Yet it is most important that the practitioner tries to keep a reflective journal in order to establish reflection as daily activity and to prepare for each guided reflection session by reflecting on the clinical experience that the practitioner intends to dialogue about with the guide. In this way the practitioner has thought through the significant issues. The practitioner can use the journal to reflect on each supervision session, noting the significant issues that arise and the actions she needs to take as a consequence. As Karen highlighted, one reason for this difficulty is the strong emotional content of experience. As Gray and Forsstrom (1991) note:

'The process of "journalling" may sound simple and easy to execute, but at times it was extremely difficult. Mostly the incidents recorded were identified because there was an affective component. This may be related to feelings of our personal inadequacy to cope with the demands of the situation. Alone, it was emotionally painful to journal events that were largely self-critical.' (p. 360)

The MSR cues are very useful to tune the guide into the practitioner. One good example is found in Chapter 7 where I use the cues to tune me into Alexia. Who is Alexia? What meaning does she give to this experience she discloses about Paul? What does she feel? Why does she feel this way? What is she hoping to achieve? Only then can I respond appropriately to her needs. In responding, I draw heavily on catharsis, drawing out Alexia's feelings into a 'space' where we can look at them. In creating this 'space' I draw a boundary so I do not absorb these feelings as my own, and yet I work towards creating a sense of trust and intimacy between us.

This is *exactly* Alexia's work with Paul. Hopefully the parallel process is evident within the text. By responding to Alexia in this way I role model ways she can be with Paul, *even* without making it explicit.

The need for guidance from another

The last point suggests that while the MSR can guide the practitioner to reflect on experience, it is not adequate in itself to facilitate deep learning. For deep learning to occur, guidance from another (suitably equipped) person is required (Gray & Forsstrom 1991; Cox *et al.* 1991; Johns 2000). Boud *et al.* (1985) describe how they constructed their model as something the student can do for themselves, but note that the 'learning process can be considerably accelerated by appropriate support' (p. 36) and that attending to feelings 'can be assisted by being encouraged' (p. 37).

The guide will enable the practitioner to reveal the way their own self-distortions and limited horizons, and those forces embodied within self and embedded within normal ways of relating, have limited their ability to know and achieve desirable practice. It is profoundly difficult to see beyond self because self is largely taken for granted. This is evident within guided reflection when a practitioner says they have no experiences to reflect on. I ask 'Have you been at work?'. They say 'Yes, but nothing has happened'. Multiple experiences are buried under a cloak of what is normal. As practitioners become more reflective then it becomes progressively easier for them to pay attention to experience both on and within practice. Just last week, I was discussing with Carmel the possibility of working with her in guided reflection. She reminisced about her recent conversion course (from enrolled nurse to registered nurse) and her difficulty with writing about experience. She had no way to access her experience. I was working as a complementary therapist at the hospice and had massaged a woman earlier in the morning. Spontaneously I began to reflect:

'Mary had fallen down the stairs that morning. She wanted a massage because she had hurt her back and felt a massage might ease her pain. I asked her about her cancer. She was having chemotherapy at present. I asked how that was going. She was optimistic despite her hair falling out. I sensed this bothered her, but didn't pick it up. I blended lavender and black pepper with grapeseed carrier oil. I quickly sensed the way stress had locked into the muscles of her right shoulder. She acknowledged this ... and I asked her how she was coping with the cancer. She made light of this but her body gave away her secret. She said she was not sleeping ... I asked her if she had repetitive thoughts at night. She said she did ... I asked her if she had had a good life ... she said she had. We were beginning to peel back the layers that masked her fears. Now I ask myself if my approach had been appropriate ... were the oils the best ones to use in this circumstance? Was it right to ask her such penetrating questions when we had just met?'

Carmel could see what I meant. Through my experience she suddenly realised how to reflect. She felt its power and its compassion. And yet it was such an ordinary moment. Kieffer (1984), in his work on citizen empowerment, noted that the greater the felt conflict the more likely people would take action. Significant in this development was the role of an external person to facilitate reflection and stoke felt conflict. This was an influential idea because I felt it went against the grain of creating 'safe' learning environments. Here we were talking about stoking conflict and pre-empting crisis. This is as true for the guide as it is for the practitioner.

However, experiencing internal conflict, the practitioner may reflect to rationalise or project against anxiety, rather than use such energy as a positive learning opportunity. It seems a natural tendency to reflect in order to defend self against anxiety. Hence the effort of reflection is to neutralise discomfort through such processes as rationalisation. Guidance can challenge and support the practitioner to explore anxiety rather than defend against it. The guide acknowledges, supports and values the practitioner, injecting (to use a medical metaphor) the practitioner with courage and resolve, especially when the practitioner feels battered or helpless. Practitioners may perceive themselves as relatively powerless to change self (Robinson 1995), and need guidance to see new ways of being and ways of taking action to achieve this. Just because we come to understand things differently doesn't mean we can act differently. Powerful forces act to sustain the status quo (Smyth 1987). Menzies-Lyth (1988) noted how nurses tend to:

'Cling to the familiar even when the familiar has obviously ceased to be appropriate or relevant.' (p. 62)

Menzies-Lyth made this deduction within the context of understanding how nurses protected themselves against anxiety.

The focus of reflection is on the person within the context of her or his practice rather than on the person per se. Of course, who the person is impacts on their practice, so making this distinction, like drawing a line in the sand, is always a question of judgement. But any line is always an illusory line. It doesn't really exist or separates the guide from the practitioner. It is like a reminder. It is the same working with patients. The practitioner learns to use herself in therapeutic ways to respond to the whole person. In doing so, the practitioner becomes sensitive to the way she perceives and responds to the other, and the impact of the other on herself. It is the same with the guide. I call it managed involvement (Johns 2000). Guided reflection is not therapy although deep personal issues may arise as a consequence of reflection or may indeed trigger reflection. The guide helps the practitioner to reflect on the impact of personal issues in the context of work related experiences. The extent that the 'personal' is explored can never be prescribed. Just as the practitioner assesses their ability to respond within situations so must the guide, and must refer the practitioner to appropriate help as required. This is also an ethical consideration of supporting the practitioner.

The practitioner may need guidance to penetrate deeper and more critical levels of reflection necessary for learning. I have often had it said to me – 'but aren't we all reflective, so what's the fuss?'. Powell (1989) demonstrated with a small group of practitioners studying at post registration diploma level that practitioners tended not to reflect at a critical consciousness level within Mezirow's (1981) levels of reflectivity. Mezirow identified that reflection could take place at a conscious level – paying attention to self – and on a critical consciousness level – critically examining conscious reactions to situations. It would seem that guidance is necessary to move across the boundary between consciousness and critical consciousness.

Fay (1987) has suggested that practitioners need to be open, curious and committed to their practice as prerequisite to reflection. Practitioners may have become used to viewing the world out of just one window and thus limiting their view of the whole landscape of practice. As O'Donohue (1997) suggests, this may have led to habitual action (which may or may not be appropriate) and complacency. The guide helps the practitioner open the shutters to all the windows in the practitioner's mind to view self and practice from new angles opening new vistas of possibility. *Opening* self engenders a curiosity – 'is there a better way of doing this?'. The guide can plant and water seeds *of doubt* in order to undermine and eventually overthrow the inappropriate dominant habits of mind that feed an accepted order of things (Margolis 1993). To be open and curious requires commitment. People pay attention to things because these matter to them. Hence the guide acts to nurture the practitioner's commitment to her practice that may have become numbed or blunted for whatever reasons (and is therefore diminishing the motivation to reflect).

Framing perspectives

Another reason the practitioner may need guidance is in order to fulfil the scope of potential learning. A comprehensive approach to scope of potential learning is offered through the use of framing perspectives. Each of these perspectives is written as a cue to challenge the practitioner to explore the reflective learning potential (Fig. 1.6).

Philosophical framing

Philosophical framing helps the practitioner to know the nature of desirable practice. Hence, when the practitioner responds to the MSR cue 'What was I trying to achieve?', the response is in terms of both functional and philosophical levels of understanding. Clearly, the effective practitioner requires a clear and *valid* vision to give purpose and direction to her practice. I emphasise *valid* because beliefs and values are confronted for their appropriateness within a wider, contemporary view of the nature of nursing and health care.

The practitioner's values are explored in each narrative in this book. In reading Chapter 8 ask yourself – What are Yvonne's values as a health visitor? Should she hold certain beliefs or values? What is her role working with the mother and her children? How does she balance the potential tension of responding in terms of what is therapeutic for the mother and safe for the children? How does she pitch herself within this tension? Should she help Helen create the conditions where child abuse will not recur, or to protect the children when it does occur?

	How has this experience enabled me to:
Philosophical	Confront and clarify my beliefs and values that constitute desirable practice?
Role	Clarify my role boundaries and authority and power relationships with others?
Theoretical	Access, critique and assimilate relevant theory within personal knowing in ways that enable me to make sense of my experience and inform my practice?
Reality perspective	Accept and understand that sometimes I cannot change things quickly because of forces within practice, whilst challenging and supporting me to become empowered to act in new, more congruent ways?
Problem	Focus, understand and explore new ways to solve particular problems in my practice?
Temporal	Make connection between the present experience and past experiences whilst anticipating how I might respond in future situations?
Parallel process	Make connections between the learning process in supervision and clinical practice?
Developmental	Become a more effective practitioner?

Fig. 1.6 Framing perspectives.

Role framing

Each experience is bounded by the practitioner's sense of role and relationships between one's role and others. Hence reflection explicitly seeks to clarify role boundaries with others and enhance the practitioner's sense of autonomy, authority and responsibility, besides developing effective ways of working with others towards mutual goals.

As with values, the exploration of role boundaries are explored in each narrative. Again, in reading Chapter 8, ask yourself – 'What are the boundaries of Yvonne's role and role relationships with social workers? Who has authority for making decisions?' In her narrative, the answer to these questions are unclear and yet are fundamental to realising desirable and effective practice. In our relationship I was conscious of enabling Yvonne to expand her sense of discretionary autonomy to take action into areas of authority traditionally claimed by other workers. Hence role is always viewed as the pattern of relating between roles.

Theoretical framing

Reflection creates the opportunity to juxtapose extant theory with personal knowing at the moment when such theory seems appropriate to inform or frame emergent issues. In this way, theory is a hook to hang upon, and can be more easily accessed and assimilated into everyday practice. From this perspective, theory is not accepted on face value but critiqued for its value to inform or frame emerging practice issues.

Realistic perspective framing

A significant aspect of learning is to understand the way things are embodied within self and embedded within social norms and reinforced within everyday patterns of relating, and the way these forces constrain the ability to realise desirable practice. Fay considered the limits of rationality for bringing about change, for example, issues around authority, prejudice, false consciousness and embodiment. Fay (1987) notes:

> 'The goal of critical social science is not only to facilitate methodical self-reflection necessary to produce rational clarity, but to dissolve those barriers which prevent people from living in accordance with their genuine will. Put another way, its aim is to help people not only become transparent to themselves but also to cease being mere objects in the world, passive victims dominated by forces external to them.' (p. 75)

Fay summarises these forces as both embodied and embedded limits to rational change:

'Epistemological limits	(1) that adequate information can be gleaned from the situation to sufficiently inform new ways of responding [opacity or self-transparency] (2) the inability to reach consensus to act [reason is clouded by self-interest]
Therapeutic limits	the inability of rational reflection to shift beliefs or patterns of normal behaviour – impervious or at least difficult to change [the impact of tradition]
Ethical limits	acknowledging the point whereby rational reflection would result in a less desirable state or chaos.
Power limits	acknowledging those forces that constrain people to be self-determining and autonomous.'

Just because we can understand something differently does not mean we can change it. In response the guide supports the practitioner to 'live with and chip away these forces' as a process over time whilst keeping in focus a strong vision of what she wants to achieve. As with the sculptor chipping away with his hammer and chisel at the slab of grey rock, every stroke is purposeful towards creating his beautiful image as a lived reality.

There is a significant ethical dimension to pushing people against barriers they cannot overcome, to which the guided reflection researcher must be sensitive. Examples of this are to be found in both Tessa's and Caitlin's narratives (Chapters 5 and 6). Both are stories that reveal the barriers that constrained achievement as if hidden monsters were lurking in the shadows.

Problem framing

As the guide pays attention and listens to the practitioner's story within guided reflection, they are listening with a view to clarifying significant issues and helping the practitioner to frame any dilemmas or problems within the particular experience. Once framed, the practitioner can see the thing for what it is and focus her mind towards resolving. In this sense guided reflection is an action research process (Kemmis 1985) of problem identification, understanding, resolution, action and evaluation – within a reflexive spiral.

Temporal framing

Consider the flow of experience within the narratives, the way experience loops together to give the narrative its distinct pattern, coherence and reflexive dimension, linking the present with the past whilst anticipating the future.

Parallel process framing

This framing pays attention to the parallel nature of guided reflection and clinical practice. For example, the plot of Yvonne's narrative (Chapter 8) is the parallel growth of her own and her client's empowerment as inter-linking spirals that weave together and unfold this realisation. Hence, the relationship between myself and Yvonne is acted out between Yvonne and Helen. The way I respond to Yvonne is a role model for the way she can respond to Helen. In parallel process framing these dynamics are surfaced and worked with consciously even though they operate on a more subliminal level.

This also reflects the way guided reflection and clinical practice mirror each other as holistic practices. Just as the practitioner needs to know what meaning the (health event) experience has for the person/family in order to respond appropriately to help that person/family make best decisions and take appropriate action to meet their health needs, so the guide responds likewise to the practitioner.

Developmental framing

Consider the way each narrative plots the practitioner's way of realising desirable practice by either constructing appropriate framing structures within the unfolding research process or by accessing and juxtaposing structures from extant theory. I often convert theory into a map (mapping techniques) to guide the practitioner to review self within the theory.

Process

The emphasis of guided reflection is on the process of development rather than on the outcome. Pirsig (1974) helps us to reflect on the meaning of process:

'Mountains should be climbed with as little effort as possible and without desire. The reality of your own nature should determine your speed. If you are restless, speed up. If you become winded slow down. You climb the mountain in an equilibrium between restlessness and exhaustion. Then, when you're no longer thinking ahead, each footstep isn't just a means to an end but a unique event in itself. This leaf has jagged edges. This rock looks loose. From this place the snow is less visible, even though closer. These are the things you should notice anyway. To live only for some future goal is shallow. It's the sides of the mountain which sustain life, not the top. Here's where things grow. But of course, without the top you can't have any sides. It's the top that defines the sides.' (p. 208)

In guided reflection, it is the day to day journey that is focused on, moving across the landscape of practice like adventurers discovering the delights and pitfalls. The metaphor of climbing the mountain seems apt to represent a journey of transformation. The guide and practitioner know what they are working towards. Yet is the attention to detail that exposes the learning opportunity of each step. Only then is the present linked to past experiences and future practice anticipated that draws out the continuity of self through consciousness. The guide like a guide wire helps the practitioner to see self unfolding, evolving within the reflexive spiral of being and becoming. I have already noted the significance of the practitioner setting the pace along this journey and the need for the guide to be tuned into this pace. This does not mean the guide has to accept the pace. They can raise it as a concern, yet at the end of the day it is the practitioner's journey. The top of the mountain, the goal, is the plot that gives direction and purpose to the journey.

Over guidance

The practitioner may need guidance to find her own way rather than follow a well-worn path. Many practitioners may prefer to follow a well-worn path because it is so well sign-posted and because they have been used to prescriptive pathways that tell them how to do something, rather than working out the best way for themselves. Again Pirsig's words (1974) give pause for reflection:

'Some people travel into the mountain accompanied by experienced guides who know the best and least dangerous routes by which they arrive at their destination. Still others, inexperienced and untrusting, attempt to make their own routes. Few of these are successful, but occasionally some, by sheer will and luck and grace, do make it. Once there, they become more aware than any of the others that there's no single or fixed number of routes.' (p. 191)

Pirsig's words are a travel warning. Guides can lead you astray. They can lead you along a familiar and safe route limiting the breadth of view and taking you away from the edges where the widest and most creative views are to be seen. The latter may be harder work and may get you into some difficulty but the rewards can be substantial. Yet climbing alone can be arduous and tricky so it's important to find the right guide who gives you enough rope to explore and yet is always at hand in case of difficulty to support the practitioner when the consequences create distress. The good guide is careful not to be directive or judgemental. Being directive and judgemental are projections of the guide's own covert agenda and imposition of values. The guide's only agenda is to enable the practitioner to learn well through reflection to realise desirable work.

'The ancient masters
Didn't try to educate people,
But kindly taught them to not-know.

When they think that they know the answers,
People are difficult to guide.
When they know they don't know,
People can find their own way.'

Lao Tzu (1999)

References

Benner, P. (1984) *From Novice to Expert*. Addison-Wesley, Menlo Park.
Bentz, V. & Shapiro, J. (1998) *Mindful Inquiry in Social Research*. Sage, Thousand Oaks.
Boud, D., Keogh, R. & Walker, D. (1985) Promoting reflection in learning: a model. In *Reflection: Turning experience into learning*. (eds Boud D., Keogh R., & Walker D.) pp. 18–40. Kogan Page, London.
Boyd, E. & Fales, A. (1983) Reflective learning: key to learning from experience. *Journal of Humanistic Pyschology*, 23, 99–117.
Buchbinder, D. (1994) *Masculinities and Identities*. Melbourne University Press, Melbourne.
Burton, A. (2000) Reflection: nursing's practice and education panacea? *Journal of Advanced Nursing*, **31**(5) 1009–17.
Cooper, M. (1991) Principle-oriented ethics and the ethic of care: a creative tension. *Advances in Nursing Science*, **14**(2) 22–31.
Cope, M. (2001) *Lead Yourself: be where others will follow*. Pearson Education Books, London.
Cox, H., Hickson, P. & Taylor, B. (1991) Exploring reflection: knowing and constructing practice. In *Towards a Discipline of Nursing* (eds Gray G. & Pratt R.). Churchill Livingstone, Melbourne.
Davies, C. & Sharp, P. (2000) The assessment and evaluation of reflection. In *Reflective Practice in Nursing* (eds Bulman C. & Burns S.). Blackwell Science, Oxford.
De Salvo, L. (1999) *Writing as a Way of Healing: how telling our stories transforms our lives*. The Women's Press, London.
Dewey, J. (1933) *How We Think*. J.C. Heath, Boston.
Dreyfus, H. & Dreyfus, S. (1986) *Mind over Machine*. Free Press, New York.
Emden, C. (1991) Becoming a reflective practitioner. In *Towards a Discipline of Nursing* (eds Gray G. & Pratt R.). Churchill Livingstone, Melbourne.
Fay, B. (1987) *Critical Social Science*. Polity Press, Cambridge.
Gibbs, G. (1988) *Learning by Doing: A guide to teaching and learning methods*. Further Education Unit, Oxford Polytechnic (now Oxford Brookes University), Oxford.
Gray, G. & Forsstrom, S. (1991)) Generating theory from practice: the reflective technique. In *Towards a Discipline of Nursing* (eds Gray G & Pratt R.). Churchill Livingstone, Melbourne.
Johns, C. (1998a) *Becoming an effective practitioner through guided reflection*. PhD thesis, The Open University.
Johns, C. (1998b) Unravelling the dilemmas of everyday nursing practice. *Nursing Ethics*, 6, 287–98.
Johns, C. (2000) *Becoming a Reflective Practitioner*. Blackwell Science, Oxford.

Johns, C. & Graham, J. (1996) Using a reflective model of nursing and guided reflection. *Nursing Standard*, **11**(2) 34–8.

Jones, Blackwolf & Jones, G. (1995) *Listen to the Drum*. Commune-A-Key, Salt Lake City.

Jourard, S. (1971) *The Transparent Self*. Van Nostrand, Norwalk.

Kemmis, S. (1985) Action research and the politics of reflection. In *Reflection: turning experience into learning* (eds Boud D., Keogh R. & Walker D.). Kogan Page, New York.

Kieffer, C. (1984) Citizen empowerment: a developmental perspective. *Prevention in Human Services*, **84**(3) 9–36.

Margolis, H. (1993) *Paradigms and Barriers: how habits of mind govern scientific beliefs*. University of Chicago Press, Chicago.

Menzies-Lyth, I. (1988) A case study in the functioning of social systems as a defence against anxiety. In *Containing Anxiety in Institutions: selected essays*, pp. 43–85. Free Association Books, London.

Mezirow, J. (1981) A critical theory of adult learning and education. *Adult Education*, 32, 3–24.

O'Donohue, J. (1997) *Anan Cara: spiritual wisdom from the Celtic world*. Bantam Press, London.

Parker, J. (1997) The body as text and the body as living flesh. In *The Body in Nursing* (ed. J. Lawler). Churchill Livingstone, Melbourne.

Pennebaker, J. (1990) *Opening Up: the healing power of confiding in others*. Morrow, New York.

Pirsig, R. (1974) *Zen and the Art of Motorcycle Maintenance*. Vintage, London.

Powell, J. (1989) The reflective practitioner in nursing. *Journal of Advanced Nursing*, 14, 824–32.

Rinpoche, S. (1992) *The Tibetan Book of Living and Dying*. Rider, London.

Robinson, A. (1995) Transformative 'cultural shifts' in nursing; participatory action research and the 'project of possibility'. *Nursing Inquiry*, 2(2) 65–74.

Rudge, T. (1997) Discourses, metaphor and bodies: boundaries and the skin. In *The Body in Nursing* (ed. Lawler J.). Churchill Livingstone, Melbourne.

Schön, D. (1987) *Educating the Reflective Practitioner*. Jossey-Bass, London.

Senge, P. (1991) *The Fifth Discipline*. Century Business, London.

Smyth, J. (1987) *A Rationale for Teachers' Critical Pedagogy*. Deakin University Press, Victoria.

Spence, D.P. (1982) *Narrative Truth and Historical Truth: meaning and interpretation in psycho-analysis*. WW Norton & Co., New York.

Street, A. (1992) *Inside Nursing: a critical ethnography of clinical nursing practice*. State University of New York Press, New York.

Tzu, L. (1999) *Tao Te Ching* (trans. Stephen Mitchell). Frances Lincoln, London.

Wilber, K. (1998) The eye of spirit: an integral vision for a world gone slightly mad. Shambhala, Boston.

Wilber, K. (2000) *Sex, Ecology, Spirituality: the spirit of evolution*. Shambhala, Boston.

Chapter 2

Collaboration, Dialogue and the Emergence of Voice

The essence of guided reflection is the dialogue between the guide and practitioner(s). Dialogue resonates with collaborative research theory. Reason (1988) refers to collaboration as a form of co-operative inquiry where all who participate are co-workers who contribute to the design and management of the research as a mutual process of co-inquiry, negotiated social action and personal development. It intends a harmonising of power within the relationship in order for dialogue to flourish. However, this may be easier said then done. People's shared backgrounds do not necessarily lend themselves to collaborative work within a prevailing bureaucratic health care service culture that is characterised by an emphasis on authoritative ways of relating (positional, sanction and rewards type of power relating) that reinforce subordination and dependency. In contrast, a collaborative culture is characterised by facilitative ways of relating (relational and expert) that reinforce agency and responsibility. (These types of leadership power are identified by French and Raven (1968) and provide a useful grid for understanding the way power is used within organisations (Johns 2000).)

Contracting the guided reflection relationship

In contracting our guided reflection relationship, Gill and I explicitly stated our intention to construct a collaborative relationship, not just for our developmental relationship, but also for our practice relationship within the philosophy of primary nursing. As we had both been socialised into our respective roles within bureaucratic organisational ways of relating, we needed to actively construct this collaborative relationship within an understanding of the authority and *relationships* between roles. As Greenwood *et al.* (1993) note:

> 'participation is a process that must be generated. It begins with participatory intent and continues by building participatory processes into the activity within the limits set by the participants and the conditions.' (p. 175).

Collaboration has to be actively constructed because it does not usually exist within normal relationships within clinical practice or academic institutions (despite rhetoric to the contrary). Inequality is normal and hence may not be perceived as a problem that needs addressing within the research relationship. In my experience, inequality often seems grounded in a need for the guide to manage her anxiety for several reasons. The guide may identify with the practitioner's performance as a reflection of her own ability. If the research project is registered as a research degree, the guide may want *her student* to achieve a high grade and may thus interfere with the agenda to manage this anxiety, especially if the practitioner is not performing well. This may encourage the guide to 'fix' problems for the practitioner rather than enable the practitioner to fix her own problems. The guide may feel constrained by the academic regulations to fit the research into some approved scheme of what a *normal* research project should look like. As a consequence the guide flips into authoritative or parental mode, either critical at her naughty or rebellious child, or nurturing towards her suffering child. Either way is a contradiction with collaboration.

Backgrounds

In our effort to establish a genuine collaborative relationship Gill and I surfaced our 'backgrounds'as a potential threat. Heidegger (1962) terms *background* as a pre-reflective state that leads people to respond to others in certain ways. Heidegger (1962) noted that the researcher's background will inevitably influence understanding simply because they exist in the world. In other words, I saw Gill's experiences through the lens of my own background, just as her background was a significant factor in the way she saw and responded to the patient or family. Hence, in order to respond to Gill's agenda, I needed to be sensitive to both hers and my own background and manage my concerns so they did not interfere with enabling Gill to see and respond to her own agenda. Spence (1982) suggests the significance of this position in an effort to see the world as the practitioner sees it:

> 'we try to imagine how the person is experiencing the world – we are then in a better position to understand her/his choice of words and to respond to his/her particular shades and colours.' (p. 112)

The guide needs to be conscious of the risk of listening through filters of their own concerns and interests, or established ways of seeing things. These may block sensitive listening, or lead the guide to project a meaning prematurely, especially when what is being said 'fits' some scheme (Spence 1982). Because Gill and I inhabited a similar social world, our backgrounds would reflect commonalties that would give me access between the lines of what she was saying but which might also tempt me to draw conclusions based on my own experiences. Street (1992) noted from her critical ethnography of nursing practice the way

> 'nurses' backgrounds shared common meanings concerning taken-for-granted knowledge about how things are understood and done. These meanings make up what it means to be a nurse and therefore powerfully and profoundly penetrate nursing culture.' (p. 30)

Whilst I could help Gill see her background, this was not necessarily reciprocated because of the intention within the relationship of roles, i.e. my role was to facilitate learning in the other's role. Hence I always needed to pay attention not to use authoritative responses such as 'I believe that...' 'I think that...' 'Read...'. This paying attention to self within relationship is a reflexive self-awareness to ensure a true working-with-type collaboration between the guide and practitioner just as there must always be that intention between the practitioner and patients within clinical practice.

The practitioner will sense when the guide is indifferent or judgemental, or imposing her own agenda. The consequence is a breakdown of 'collaboration'. Under these conditions, it might be hoped that the practitioner will raise her concern at this breakdown or even terminate the relationship. However, this may be difficult for the practitioner, especially if the guide has (unwittingly) assumed an authoritative role. I say unwittingly because even with good intent, people can slip into subordinate or authoritative modes of being. The practitioner may feel constrained in tackling inter-personal issues with the guide because she feels intimidated or has a misplaced concern about upsetting the guide or inviting sanction. Collaboration represents an equality of power and mutual responsibility.

Contracting is the formal negotiation to establish the conditions for collaboration between the guide and practitioner. So, what makes a good guide? Because guided reflection is an intensely inter-personal process grounded in practitioner disclosure, the guide is someone whom the practitioner *must* trust and feel confident in. Some degree of mutual attraction may be helpful. Ask yourself – what would attract you to a guide? Attraction is a deeply subjective experience. It is interesting to speculate whether it is important that the guide has an appropriate clinical background. As the reader will note in the narratives, the focus of reflection is rarely on the 'technical' aspects of everyday practice. A good guide will always challenge the practitioner to access an appropriate technical literature or steer the practitioner to access relevant sources for such information. Indeed, the resourceful guide can ask for copies of such material in order to expand her background, and then use this literature to challenge the practitioner as appropriate. A guide with a similar background may be at a disadvantage if the guide subsequently over-identifies with the practitioner's experiences or responds in light of their own experiences. A lack of shared background will enable the guide to ask more naive questions which may otherwise be taken for granted within a shared background. The guide's mind is less crowded with her own ideas.

On a more practical level can the guide (and practitioner) make the commitment to meet for regular sessions? Dedicated time is essential to sustain guided reflection relationships. I work with both individuals and groups. With individuals, I find a meeting for one hour every four weeks is adequate over the period of the research. The advantage of individual meetings is that the work is very focused and the sessions flexible to fit in with practitioners' own agendas. I always work individually with practitioners when I intend to write the narrative. I organise group guided reflection as a 'research school', which meets for three hours every three weeks. Practitioners who register for dissertations or research degrees are supervised through this school which is supplemented by individual tutorials as required. The major advantage of a research school is that collaboration extends between students. Without doubt, mutual support from other practitioners is probably the most sustaining force.

The good guide is sensitive to the unfolding dynamics of the guided reflection relationship and able to surface any tension – what I term as 'pricking the bubble' – and resolve tension. Otherwise the practitioner or the guide may become defensive and resort to game playing that undermines collaboration (Kadushin 1968). As you review the narrative dialogue, ask yourself to what extent collaboration was constructed? Who controlled the agenda? Were dominant meanings imposed? Is my influence evident and is there potential for this to be abused by asserting my own perspectives? As a guide, I must always have a conscious mind-set to create the conditions for genuine collaboration within the guided reflection relationship and tuned into spotting what Whitehead (2000) terms *living contradictions*.

To reiterate, collaborative relationships are implicit within guided reflection. There can be no compromise. Failure to achieve collaboration must always be a contradiction that needs resolving. This is in line with Freire's (1972) belief that empowerment should be a process of collaboration between groups rather than an outcome achieved by one powerful group for another less powerful group, or, in other words, where the powerful group retain control. Within a collaborative relationship the researcher cannot adopt a detached or objective position. That the researcher can be objective is itself a distortion because of the way people always respond from a pre-reflective state (Heidegger in Dreyfus 1991, pp. 82–3). Hence, 'who I was' as a researcher could not be separated from 'who I was' as a manager and supervisor. This point has widespread acceptance within collaborative research theory (Heron 1981) and feminist theory (see Acker *et al.* 1983 and Paget 1983). Paget (1983) recognised how the similarity between her own and her interviewees' life experiences influenced questions she asked and entered into her understanding and interpretation of the story being told. Paget points out her approach, which gave control of the interview process to the interviewee, establishing solidarity between them as they engaged in the shared task of trying to understand important life experiences.

Ultimately there is no formula for the practitioner to choose a guide. Perhaps it is no more than an act of faith, but if that is so, the practitioner and guide need to carefully contract their working relationship and establish the conditions where they can openly discuss the dynamics of their relationship.

Dialogue

Dialogue is the flow of guided reflection. The following Zen poem captures this sense of flow:

> Be soft in your practice. Think of the method as a fine silvery stream, not a raging waterfall. Follow the stream, have faith in its course. It will go its own way, meandering here, trickling there. It will find grooves, the cracks, the crevices. Just follow it. Never let it out of your sight. It will take you.
>
> Sheng-yen – in Zen (Levering 2000, p. 69)

The poem's message is clear to those who are open to it. Dialogue is the fine silvery stream; it needs to flow and find its own levels, essentially unpredictable. The researchers pay attention to its flow and chart its course, confident in its ability to transport and transform self to new, more enlightened levels of being.

The influence of David Bohm

My view of dialogue is strongly influenced by the work of David Bohm (1996). Bohm's ideas on dialogue were strongly influenced by Krishnamurti's belief that dialogue could penetrate and transform the way people thought about issues, enabling new ways of seeing and responding to issues that could uproot the old ways of thought, freeing the mind from traditions and habits. In Krishnamurti's (1996) words:

'To inquire and to learn is the function of the mind. By learning I do not mean the mere cultivation of memory or the accumulation of knowledge, but the capacity to think clearly without illusion.' (p. 93)

As such, the foremost intention of dialogue is the process of dialogue itself rather than its results. This requires careful listening. Yet to listen requires an awareness and suspension of personal ambition, dominant perspectives, values, defensiveness and weight of tradition (Krishnamurti 1996, p. viii). As Bohm notes, thought is infiltrated with these notions. Dialogue requires people to be critically conscious of their own thinking so this does not corrupt the effort to find true meaning. Bohm calls this proprioception of thought in much the same way that the body is aware of itself in space. This does not mean the listener has to agree with what is being said, but they have to understand what is being said without a sense of judgement in order to allow the dialogue to flow. Reflection is the way to access one's assumptions and see them for what they are. Yet this is profoundly difficult because our assumptions reflect 'who I am', and, as such, are taken for granted. Yet they are apparent as the root of all contradiction and contradiction is at the root of anxiety and emotion. This is the same for both guide and practitioner. The guide does not impose a meaning on the practitioner from his or her authoritative advantage. Yet neither does the guide simply accept the practitioner's interpretation. The aim of dialogue is to understand and challenge the perspective of others but always with the intention of moving towards a greater understanding that benefits humanity. Hence dialogue is always a movement towards consensus and harmony. Bohm notes:

'it is clear that if we are to live in harmony with ourselves and with nature, we need to be able to communicate freely in a creative movement in which no one permanently holds to or otherwise defends his own ideas.' (p. 4)

Fusion of horizons

People in dialogue need to be ready to drop old ideas and intentions towards making something in common or 'co-creating meaning'. The practitioner and guide each brings to the dialogue their own perspective, or what Gadamer (1975) referred to as *horizon*. *Horizon* is a metaphor to represent the person's normal vision and understanding. As practitioners learn through experience, their horizons are constantly shifting, as in a developmental process of moving forward. Gadamer considers that people are always understanding and interpreting themselves in the context of their worlds and in light of their fore-knowledge, which, from the reflexive viewpoint, is always changing through experience. This looking back and seeing self as a changed person is the essential nature of reflexivity. It is not as some end-point, but is always open and anticipatory to future experiences. Gadamer (1975) notes:

> 'every experience has implicit horizons before and after, and fuses finally with the continuum of experiences that are present before and after into the unity of the flow of experience.' (cited in Weinsheimer 1985, p. 157)

The aim of dialogue is to reveal the paradoxes that exist within everyday practice, or what I describe as the contradictions between what it is desirable to achieve and everyday reality. Bohm refers to 'paradox' as the contradictions that exist in thought. For example, a practitioner may think she is good at listening to patients' problems. Indeed she has internalised this as a characteristic of a good nurse. Yet she is often intolerant of patients, which she rationalises in terms of being busy in order to deceive herself that she is indeed a caring practitioner. Bohm's argument is that the practitioner's thinking is dominated by a set of self-contradictory demands and needs that impede a solution. By paradox, Bohm suggests the self-contradictory thinking is exposed for what it is. This requires the suspension of the forces that govern the paradox, and highlights the fundamental need to set up conditions of trust in order for people to let go of defences that sustain the paradox. This is to take people back to their values and the way values are contradicted within everyday practice because of competing values inherited through social processes. For example, Karen, one practitioner at Burford, believed she should have a positive regard for all patients and families and yet on a subconscious level she could not tolerate women who wanted to mother her. Dialogue, in pursuing the underlying reasons, takes the person into deeper realms of self (Johns 2000). Bohm's work on dialogue reinforces the notion that who we are is embodied and governed by tradition over which people have little conscious control and that the work of reflection is to reveal these conditions that lead to self-contradiction and paradox. As Bohm says:

> 'What is called for, then, is a deep and intense awareness, going beyond the imagery and intellectual analysis of our confused process of thought, and capable of penetrating to the contradictory presuppositions and states of feelings in which the confusion exists.' (p. 67)

And, of course, it is the same for all people within the dialogue situation, reinforcing the view that the guide needs to be aware of her or his own background, and the prejudices that govern and dominate the way they respond to specific situations. It is the practitioner who is the expert of his own condition. The guide adopts a position of not knowing.

Tradition

The suspension of beliefs, judgements, prejudices and the like within dialogue reflects what Gadamer (1975) refers to as pre-knowledge – the way people dialogue through a lens of personal concerns. These personal concerns are shared within a *tradition* that characterises society. Bernstein (1991) notes:

> 'As Gadamer sees it we belong to a tradition before it belongs to us; tradition, through its sedimentation, has a power which is constantly determining what we are in the process of becoming. We are always 'thrown' into a tradition, what we are, whether we are explicitly aware of it or not, is always being influenced by tradition, even when we think we are most free of it. It is important to [reiterate] that a tradition is not something 'nature-like', something 'given' that stands over against us. It is always 'part of us' and works through its effective-history. (p. 142)

Tradition has a powerful impact on the way people view the world, largely because it is pre-reflective. It is most powerfully reflected in the prejudices people hold, which govern their responses to the world. Gadamer notes:

> 'We do not choose our prejudices, for we discover them in ourselves as things that exist prior to conscious choice. Yet this priority to consciousness does not make them subjective either, for prejudices do not derive from a private subconscious but from a communal tradition.' (Gadamer 1975, p. 261, cited in Weinsheimer p. 169/176)

Given the powerful impact of prejudice and tradition on the way people respond to the world, the effort of dialogue is to surface and understand the way the practitioner's prejudices create contradiction with what is desirable. However, prejudices are deeply embodied and not so easily shifted for both the practitioner and guide. However, this does not mean becoming 'objective' in the sense of putting aside one's prejudices. This is a form of disassociation where the person tries to split off and control unacceptable parts of self. Rather it requires a transformation of one's prejudices towards a radically transformed view of the world. Weinsheimer's interpretation of Gadamer makes the point eloquently:

> 'Understanding is projection and what it projects are expectations that precede the text. They "jump the gun" as it were because they anticipate meaning before arriving at it. What the interpreter projects in advance is what he understands already – that is, before beginning. He tries out meaning already familiar to him and proposes it as a possibility. This projected meaning is his own possibility in that he has projected it; it is part of the world he already knows his way around, and it is something he can and does understand … yet since we are prepared for the text to say something new, we read with an openness to the unexpected. Rather than stubbornly persisting in our preconceptions, we stand ready to revise them – and not because we are prepared to believe anything, nor because we merely want to know what the author has to say on the topic, but instead because we want to know and learn about it … we hold our own opinions open to disconfirmation and place them at risk not because we are neutral but, quite the opposite, because we too are interested … Because we are concerned and interested, our receptivity implies that we are willing to integrate the meaning of the text with our previous preconceptions by making them conscious, bringing them into view, and assimilating them to what the text reveals.' (p. 166–7)

From this perspective the guide reads the practitioner's experience as 'text'. This is the fertile ground of dialogue, the fusion of horizons whereby the practitioner's and the

guide's perspectives are transformed through dialogue through reaching understanding between them. It is also the ground between the narrative and the narrative
reader. It is 'this between' Gadamer writes that 'is the true locus of hermeneutics'
(p. 279).

Reflection as empowerment

The work of Freire (1972) challenged me to consider any taken-for-granted authority
of the guide (no matter its benevolent intent), and the ensuing intrinsic threat of the
guide imposing an agenda and dominant meanings. That thought forced me to ask
myself 'What is my agenda?'. Whilst I might claim to enable Gill to realise desirable
and effective practice, who defined and judged this realisation? Whilst I might also
claim that Gill contributed to the Burford Unit philosophy, how much of her contribution was compliance with my persuasive leadership? And how well informed was
she to make a contribution? Such questions taunt yet are fundamental to establishing
a genuine collaborative relationship between the practitioner and guide.

Critical social science

Alongside the work of Freire I became immersed in the ideas of critical social science
(Fay 1987), notably the idea of reflection being a process of enlightenment,
empowerment and emancipation. Enlightenment is understanding why things are as
they are. It is a critical process of deconstruction, of peeling away the layers of
experience to reveal the conditions that govern why people respond as they do. These
conditions are embodied within self and embedded within the fabric of practice in
ways that reinforce the embodied conditions through ways of relating. Empowerment
is having the knowledge and courage to take appropriate action towards changing the
way things are in order to realise self's own interests. Empowerment acknowledges
the limits of rationality to bring about change, and the positive energy required to take
appropriate action in ways that may incur resistance from more powerful others
whose interests may be threatened. Emancipation is the realisation of self's best
interests through appropriate action.

Fay's work enabled me to cross the critical threshold and pay attention to the
conditions of practice and the way oppressive forces embedded in 'tradition' or what
Fay himself terms as *authority*, come to constrain practitioners from realising desirable work – not only that, but also constrain people from learning through experience. From this perspective, empowerment *is* the cornerstone of reflection, the critical
edge to reflection to free ourselves from oppressive forces in order to relieve our
misery. Perhaps in our frantic world it is easier to defend against anxiety than face up
to such strong emotions where there are no easy answers. As such, reflection may
create a crisis for practitioners as normal coping mechanisms are exposed as incongruent with achieving desirable work. Insight into 'their condition' may exacerbate a
sense of frustration ultimately leading to a personal crisis where self doubt about
competence and de-masked ways of coping become redundant. Yet with enlighten-

ment the practitioner can view the scenario unfolding, almost as an observer, and accept that things do not necessarily change quickly. Cox *et al.* (1991) note:

> 'As we come to expose these self-imposed limitations, then the focus of our reflection shifts towards new action, towards the ways in which we might begin to reconstruct and act differently within our worlds.' (p. 387)

However, exposing these 'self-imposed limitations' may not necessarily be easy or comfortable. It may be difficult for practitioners to see beyond themselves because of 'habits of mind' that act as barriers (Margolis 1993). Margolis refers to the way paradigms are maintained and shifted. Where particular habits of mind need to be shifted for change to take place, they constitute a barrier. However, the practitioner's own best interests may be distorted because of competing dominant power discourses that she has internalised and taken for granted as normal. This is perhaps particularly significant for nurses whose own nursing discourse has been dominated within the discourses of medicine and managerialism. Practitioners may feel more comfortable adhering to false beliefs or 'false consciousness'. Lather (1986) defined this as:

> 'the denial of how our common-sense ways of looking at the world are permeated with meanings that sustain our disempowerment.' (p. 264)

Mezirow (1981) viewed reflection as the means to enable practitioners to penetrate 'false consciousness' through perspective transformation. He defined this as:

> 'The emancipatory process of becoming critically aware of how and why the structure of psycho-cultural assumptions has come to constrain the way we see ourselves and our relationships, reconstituting this structure to permit a more inclusive and discriminating integration of experience and acting upon these new understandings.' (p. 6)

Psycho-cultural assumptions are those norms and prejudices embodied within individuals and embedded within practice settings that lead people to see and act in the world in certain ways. Mezirow sees reflection as the means to access and transform these norms and prejudices to enable them to fulfil their own best (emancipatory) interests. Mezirow talks about 'disorienting dilemmas' and how the 'traumatic severity of the disorienting dilemma is clearly a factor in establishing the probability of a transformation' (p. 7). It is this sense of disorientation or trauma that brings the person to pay attention to the experience, although a more deliberative stance can be developed as the practitioner becomes increasingly sensitive to herself in the context of what they are trying to achieve. Street (1992) drew the conclusion from her critical ethnography of nursing practice that:

> 'The confrontation with experience through reflection and of the meanings and assumptions which surround it, can form a foundation upon which to make choices about future actions based on chosen value systems and new ways of thinking about and understanding nursing practice.' (p. 16)

Through reflection, the practitioner is guided to reveal the contradictions between ideal and real value systems. Because beliefs and values matter to practitioners, failure to live these values in practice creates anxiety. Anxiety, because of its discomfort, tends to make itself conscious and becomes a focus for reflection. It is the felt degree of conflict within contradiction that propels practitioners towards taking action to remedy the anxiety and, as a consequence, to resolve the contradiction (Kieffer 1984). Kieffer studied 15 people who were active in grassroots political and community leadership roles and who could self-acknowledge personal transformation. Kieffer chose these 'experts' to analyse and construct a model of empowerment as a developmental process. In considering the implication for practice Kieffer noted:

> 'In becoming empowered individuals are not merely acquiring new practical skills; they are reconstructing and re-orienting deeply ingrained personal systems of social relations. Moreover, they confront these tasks in an environment which historically has enforced their political repression, and which continues its active and implicit attempts at subversion of constructive change.' (p. 27)

Individuals can be replaced by *nurses*, and *political repression* with *professional and organisational repression*. Kieffer emphasised how reflective experience was the irreducible source of empowerment and growth. Kieffer plotted the development or empowerment of community leaders through four eras of involvement: era of entry, era of advancement, era of incorporation and era of commitment. In their narratives, Yvonne (Chapter 8) and Jane (Chapter 9) use these *eras* to plot their journeys of becoming empowered. The era of entry is characterised by a sense of 'one's integrity being violated' and that it cannot be tolerated. In terms of narrative, it sets the plot – a journey to overthrow the forces that violate until self emerges triumphant in realising desirable practice. Dramatic stuff!

Voice as metaphor

Voice is a metaphor for empowerment (Belenky *et al.* 1986). The majority of nurses I have worked with have been women, and as such, it is crucial to pay attention to the struggle women have within patriarchal dominated organisations such as the Health Care Service (Watson 1990) to have their voice heard and valued. This is, of course, the theme of a critical social science – the struggle to throw off the forces of oppression that deny 'voice' and realisation of self's best interests. Undoubtedly this is the major plot of guided reflection narrative. Belenky *et al.* (1986) identified five stages of developing voice from listening to the experiences of groups of women; silence, received voice, subjective voice, procedural voice (connected and separate), and constructed voice.

The level of *silence* represents women who have no voice, dominated by the authoritative voices of others. Reflection gives the person a *potential* voice to write her journal or share her story, to ask self 'who am I?'. *Potential*, because the forces that keep women/nurses silent may shut off even this possibility. I have often asked people to write a brief description of a recent experience and it is beyond them to do this. I have noted two reasons why nurses struggle with this activity. The first is a technical reason – they do not know how to reflect, and this reflects the way that they can only speak with the voices of others to the extent that they deny their own intuitive sense. The second is more profound – they do not know who they are and have no way of expressing self. Of course this raises all sorts of dilemmas in using reflection as a developmental process in that the very tool of empowerment may serve to disempower (Johns 1999). Aileen's story (Chapter 4) is included in the book as an exemplar of her struggle to find a voice to reflect. It is an important story because she is a mature and intelligent woman yet found herself feeling increasingly helpless and powerless to change her predicament yet unable to express this predicament in any coherent way. She had descended into self-alienation whereby she felt she was clinging on to remnants of her real self. She felt she was going to fragment. Her brief narrative plots her journey to recover herself.

The level of *received voice* is listening and speaking with the voice of others. Women conceive themselves as capable of receiving, even reproducing knowledge from all knowing external authorities but not capable of creating knowledge of their own, reflected in the way the practitioner speaks as if filled with the words of others yet without any critical understanding. It is profoundly difficult to reflect on this level because the person cannot respond to the reflective cues beyond simple description. They lack the resources to be critical of self. Reflection is experienced as confrontational and threatening. At this level practitioners want a didactic style of guidance that fits with the experience of being filled up. Yet they also resist being emptied because the words of others have become embodied. On this level reflection proceeds with a gentle inquiring light to plant the seeds of doubt. The typical response of the received knower is 'don't know', for example: 'Why do you feel that way?' – 'I don't know.' 'Could you respond in different ways?' – 'I don't know'.

At the level of *subjective* voice reflection is perceived as permission to have and voice opinions and feelings, to express outrage, to shed tears, to rant against injustice, and most importantly to connect with others and form a caring community where people, perhaps for the first time, can express themselves with a sense of freedom. On this level feminist strategies such as the Peace and Power feminist process (Wheeler & Chinn 1991) offer practitioners a mirror to see themselves within this process. The group process is explicitly about valuing self and taking power, yet in peaceful ways. However, at the subjective level, the practitioner's voice is unsubstantiated.

At the level of *procedural* voice the practitioner is able to realise self within the simultaneous and complementary processes of separate and connected knowing. Separate knowing is the ability to critically apply theory to practice in meaningful ways. Connected knowing is the ability to know and connect self with the experiences of others. In other words, in order to know the other, one has to know self so connection can be made in terms of the meanings the other gives to a situation. People who experience self as predominantly separate tend to espouse a morality based on impersonal procedures for establishing justice, whilst people who experience the self as predominantly connected tend to espouse a morality based on care.

The level of *constructed* voice is the weaving of the subjective and procedural voices into a coherent whole whereby the practitioner can speak with an informed, passionate and assertive voice. From this perspective women view all knowledge as contextual, experience themselves as creators of knowledge, and value both subjective and objective strategies for knowing. Developing the practitioner's *constructed voice* is always the intent of guided reflection expressed in narrative form.

Yvonne (Chapter 8) explicitly uses the metaphor of voice to mark her own and other's empowerment, and in particular the sense of connected knowing – where each other's empowerment is a reflection of the other.

A feminist slant

Valerie Young introduced me to the perspective of masculine and feminine in narrative through the work of Virginia Woolf. Belenky *et al.* (1986) wrote from a feminist perspective. Virginia Woolf, in her lecture *A room of one's own* given at Girton College, Cambridge in 1928 deepens this perspective. Woolf had been asked to speak about women and fiction. Woolf presented *A room of one's own* as a metaphor for creating space to write a story – a space that had been foreclosed within a society that had not valued women in terms of the way women view the world. Indeed, the dominant stories of nursing tend to reflect the way medicine and organisation value nursing – stories of the nurse valiantly assisting the intrepid doctor in his (sic) technological battle against disease and death. As a way of viewing this dissonance of values Virginia Woolf posited a dichotomy between the masculine and feminine. She reflected the way women's fiction had reflected social values as to what counts as significant (Woolf 1945):

> 'This is an important book, the critic assumes, because it deals with war. This is an insignificant book because it deals with the feelings of women in the drawing room. A scene in a battlefield is more important than a scene in a shop.' (p. 74)

Woolf suggested that, through history, masculine values had tended to be viewed as more significant – the triumph of the masculine rational mind and reason over the female emotional body. By drawing a contemporary comparison, her words can be construed to reflect professional values and draw a distinction between *feminine* nursing values and *masculine* nursing values. So I can rewrite Woolf's words:

> 'This is an important book, the critic assumes, because it deals with the high technology of nursing practice. This is an insignificant book because it deals with the feelings of patients and families in the health care setting.'

The challenge through story is not to de-emphasise the drama and technology of nursing practice *qua* medical practice, but to emphasise the exquisite nature of caring and the profound significance caring has on the lives of patients and families, and to value the mundane that takes place between women as if in the drawing room or as if a scene within a shop; so mundane that it can be so easily dismissed with the raging war all around to save lives. It is through story that the mundane and the profane can become sacred. It is through story that nurses can make visible, find meaning in, and value this quintessential essence of nursing. And as if to prove the point, it is rarely the high technology that practitioners reflect on. Yet a shadow dims the light to thwart this enterprise. Within the masculine dominated world, some nurses aspire to have masculine values, whilst others do not assert their values of caring, their voices silenced under the weight of dominant values and the organisation of health care whereby the dominant values attain priority, making little allowance for what might be construed as caring. Such tensions ripple through the narratives in this book, tensions born out of the struggle to assert the feminine perspective within a masculine world – the most ironic and most significant contradiction that faces nurses – the continual denial of self, the continual suppression of voice even within nursing itself. I felt strangely uncomfortable when I read:

> 'When a woman speaks to woman she should have something very unpleasant up her sleeve. Women are hard on women. Women dislike women.' (Woolf 1945, p. 109)

But why should I feel strangely uncomfortable about this? That women purport to care for each other, yet fail? Indeed worse, project their frustration into each other – unable to project it into the 'masculine' of those who oppress. The sense of horizontal violence that spills over the top of the water-butt, that leaks along the seams of teamwork. Is it for the desire to become masculine that women sacrifice each other and in doing so lose touch with their feminine and so alienate themselves from who they are? Visions of caring spiralling down the plughole. It is this tension and struggle that sets up contradiction and plots the stories that nurses share, stories that highlight the possibility of caring yet are shipwrecked against the reef of masculinity. Woolf (1945) puts it like this:

> 'Everywhere and much more subtly the difference of values persist. The whole structure, therefore, of the early nineteenth century novel was raised, if one was a woman, by a mind which was slightly pulled from the straight, and made to alter its clear vision in deference to external authority [p. 74] ... she had altered her values in deference to the opinion of others. [p. 75] ... Moreover, a book is not made of sentences laid end to end, but of sentences built, if an image helps, into arcades and domes. And this shape too has been made by men of their own needs for their own uses.' (p. 77)

Woolf suggests that the shape of narrative has been determined by man built upon a masculine tradition of the way a narrative should be fashioned. As such, women (nurses) may struggle to find an adequate form to shape their stories because there is no tradition for doing this. When I first ask practitioners to write about an experience using 'I' they stumble, for it is often the first time they have tried to express 'I'. It is as if they try and position themselves outside their experience, to turn themselves into objects to gaze at. When they are enabled to focus on self, the self is often deprecated, diminished, reflecting the way these practitioners tend not to value their experience. And in not valuing their experiences they do not value themselves. In shrugging aside their values they alienate themselves from self as reflected in the struggle to know how to adequately express their experiences or stories.

In her lecture Woolf drew on the novel *Life's Adventure* by Mary Carmichael to reflect on the development of women's fiction from the early nineteenth century pioneering work of Charlotte Bronte and Jane Austen to contemporary twentieth century work. From the novel Woolf (1945) cites:

' "Chloe liked Olivia" … let's admit in the privacy of our own society that these things sometimes happen. Sometimes women like women.' (p. 81)

Woolf (1945) urged her listeners not to blush and goes on to reflect:

'For if Chloe likes Olivia and Mary Carmichael knows how to express it, she will light a torch in that vast chamber where nobody has yet been. It is all half lights and profound shadows like those serpentine caves where one goes with a candle peering up and down, not knowing where one is stepping. And I read the book again, and read how Chloe watched Olivia put a jar on a shelf and say how it was time to go home to her children.' (pp. 83–4)

Knowing how to express it is the key to narrative, to light a torch in that vast chamber of practice where nobody has yet been. Each experience, each human-to-human encounter is unique. It has never been enacted before and yet readers will identify with the experience because they are familiar with the vast chamber where they have had similar experiences. The narrative is itself a torch to help the reader shine a light on self and these experiences, and written in such a way the reader can trigger and relate to her own experiences. To adequately do this the reader needs to be able to grasp the pattern of the writer's experience so she can interpret it in her own terms. The writer's pattern contains the threads of her own interpretation, yet without imposing this meaning on the reader as the way the narrative should be read. '…*how Chloe watched Olivia put a jar on a shelf*' – the profound buried within the mundane yet when watched, lifts it into immense significance, valued in its unfolding moment, a light across the reader's soul. The word profound is used by Woolf (1945):

'One has a profound, if irrational instinct in favour of a theory that the union of man and woman makes for the greatest satisfaction. [p. 96] … And I went on amateurishly to sketch a plan of the soul so that in each of us two powers preside, one male and one female; and in the man's brain the man predominates over the woman, and in the woman's brain, the woman predominates over the man. The normal and comfortable state of being is that when the two live in harmony together, spiritually co-operating … It is when this fusion takes place that the mind is fully fertilised and uses all of its facilities. (96–7)

Of course what is profound is rarely rational within the unique human–human encounter of nursing practice. It follows from Woolf's reflection that texts written from a masculine-type brain fall upon the woman's deaf ears and vice versa. To this I would add blind eyes. Indeed all the senses are depressed, and even deny the feminine's fundamental intuitive and empathic sense. Perhaps this is why so many nurses struggle with theory? They simply cannot relate to it, written as it is from this masculinity with such depressed senses clinging to an illusion that they need only be rational. It is not an appeal to reason that counts, but an appeal to sensitivity. Women may need permission and empowerment to listen to their own senses and souls in order to listen to the sense and souls of others – the empathic sense that is vital to connect with and know the experience of the other (Belenky *et al.* 1986).

My fear is that women/nurses have been disempowered through being encouraged to listen with the ears of men, denying the sensitivity of their senses. This may be difficult if such sensitivity has become crusted and buried along the edge of rationality, where the description and significance of the everyday subtlety of the emotions may not be recognised or valued by nurses. Woolf (1945) writes:

'It is fatal for anyone who writes to think of their sex. It is fatal to be a man or woman pure and simple; one must be womanly-manly or manly-womanly. It is fatal for a woman to lay the least stress on any grievance; to plead even with justice any cause; in any way to speak consciously as a woman. And fatal is no figure of speech; for anything written with that conscious bias is doomed to death. It ceases to be fertilised. Brilliant and effective, powerful and masterly, as it may appear for a day or two, it must wither at nightfall; it cannot grow in the mind of others. Some collaboration has to take place in the mind between the woman and the man before the art of creation can be accomplished. Some marriage of opposites has to be consummated. (pp. 102–3)

To return to the metaphor of *a room of one's own*, Woolf suggests the room will need a lock on the door. Woolf throws down a challenge to nurses (and women everywhere) to throw off their cloaks that wrap their feminism and to synthesise the feminine with the masculine – a marriage of souls that finds its fullest expression. Perhaps before such marriage can be consummated, to give rein to the feminine simply so that the feminine can be known. As Woolf (1945) puts it:

'So long as you write what you wish to write that is all that matters; and whether it matters for ages or only for hours, nobody can say. But to sacrifice a hair of the head of your vision, a shade of its colour, in deference to some ... professor with a measuring rod up his sleeve is the most abject treachery. (p. 105)

The narratives written in this book are written by women either by themselves or in collaboration with me. Madden (2001) wrote in her dissertation:

'In a simple way, my feminism finds expression in my dissatisfactions and frustrations as a practising midwife. This research is an exploration of those frustrations – teasing out the elements of constraint upon me to practise in ways congruent with my beliefs and ideals. I have already said that the writing of this project is its creation, but I am concerned that I find it so difficult to mould this dissertation into a compact, recognisable, academic piece of work. I search for the freedom to let it develop devoid of predetermined chapters and sections, finding it difficult to think in terms of self-contained, clearly demarcated issues and arguments. I tell myself this is laziness, that what results must be logical, progressive and complete: beginning, middle, end. I worry about assessment, and the need to gain accreditation. But Cixous (1996) challenges us to write our femininity, "it is the whole that makes sense", and for a while I worry less about the format of the fragmentation. Cixous objects to what she sees as masculine writing, because it is cast in oppositions – it relies on reason and logic for its validity. She identifies women's writing as much more fluid, "marking, scratching, scribbling, jotting down," and argues that it is this flexibility that makes feminine writing potentially subversive and transformative. I am after all writing a story about myself here, surely that is not too difficult? But I am ever worried about the validity of the exercise, how can I make this academic? How can I turn this into knowledge that is "worth something"? Just as I seek the discourse of resistance in women's narratives, so I resist the patriarchal, rational discourse of academic writing at the same time as attempting to gain by it. How can I reconcile these tensions, or live with them?' (pp. 25–6)

Cixous's work legitimises (as if I needed permission) writing from the body, unwrapping self from a logocentrism and phallocentrism that has dominated everyday life, reflected through language. To quote Cixous (1996):

> 'Woman, writing herself, will go back to this body that has been more than confiscated, a body replaced with a disturbing stranger, sick or dead, who so often is a bad influence, the cause and location of inhibitions. By censoring the body, breath and speech are censored at the same time. To write – giving her back access to her own forces; that will return her goods, her pleasures, her organs, her immense bodily territories which have been kept under seal; it will tear her out of the superegoed, where the same position of guilt is always reserved for her. Write yourself: your body must make itself heard. Then the huge resources of the unconscious will burst out.' (p. 97)

Deep breath. Vapourised trails that mark such journeys into the unknown. Have the authors in this book, all women except myself, been liberated to express their feminine side in balance with their masculine side to create a creative fusion? This is an important question within a narrative tradition grounded in caring. Both Woolf and Cixous help to balance the feminine and masculine perspectives, in particular to unwrap the more masculine perspectives that have dominated patterns of thinking and writing. Yet, as Mayeroff (1971) says of the nature of caring, it takes courage to step into the unknown. Only by stepping into the unknown with pen poised over paper, can the unknown be revealed. Cixous's words inspire the journey and give courage.

An evolutionary slant

When a practitioner shares an experience she is always throwing out cues that are signs to deeper issues. The guide working with the practitioner pursues these signs for deeper significance within the whole, piecing together the whole pattern. The idea that the self ripples along its surface and can be read as signs to the deeper self is given substance within Newman's (1994) *theory of health as expanded consciousness*. Newman viewed nursing in terms of the way practitioners can work with patients to reflect on the meaning of health events so as to re-pattern their lives in more meaningful ways that lead to a new expanded sense of self and harmony. This theory is equally applicable to practitioners presenting in guided reflection with their own sense of overt or muted crisis. In her theory Newman linked together evolutionary theories including Prigonine and Stengers' (1984) *theory of dissipative structures*. In this theory, people or systems (of people) operate in a rhythmic and predictable fashion until some event or fluctuation occurs that throws the system off balance leading to crisis. In guided reflection, the practitioner may experience a sense of crisis signalled by anxiety, uncertainty or strong feelings. Heidegger (1962) noted that many breakdowns are like blips that the practitioner can subconsciously adjust to. However larger breakdowns create a crisis within the experience. Guided reflection is an 'environment' that facilitates energy exchange. Negative feelings are validated and explored to pinpoint the cause of fluctuations that have thrown the person out of balance. Through understanding and contemplating new ways of being, the practitioner dissipates the negative energy into positive energy necessary to take positive action to re-pattern the disorganisation of self to emerge on an expanded level of consciousness. The idea of dissipating negative energy highlights reflection as a deeply cathartic and healing experience for both patients and practitioners.

Young's (1976) *theory of evolutionary consciousness* guides the practitioner to plot a slightly different yet complementary pathway by viewing self along life's journey from a point of potential freedom towards real freedom. The pivotal point of the journey is the practitioner's realisation of a self-consciousness, when she comes to realise herself as self-determining through her responsibilities and the subsequent choices she is faced with. Young considers that people are born with potential freedom yet become socialised in ways that bind them to cultural norms of feeling, thinking and behaving in the world. As people develop they come to see themselves as individuals with distinct identities able to make and act on choices about themselves towards realising their potential as human beings. This means confronting who self is in order to change or transform self in tune with values. She comes to see that it is her *situation* which limits possibilities and that old ways no longer work, and that beliefs strongly held are misguided. Such knowledge enables her to open herself to possibilities freed from the constraints of previously held mental models that had freeze dried her flow of experience (Levine 1986). As Levine notes:

> 'Our models are a prison. They are the limit to which we can accept the molten flow of change. They act as filters that accept what we believe and reject what seems otherwise.' (p. 53)

The practitioner, like the researcher, needs to see models for what they are, as a sense-making tool rather than as a thought prison. She needs to ask herself: 'How open am I to new ideas?' 'How do my "models" constrain the way I view the world?' 'How do my models create suffering for those I work with and for myself?'

Managing chaos

On a deeper level the practitioner reflects to give herself feedback of her ability to bring order to chaos within her self-mastery and mental systems for viewing and responding to the world (Senge 1991). Much of practice is complex and indeterminate without easy solutions. The practitioner often feels she is trying to tread gingerly through a sense of chaos. I will assume that the reflective (and effective) practitioner is someone who is always seeking to stretch and move beyond personal and organisational boundaries in the quest to realise self. As we move away from the centre where it feels safe and secure because things do not change, the practitioner comes to realise that practice is chaotic and that chaos does not go away. Indeed it becomes manifest as everyday lived experience.

The difference is that the practitioner now has the means to work with it rather than push it away as threatening, even though chaos may have initially been perceived as destructive. Indeed, guided reflection may precipitate chaos and crisis. However, chaos is also the creative edge, the frontier of innovative change. Stable systems are generally stable because they resist change and new ideas. Available energy is used to maintain stability by resisting change. However, innovative systems are always unstable because they are always challenging the boundaries. The effective practitioner must inevitably move away from the stable centre towards the creative edge simply because staying in the centre becomes untenable. As a consequence, the practitioner may feel that reflection spirals her out of control into a crisis that always ripples just below the surface. It feels as if a thin veneer of protection is about to peel off and spiral the self into a chaotic void.

Uncertainty brings with it a degree of risk because the outcomes within innovative systems are no longer predictable. Reflection offers a sanctuary because it offers both high challenge to move towards the creative edge and high support to live and thrive within the creative pull of chaos. Then both practice and reflection become invigorating.

Taking notes

To finish on a practical note, I record dialogue and encourage practitioners to record dialogue either verbatim or in note form. Taking notes:

- Enables the practitioner or guide (depending who has taken responsibility for doing this – usually the person who intends to write the narrative) to record dialogue or the content of the session in note form
- Enables the continuity of the sessions by issues being picked up from the notes in subsequent sessions
- Facilitates a deeper reflection on issues simply because it is written and read after the session
- Drafts the unfolding narrative.

Notes can be structured through three headings:

- Description of experiences/issues shared during the session
- What has been significant about these experiences (insights)
- What actions need to be taken as a consequence (action).

At the subsequent session, the practitioner and guide commence the session by revisiting the notes and continue the unfolding narrative by picking up what was significant and actions taken. If actions were not taken then why not? This leads to an exploration of the factors that constrained the practitioner from taking desirable action. If actions were taken as agreed, or different actions, then their consequences are explored: Did they lead to desired outcomes? What new issues arise as a consequence?

In the projects where I intend to write the narrative, I word-process the notes I have taken within 24 hours of the session and give a copy to the practitioner. From a one hour session I word-process around 1500 words, which takes between one and two hours to accomplish. Practitioners quickly get used to my prolific note-taking during the session and the guide quickly learns to manage space within the session to ensure notes are adequately taken. For example I might say 'Can we just clarify what you have said?' or 'That's interesting – I need to write that down?'. Word-processing expands the notes into a narrative format, so my notes have to be adequate at the time of writing for me to get the gist later. That's why 24 hours is critical in order to accurately relate the notes to the session. It is best done the same day. An alternative is to audio-tape, which I have done in order to validate the adequacy of my note-taking (Johns 1998). However, to transcribe a one hour tape takes me approximately six hours and then I have to deal with the data. Hence it is not practical and serves little purpose when handwritten notes have proved to be adequate. Researchers will obviously experiment with recording notes adequately.

References

Acker, J., Barry, K. & Esseveld, J. (1983) Objectivity and truth: problems in doing feminist research. *Women Studies International Forum*, 6(4) 423–35.

Belenky, M., Clinchy, B., Goldberger, N. & Tarule, J. (1986) *Women's Ways of Knowing: the development of self, voice and mind*. Basic Books, New York.

Bernstein, R. (1991) *Beyond Objectivism and Relativism: science, hermeneutics and praxis*. University of Pennsylvania Press, Philadelphia.

Bohm, D. (1996) *On Dialogue* (ed. L. Nichol). Routledge, London.

Cixous, H. (1996) Sorties: Out and out: attacks/ways out/forays. In *The Newly Born Woman* (eds H. Cixous & C. Clément). Tauris, London.

Cox, H., Hickson, P. & Taylor, B. (1991) Exploring reflection: knowing and constructing practice. In *Towards a Discipline of Nursing* (eds Gray G. & Pratt R.). Churchill Livingstone, Melbourne.

Dreyfus, H. (1991) *Being-in-the-world*. A commentary on Heidegger's *Being & Time*. The MIT Press, Cambridge, MA.

Fay, B. (1987) *Critical Social Science*. Polity Press, Cambridge.

Freire, P. (1972) *Pedagogy of the Oppressed*. Penguin Books. Harmondsworth.

French, F. & Raven, B. (1968) The bases of social power. In *Group Dynamics: research and theory* 3rd edn (eds D. Cartwright & A. Zander). Harper & Row, New York.

Gadamer, H-G. (1975) *Truth and Method*. Seabury Press, New York.

Greenwood, D., Whyte, W. & Harkavy, I. (1993) Participatory action research as a process and as a goal. *Human Relations*, 46(2) 175–92.

Heidegger, M. (1962) *Being and Time* (Trans. Macquarrie J. & Robinson E.). Harper & Row, New York.

Heron, J. (1981) Philosophical basis for a new paradigm. In *Human Inquiry* (eds Reason P. & Rowan J.). John Wiley, Chichester.

Johns, C. (1998) *Becoming an effective practitioner through guided reflection*. PhD thesis. The Open University.

Johns, C. (1999) Reflection as empowerment? *Nursing Inquiry*, 6(4) 241–9.

Johns, C. (2000) *Becoming a Reflective Practitioner*. Blackwell Science, Oxford.

Kadushin, A. (1968) Games people play in supervision. *Social Work*, 13, 23–32.

Kieffer, C. (1984) Citizen empowerment: a developmental perspective. *Prevention in Human Services*, 84(3) 9–36.

Krishnamurti, J. (1996) *Total Freedom: the essential Krishnamurti*. Harper Collins, San Francisco.

Lather, P. (1986) Research as praxis. *Harvard Educational Review*, 56(3) 257–77.

Levering, M. (2000) *Zen. Images, texts and teachings*. Duncan Baird Publishers, London.

Levine, S. (1986) *Who Dies? An investigation of conscious living and conscious dying*. Gateway Books, Bath.

Madden, B. (2001) *Working with women following traumatic child birth*. MSc dissertation, University of Luton.

Margolis, H. (1993) *Paradigms and Barriers: how habits of mind govern scientific beliefs*. University of Chicago Press, Chicago.

Mayeroff, M. (1971) *On Caring*. Harper Perennial, New York.

Mezirow, J. (1981) A critical theory of adult learning and education. *Adult Education*, 32, 3–24.

Newman, M. (1994) *Health as Expanded Consciousness*. National League for Nursing, New York.

Paget, M. (1983) Experience and knowledge. *Human Studies*, **6**(2) 67–90.

Prigonine, I. & Stengers, I. (1984) *Order Out of Chaos*. Bantam, New York.

Reason, P. (1988) *Human Inquiry in Action. Developments in new paradigm research*. Sage, London.

Senge, P. (1991) *The Fifth Discipline*. Century Business, London.

Spence, D.P. (1982) *Narrative Truth and Historical Truth: meaning and interpretation in psycho-analysis*. W.W. Norton & Co, New York.

Street, A. (1992) *Inside Nursing: a critical ethnography of clinical nursing practice*. State University of New York Press, New York.

Watson, J. (1990) The moral failure of the hierarchy. *Nursing Outlook*, **38**(2) 62–6.

Weinsheimer, J. (1985) *Gadamer's Hermeneutics. A reading of Truth and Method*. Yale University Press, New Haven.

Wheeler, C. & Chinn, P. (1991) *Peace & Power. A handbook of feminist process*, 3rd edn. National League for Nursing, New York.

Whitehead, J. (2000) How do I improve my practice? Creating and legimating an epistemology of practice. *Reflective Practice*, 1, 91–104, 105–12 (reply).

Woolf, V. (1945) *A Room of One's Own*. Penguin Books, London.

Young, A. (1976) *The Reflexive Universe: evolution of consciousness*. Robert Briggs, San Francisco.

Chapter 3
Unfolding the Reflexive Narrative

'Like the gradual shading of blue to green, we become, we live the transformations. It is as though we are in a cocoon, within a cocoon, within a cocoon. The more truth we experience, the more we are set free in colourful flight. Always in movement, the different levels of consciousness we experience lead us to the next level. This is how we come to soar.'

(Blackwolf and Gina Jones 1998)

Narrative

Narrative is the written account that tells the story of the practitioner's reflexive spiral of being and becoming. The narrative traces the practitioner's unfolding journey, paying close attention to the steps along the way for their significance within the whole journey. Narrative, like any good drama, is essentially anticipatory and as such indeterminate. There are no absolute beginnings and no absolute endings; there is no closure when we can know for certain who we are and what we have done. The process of understanding ourselves can never achieve finality but is always unfolding and always being revised. There is no genuine narrative that will definitely reveal our true identity (Fay 1987, p. 140). To construct an adequate narrative is to weave an unfolding pattern. This pattern becomes the plot of the narrative (Fay 1987). Spence (1982) noted how the 'narrative fit' is significantly enhanced by the discovery of a pattern match. The more comprehensive, coherent, and self-consistent the narrative is, the more adequate the explanation becomes both for the practitioner and the reader. Robinson and Hawpe (1986) note:

'In order to perceive order and recognise repetition and similarity we must go beyond the surface features in dealing with the world of concrete objects and human social interactions. A story provides the right balance between uniqueness and universality. Because stories are contextualised accounts they can convey the particularity of any episode. But because they are built upon a generic set of categories and relationships each story resembles other stories to varying degrees. A sense of familiarity is the result of this underlying similarity.' (pp. 113–14)

Narrative is persuasive because it *can* accommodate contradictory experience and the complexity of experience. The structure cannot be static or immutable, it needs to be a reflexive structure, responding to new interpretations that emerged from the constant dialectical process of deconstructing shared experiences and constructing coherent narrative form whereby the practitioners' learning remains at the centre of the narrative (Giorgi 1985; Van Manen 1990). The challenge is not to de-contextualise and reduce experience into categories, but to construct a structure through which experience can be most meaningfully communicated, whereby the meaning of experience from the practitioner's viewpoint can be heard.

Plot

The narrative plot is to realise desirable and effective practice. Plot gives narrative direction and focus (Mattingly 1994). Mattingly notes:

> 'It is the plot that makes individual events understandable as part of a coherent whole, one which leads compellingly towards a particular ending... Any particular event gains its meanings by its place within this narrative configuration, as a contribution to the plot. This configuration makes a whole such that we can speak of the point of the story. Yet this is an always shifting configuration for we live in the midst of unfolding stories over which we have a very partial control.' (p. 813)

The plot can be focused on specific aspects of desirable practice as with Jane's narrative on working with suicidal patients in an A&E department (Chapter 9) or Tessa's narrative on becoming an effective clinical leader (Chapter 5). Whilst the collection of narratives in this book offered as examples of the genre portray narrative in the form of cognitive structures, narrative can legimately be presented using a variety of media: poetry, analogy, film, painting, photography, play, etc., whatever feels most appropriate. For example Wagner (2000) creates poems from her patients' experiences to express meaning. Martin (1998), who takes a powerful eco-feminist perspective, uses analogy with nature to express stories of caring and being caring. In other words, the way people tell stories and the way narratives are constructed are concerned with releasing and honouring the creative imagination. The fusion of the left and right brain – Woolf's androgynous mind.

Reflexivity

To reiterate, guided reflection is a reflexive spiral of being and becoming; of enabling the practitioner to realise desirable work by looking back at seeing herself as a transformed person through a series of unfolding experiences. Each subsequent experience applies and reflects on the insights gained from the previous experience. Hence, reflexivity is this looking back activity. Gergen and Gergen (1991) make a distinction between inward looking reflexivity which seeks feedback to reinforce and sustain a particular world view, and outward looking reflexivity which draws on multiple perspectives to challenge a world view. The former might be called a 'closed' or single loop system whilst the latter might be called an 'open' or double loop system (Argyris and Schön 1974) whereby the self is open to critique and transformation of one's actions congruent with beliefs about the nature of practice. It is double feedback that is characteristic of learning through guided reflection. The reflexive spiral of being and becoming is sometimes a dramatic moment of revelation or it is a gradual almost subliminal unfolding moment by moment. Dewey noted (1933):

> 'The successive portions of a reflective thought grow out of one another and support one another; they do not come and go in medley. Each phase is a step from something to something – technically speaking, it is a term of thought. Each term leaves a deposit that is utilised in the next term. The stream or flow becomes a train or chain. There are in any reflective thought definite units that are linked together so that there is sustained movement to a common end.' (pp. 4–5)

It is these definite units that mark the reflexive developmental journey and give shape to the narrative form.

Framing effective practice

As the narratives in Chapters 4–10 illuminate, there are many theoretical frameworks that can be used for framing and monitoring the practitioner's development. Such frameworks can focus on discrete aspects of practice, such as conflict management, or more global structures that attempt to capture the whole essence of practice, such as the being available template. Frameworks can be imported from extant theory or constructed within the analysis of experience as the research process unfolds. This is the reflexive nature of guided reflection research, to construct and subsequently test interpretative frameworks for their adequacy to represent transformation of practice. Such frameworks must be sensitive enough to portray the nuances, subtleties, complexities and contradictions of everyday practice, yet robust enough to reflect the practitioner's journey of realisation in ways that enable the reader to follow the trail and be convinced of its authenticity.

The being available template

The being available template is an example of a global framing structure to mark the developmental journey of becoming. The template was reflexively constructed through engaging with practice as a process of thematic reduction to find a framework that adequately reflected the essential nature of desirable practice (Johns 1998). It asserts that the core therapeutic is the practitioner *being available* to work with the person and family to help them find meaning in the health event and make good decisions about their lives, and take appropriate action to meet their health needs. (Johns 2000, p. 68). The extent to which the practitioner can be available is determined by six inter-related factors (Fig. 3.1).

As with using any framework, there is always the risk of fitting the practitioner's development to the framework. Offsetting this risk requires a sceptical attitude to challenge the adequacy of any framing device and to work towards constructing more valid frameworks. Remember that developmental frameworks are only heuristics to frame development, not a rigid structure to force-fit experience. As such they can be used creatively to expand understanding rather than being used in a rigid reductionist way.

The practitioner knows what is desirable	Knowing what is desirable gives meaning and purpose to practice and focuses concern and action.
The practitioner knows the person	Knowing the person/family in the context of the meanings they give to the health event. The practitioner must tune into the patient's wave-length, connect and establish a dialogue with the patient and family where meaning and needs are constantly interpreted within the unfolding moment.
The practitioner is concerned for the person	Concern is the motivational expression of caring that creates possibility within the caring relationship. The greater the practitioner's concern the greater the possibilities within her relationship with the patient and family.
The aesthetic response	The practitioner grasps and interprets what is unfolding, envisages possibility, and responds with appropriate and effective action.
The practitioner knows and manages herself within relationships	The practitioner stays in tune with the patient by paying attention to and managing any personal concerns that create resistance.
The practitioner can create and sustain an environment where being available is possible	The relationship between the practitioner and the patient/family takes place within a specific organisational and professional context, which may constrain her being available to the patient and family. Constraining factors may also be embodied within self.

Fig. 3.1   The extent to which the practitioner can be available – 'being available template'.

Of course, readers will judge for themselves the extent to which the narratives in Chapters 4–10 are fitted into the developmental frameworks and the extent to which the practitioners have critiqued the coherence of such frameworks to justify their use. It is relevant to pose a number of questions: Are such frameworks merited? Doesn't the use of such frameworks inevitably reduce and fragment the holistic nature of experience rather in the genre of phenomenological reduction? Yet if the purpose of the research is to enable the practitioner to realise desirable work, then should this unfolding process and subsequent outcome be monitored in valid ways? These are tricky questions that I will return to in terms of narrative construction and validity.

Agency and victimicy

Another approach to frame development congruent with empowerment, is to view experience in terms of victimicy and agency and to plot the development of agency through the signs that represent agency. The effort to challenge and rebalance power relationships that constrain the realisation of desirable practice can be viewed as the effort to assert agency over victimicy. Bruner (1994) asks 'what sorts of criteria guide the selectivity of memory retrieval?'. He asserts that 'one of them must surely be derived from some sort of need to emphasise agency, the flip side of which might be called 'victimicy'. Bruner notes:

> 'Agency is an affirmation of the triumph of the autonomous self in realising aspirations, whilst victimicy is a negation of this process, a reflection on those forces that have constrained this in some way.' (p. 42)

Triumph is the realisation of realigning power relationships in the best interests of patients and families, a new collaborative alliance based on mutual respect and understanding of roles. Autonomy is always contextual. Within collaborative relationships, power is liberated from the shackles of domination for both self and other to use in therapeutic ways. However power ways of relating are deeply embodied and reinforced in daily ways of relating. The guide helps the practitioner to see self as a victim and simultaneously to envisage agency – what must I do to shift my perception of self? Narrative is the transformational movement to power this shift of perception reinforced through reflection on new ways of relating within practice.

As such, the narrative is a critical description of the practitioner's effort to realise the agentic self and conquer the forces of victimicy. Polkinghorne (1996), developing Bruner's ideas of agentic and victimic plot, cites the work of Cochran and Laub (1994) who explored the transformation from a victimic to an agentic life plot developed from studying the rehabilitation of persons who had been severely injured. Cochran and Laub concluded that the change in identity from victimic to agentic consisted of two correlative movements: the progressive construction of a new agentic life story, and the destruction and detachment from the victimic life story. The victimic plot does not simply fade away, it has to be actively confronted. As with Kieffer's (1984) emergence of community leaders, it is a movement away from victimicy to agency, a process of empowerment. For Tessa (Chapter 5) to succeed she must become empowered in order to break away from those forces that constrain her. Fundamentally she must shed her self-perception of subordinate and therefore powerless, and the consequent fear that action will inevitably result in conflict which she cannot win because she is gripped by the fear of sanction or loss of reward. Such fear paralyses and leads to a failure of integrity to act in the patient's and family's best interests. Instead the practitioner feels 'forced' to be loyal to her 'masters'. When dominated by fear the practitioner has no control and cannot take action. Through reflection the way the organisation projected their anxiety that things go smoothly into ward managers such as Tessa, became evident. To take control, Tessa needed to learn to see and resist this projection in appropriate ways.

Narrative thread

A narrative has a coherent organisational structure that successfully weaves its parts into a meaningful whole. Guided reflection narrative is characterised by an unfolding sequence of experiences that adequately illuminates the practitioner's reflexive effort to realise desirable and effective practice.

Guided reflection narrative can be structured in various ways:

- Chronologically through each theme of the chosen monitoring/interpretative framework(s)
- Chronologically through each guided reflection session in which the various parts of the whole framework are pursued
- Chronologically through each unfolding experience.

With the exception of Madden's narrative, the narratives in Part 2 are structured chronologically through successive guided reflection sessions, whereby each session is a reflexive transition point. Madden's narrative is an exception whereby she merely comments she shared ideas within guided reflection that influenced her future visits. However, the first narratives I constructed pursued each theme chronologically through each guided reflection session. This approach was limited because it resembled a phenomenological approach of thematising experience, fragmenting the whole experience by reducing into 'bits' of dialogue, to justify the existence of the themes, as if the themes were concrete realities. As Paget (1983) noted:

> 'An exchange cannot be severed from the shared historical understanding which it pre-supposes without radically shattering its meanings. An exchange contains the meanings of what has already been said … isolating an exchange from its antecedents, those exchanges which already occurred and are pre-supposed, shatters a discourse process and undermines the unfolding complex and multi-meaninged construction of experience.' (p. 79)

In contrast, the chronological approach of unfolding the narrative through each subsequent guided reflection session enabled the whole experience (whole chunks of dialogue), and then for it to be reflected as a whole using the domains as a reflective framework. This approach created a gestalt view of the practitioner's *whole* experience unfolding over time, whereby aspects of experience can be viewed against a background of the whole, and it is this understanding that supported the latter view. In reducing Gill's narrative to an elaborate scheme of categories and themes, I was unwittingly influenced by phenomenology as a way of representing and explaining lived experience. I believe it was an unwitting need to control the developmental process that led me to view subsequent narratives through this framework. The reader may argue that to some extent Alexia's experiences (Chapter 7) were fitted into the being available template. To some extent this is true although, in the spirit of dialogue, I am conscious of suspending my viewing lenses in order to keep an open mind.

I have a deep disquiet about the way phenomenology reduces experience into discrete categories, uses fragments of people's narratives to support each theme, and then claims to be representative of lived experience. Likewise Thorne (1997) has raised concerns of a slippage from the original objectives of the qualitative research enterprise into some form of pseudo-objective version of reality – in other words a contradiction between the ideals of an existential philosophical approach and actual practice, a contradiction deeply embodied within the nursing psyche. As Lawler (1998) points out:

'nurses as researchers have not always paid due regard to what might be considered sacrosanct or methodologically pure' (p. 105) especially with regard to 'phenomenologies and other interpretative approaches in which the design characteristics are not so tightly prescribed.' (p. 105)

Whilst most phenomenologists would decry a positivist world viewpoint, I wonder to what extent such thinking does determine this approach, even unwittingly as a left-over brain trace. If such researchers were truly interested in the nature of lived experience they would need to tell the whole story rather than fragments split into different parts. Without doubt phenomenological studies are valuable sources to inform and challenge the practitioner to reflect on the meanings people give to events. As with all theory, the reader must carefully distil the 'phenomenological' study to render the validity of the methodological approach in terms of its outcomes. However, this is not to diminish the responsibility of researchers to make such issues clear within their studies (Borbasi 1995).

Frameworks can give the impression that experience is more orderly than it really is. In other words they impose an illusionary order. Experience is not an orderly affair with neat beginnings and endings amidst a smooth flow of logic. It is complex and contradictory. To adequately reflect experience, narrative must itself be a complex and contradictory affair, an unfolding drama of stories within stories. Hence narrative can only be constructed as an unfolding story rather than constructed at the end. As such, the guide and practitioner consciously construct the narrative by recording the dialogue of each session evolving from the previous session, layers upon layers woven together through the series of unfolding experiences, drawn together by the plot and the markers that monitor the journey of self being and becoming.

The effort to reduce the complexity of experience into themes or categories reflects the positivist, masculine concern, to order, predict and control life. And yet, in our ordered lives, for others to feel confident in such research, a compromise may need to be made to see a path through the complexity. People are so used to speaking with received voices that they are unable to unravel their own meanings from such texts, but then perhaps teachers, writers and researchers of nursing have not encouraged or facilitated such personal adventures. Narratives can never tell the whole story but they give glimpses to other dimensions not overtly addressed, the gestalt relationship between foreground and background.

Paget (1983) led me to recognise the need to use adequate dialogue to support 'proof' of practitioner development *and* to portray the subtlety, complexity, context and subjectivity of experience. In my PhD narratives (Johns 1998) I increasingly used more dialogue taken from guided reflection sessions, until approximately 60% of the narrative was constructed from dialogue because I felt that such dialogue best captured the spirit of the work rather than the language of interpretation 'that flattens rather than deepens our understanding of human life' (Van Manen 1990, p. 17). Because much of the dialogue was led by the practitioner, it seemed natural to use dialogue as the primary source of description (Agar & Hobbs 1982). Using dialogue as central to the narrative construction inevitably incorporated the feelings, goals, needs, and values of the people who created it (Robinson & Hawpe 1986) because these are always implicit within dialogue. The narrative writer(s) make explicit the significant issues within the dialogue and fashion these fragments into a whole whose integrity is in its presentation in narrative form (Gergen & Gergen 1986).

One consequence of using substantial chunks of dialogue to construct narrative is that narratives are likely to become very long. The narratives presented in this book are relatively short in terms of the number of sessions. Narratives that span 30 sessions have been 30 000 words. For example, in a two year study of working with four surgical ward sisters within guided reflection, the approximate length of each narrative was Shirley (34 sessions) 30 000 words; Claire (29 sessions) 25 000 words; Saskia (26 sessions) 24 000 words; Jenny (22 sessions) 20 000 words. In terms of report writing and publication, this requires a rethink about the nature of a thesis and subsequent publications. The narratives presented in this book vary in length between 11 000 and 12 000 words. Are these narratives too long? Could they be more parsimonious? Yet they have been edited *to the bone* without losing their coherence.

Narrative style

This book contains seven narratives, each presenting contrasting ways in which dialogue has been used. Of these I wrote Tessa's, Caitlin's and Alexia's narratives (Chapters 5, 6 and 7) based on extensive notes taken during the guided reflection sessions and word-processed within 24 hours. The reader will note that these particular narratives are predominantly written using guided reflection dialogue. Of the remaining narratives, I edited Aileen's written assignments for her degree course (Chapter 4). Yvonne, Jane and Bella (Chapters 8, 9 and 10) wrote their narratives as fulfilment of their degree courses. My role was to guide their writing and edit the narratives for inclusion in the book. The reader will note the diversity of style. There is no best 'style' of narrative provided all styles are coherent (see discussion later in this chapter). In these latter narratives my presence within the narrative is at the discretion of the practitioner. I have a lesser presence in Bella's narrative, reflecting my relative lack of involvement as her guide.

Positioning of the guide within the narratives

In the narratives I have written, as opposed to those I have edited, it is interesting to ask the question: Who's narrative is it? Clearly whoever constructs the narratives reflects their particular view, even though co-creation of meaning is intended. In other words the narrative must inevitably be skewed towards the writer's perspective. How would Jane Groom's narrative (Chapter 9) have looked if I had recorded extensive dialogue from our guided reflections sessions and applied the interpretative frameworks? Would she have agreed with my record as being representational of what took place? Evidence suggests she would have done so, trusting in my integrity to represent what took place adequately. Perhaps the content and certainly the style would be different. Two views on what took place. Perhaps the narratives I construct are my own narratives of guiding the practitioner to realise desirable practice, rather than their narratives. Reading Jane's and Yvonne's narrative, they pay attention to the process of guidance but my presence within these narratives is not significant in comparison to the ones I constructed. Does it matter? Is there a deeper issue of validity here that needs attention? I do not think so. The narratives are what they are and as long as they are transparent in terms of their integrity then all well and good.

The influence of Ben Okri

Ben Okri in his book *A way of being free* (1997) inspired me to grasp a literary perspective on narrative. Narrative refocuses the self at the centre in ways that honour and mend the fractured nature of reality, yet in ways whereby a temporal unity or plot is established not just in a written form but within life itself. The art of storytelling challenges the narrative writer to write accounts that can capture the imagination. Okri (1997) notes:

'Even when it is tragic, storytelling is always beautiful. It tells us that all fates can be ours. It wraps up our lives with the magic which we only see long afterwards. Storytelling reconnects us to the great sea of human destiny, human suffering, and human transcendence.' (p. 47)

What images are conjured by the stories, as if the stories are magical tales. Yet within the stories lies the truth of the nursing, or any other tradition. The stories shed a light on everyday practice in ways that mean the very roots of the tradition are revealed. The stories are beacons of the effort to realise self as caring. In this sense they are poignant, both wonderful and terrible, wonderful through the caring effort to respond to the suffering of others and terrible through the ways the caring effort is constantly thwarted. Again Okri (1997) notes:

'The joy of transgressing beautifully, of taking readers to places they wouldn't willingly go, this joy of seducing or dragging readers in spite of themselves to places deep in them where wonders lurk besides terrors, this delicate art of planting delayed repeated explosions and revelations in the reader's mind, and doing this while enchanting them – this is one of the most mysterious joys of all.' (p. 65)

Stories must always be challenging, unsettling. As you feel the struggle of the story-tellers you begin to absorb the tensions within as you begin to relate the story to your own experiences and then the story begins to live within you, being changed and in the process changing you. Again, Okri writes:

'Storytelling is always, quietly, subversive ... when you think it is harmless, that is when it springs its hidden truths, its uncomfortable truths, on you. It startles your complacency. And when you no longer listen, it lies silently in your brain, waiting. Stories are very patient things. They drift quietly in your soul. They infect your dreams and perceptions, occupying your spirit. Stories are living things; and their real life begins when they start to live in you. Then they never stop living, or growing, or mutating, or feeding the groundswell of imagi-nation, sensibility, and character. Stories are subversive because they always remind us of our fallibility. The subversion in storytelling is an important part of the transformation of human beings into higher possibilities. (pp. 43–5)

The power of the stories is the truth they speak to the reader. The stories are both a window for the reader to view the lives of those within the stories and also a window or mirror to her or his own soul. The stories are compelling because they capture the complexity of everyday practice without essentially fragmenting it. Perhaps the stories seem unnecessarily long to those readers used to being presented with the facts. Yet stories have no facts; nothing can be presented with any certainty. Indeed the stories are a testament of uncertainty; within the apparent fragmentation of everyday life is found the wholeness of experience. The facts are those perceived by the reader to be open to her experience in the juxtaposition of self and other's own experiences, a fusion of horizons. The stories are truthful renditions of experience. They may not be historically accurate in terms of detail. They may be distorted in the self's need to perceive self in certain sorts of ways. Yet, it is still a valid story because people need to distort things for reasons which themselves become a focus for understanding and revealing the true self beneath the layers of distortion that mask the therapeutic self. The purpose of narrative is to reveal self and the layers that obscure self because if we cannot reveal the true self then the self cannot be available to achieve desirable and effective work.

Academic presentation

How might a student present her narrative within a dissertation or thesis? Many practitioners who use guided reflection are likely to do so in order to meet the requirements of an award whether at undergraduate, taught masters' or MPhil/PhD level. Yvonne Latchford and Jane Groom's narratives were part of their dissertations for the award of a BA Health Care honours degree. Bella Madden's narrative was part of her dissertation for the award of a masters degree in Research and Evaluation. In each case I guided them to construct the dissertation in five chapters (Fig. 3.2), although I want to emphasise that this format is not a prescription. Practitioners who completed their narratives as undergraduate dissertations required 50% more words than the criteria which were written for more 'conventional' type research reports. Fulfilling criteria can be a thorny issues for such aspects as ethics and validity, which I consider next.

Ethics

Researching and developing self in the context of self's own practice demands no ethical approval from others. Indeed it is a mark of responsibility to take self so seriously and develop self's potential to realise desirable practice. However, self is always viewed in relationship with others, as illustrated through the narratives. As such, others become visible within the narrative, and because the narrative is subjective and contextualised, the other is more easily recognised. Where the relationship is critical of others, they may recoil from the light, unable to tolerate being seen in a 'bad light'. Where others are generally perceived as more powerful, such exposure is likely not to be tolerated. Such is the abuse of patriarchal power that the 'research' is suppressed because the views expressed are 'subjective' and therefore are less easy to justify as factual.

Chapter 1 – Beginnings	The function of this chapter is to set the scene for the project. Key issues that seemed important to address were: • Who is the practitioner? • From what perspective do they approach this project of self-inquiry? • How do they view the nature of desirable practice? • How did they come to focus on the researched aspect of self, for example Jane Groom working with DSH patients in an Accident & Emergency Department (Chapter 9).
Chapter 2 – Methodology	In this chapter the practitioner sets out their understanding of the nature of guided reflection. The chapter should not be a faithful rendition of previous studies, but an effort to expand the known boundaries of guided reflection methodology, especially for practitioners working at higher degree levels of study.
Chapter 3 – Method	In this chapter the practitioner sets out the way she and the guide went about the research, picking up and developing issues introduced in Chapters 1 and 2. It is the nuts and bolts of how the methodology was put into action, for example keeping a journal, guided reflection sessions, narrative construction, etc.
Chapter 4 – The narrative	In this chapter the practitioner presents her narrative in her own style.
Chapter 5 – Reflection	In this chapter the practitioner highlights the significance of her reflection and draws conclusions for its wider significance in terms of clinical practice, education, research and society. On another level of reflection, the guide and practitioner might consider the congruence of the research, notably dilemmas and contradictions they faced within the process.

Fig. 3.2 A potential academic structure for constructing a guided reflection thesis.

In terms of protecting patients and families, the use of pseudonym is adequate because the intent is always to realise caring and that such stories are valuable to others to learn from. I do not feel it necessary to seek permission from patients and families that I am writing about them in my reflective journal and talking about them within guided reflection, and researching my relationship with them in narrative form. However, from a holistic perspective I am in dialogue with them and, as such, it is possible to involve them in the study or to express their viewpoints more accurately.

Wearing my critical social science hat, the narrative is an expression of emancipation yet always with good intent to realise caring in practice. As such I have no hesitation in exposing conditions of practice that constrain this realisation, and would indeed hope that organisations would appreciate this feedback if they are truly patient centred. In other words, complaint that such research breaches ethical codes of research conduct is merely another constraint on practitioners to have a voice.

Madden (2001) considered the moral positioning of women's voices within her narrative:

'Miller (2000), argues that our lives are given continuity through narrative construction and reconstruction. Without the opportunity to consolidate and build our own narratives, women, particularly new mothers, literally run the risk of "losing the plot" of their own life history. As clinical researchers, we have unique access to this interface between the public and private spheres of life, and therefore have a duty if we research it at all, to do so with respect and sensitivity. May and Fleming (1997) argue that there is a moral imperative within nursing research, that demands that we not only look at what is, but also at what ought to be, and that narratives offer such an opportunity, as they are reflections of both ourselves as practitioners and the occupation of nursing/midwifery in general.

De Francisco (1997) feels that to attempt liberating research, we must place the non-dominant group at the centre of our study, and we must force ourselves as researchers out of 'ethical objectivity' which only serves to deny the real affective aspects of our lives and oppression. Our methodology must think globally, that is, it must be rooted in ideas of social structure, and the wider forces of society; but act locally by looking at what is happening within the smaller picture of people's lives. The point is to make acts of resistance visible, and facilitate their spread. In this way, the concept of power at a societal or interpersonal level is also a positive one – it is not inevitably about oppression. There are echoes of Fay's (1987) warning here as to the danger of replacing one dogma with another – De Francisco argues that we must move away from tendencies to overgeneralise behaviour, as well as studying the power differentials between researcher and researched. This is very self-conscious research she is proposing, and it is interesting to note that other feminists see our modern task connected to that of reconstructing our sense of self and identity.

Weir (1995) sees the problem of self-identity as the capacity to sustain and resolve, often conflicting, identities, and that to do this we need high degrees of self awareness and self-direction. However, the down side to this is that we are burdened by our own insights, as every act becomes one of self-definition, and every meaning problematic. This is balanced by the knowledge that we are, through the process of self-realisation, affecting our world and our place in it. We are awake to the buzz at the intersection of the individual and social forces, and feel the powers exerted on us, our acquiescence and resistance.

But nurses and midwives have traditionally been wary both of feminist thought (Doran & Cameron 1998) and reflexive research. Stereotypes of feminists abound, and are usually negative in the minds of many women. However, as De Francisco (1997) argues, when we stop concentrating on gender differences and look instead to the exercise and expression of power as both a negative and positive force, then our feminism takes a less dogmatic form than many expect.

This requires us to move further than the qualitative/quantitative split – much 'qualitative' research appears to be positivist in its orientation when it stresses objectivity. The basic conundrum here is that such research becomes respectable because it mirrors the concerns of empirical, scientific rational enquiry, and so all researchers adopt the language of value-neutrality in an effort to get published and be taken seriously. Wainwright (1997) argues that one of the consequences of this is to deprive research of its critical nature, on the assumption that qualitative research can be critical or valid but not both. Just as we risk losing our 'caring' focus when we strive for professional status, so may we lose our intuitive, affective knowledge if we uncritically accept such definitions of validity. The only response is to plough the furrow that means the most to us as midwives and women – to go on regardless, and take the attendant risks of ambivalent status.

A process of deconstruction is therefore required, in order that we know what it is that we know, and its origin. If midwifery is to remain focused on women, and not medicine, then some introspection is required. Chenail and Maione (1997) have argued that when clinicians turn researchers, they already have a strong sense of the 'other', the patient or client they are researching. They need, therefore, to face their 'sensemaking' by deconstructing this using three reference points: the literature of others (what is already said); their own reflections on the phenomenon (examining forestructures); and reflexivity within the research process itself (awareness of ongoing dialogue). Thus a critical methodology is turned also on the self, and the political force of the knowledge being created.' (pp. 75–8)

Madden illuminates a real tension of positioning voices within the narrative that are acceptable to the diverse gaze of actors. Perhaps Madden is more sensitive about this positioning because of the tension in her role of listening to women's stories that inevitably reveal poor practice. The risk of compromise to make narratives acceptable is to sanitise them and risk their potency. Without doubt, as all the narratives reveal, we live in a world where issues are not determined in patients' best interests. Although this world view is shifting, it is a prevailing legacy of patriarchy that doctors and managers can determine what is best for patients. In response, the narrative writer needs to pay careful attention to being negatively critical about another colleague, especially where criticism implies negligence, and even where the people involved are masked behind pseudonym. For those involved within stories it is not so difficult to penetrate identity. The key is to word criticism in ways which are non-threatening. It's akin to walking a fine line between asserting self and marginalising self. It may be difficult in a libel case to convince that the reflection is adequate evidence of fact. This can only be a question of judgement. Asking someone to read the narrative with a legal eye is also wise. However, I do not suggest people seek permission to publish their narratives from the organisation, which may have a vested interested in keeping invisible practice that might be construed as less than desirable.

Congruence and validity

What makes a reader feel confident that a narrative adequately represents the practitioner's journey in being and becoming an effective practitioner? In other words, what makes a narrative congruent? Reason and Rowan (1981) suggest that congruence is a more appropriate word than validity in an attempt to move away from the meanings generally associated with 'validity' in terms of an empiricist paradigm. Hence the idea of a 'new' paradigm that explicitly seeks to know subjective experience. A dictionary definition of congruence is 'suitableness, fitness, agreement between things, consistency'. To return to Wilber's (1998) ideas, perhaps genuineness, integrity, trust and authenticity are the key words to test the truthfulness of practitioner reflection.

By congruent I do not mean that these influences are not contradictory. There are no straight lines in nature and the idea that perfection exists in methodology is a fallacy. Congruence is important to establish because it suggests a philosophical compatibility rather than a sharp edge. There are always different perspectives both within the thoughts of writers and in the way readers interpret writing. Things find their own rhythms and the researcher must learn to tune in and flow without seeking absolute explanations for why things are as they are.

Eyes of knowing

I am conscious of an inherent threat that the adequacy of narratives will fall on the stony ground of empiricist dogma. To put narrative knowing into a paradigmatic perspective, Wilber's view (1998) of an integral view of consciousness is useful. As I outlined in Chapter 1, Wilber differentiated knowledge into four quadrants, divided into subjective and objective, and individual and collective.

Each quadrant or conception of truth has its own paradigmatic injunctions or what Wilber called the *eyes of knowing*. He argued that people have available to them a spectrum of different modes of knowing, each of which discloses a different type of experience – the eye of flesh, the eye of mind, and the eye of contemplation. Wilber considered the way each type of knowing can be apprehended as valid. He suggests that all valid knowledge has the following strands:

Instrumental injunction	This is always the form – if you want to know this, do this.
Intuitive apprehension (illumination)	This is an immediate experience of the domain disclosed by the injunction; that is, a direct experience or data apprehension.
Communal confirmation	This is checking of the results – the data, the evidence – with others who have adequately completed the injunctive and apprehensive strands.

As Wilber notes:

> 'The strength of empiricism is its demand that all genuine knowledge be grounded in experiential evidence. But not only is there sensory experience, there is mental experience and spiritual experience... And thus, if we use experience in its proper sense as direct apprehension, then we can firmly honour the empiricist demand that all genuine knowledge is grounded in experience, in data, in evidence. But data and evidence are not simply lying around waiting for anybody to see, but are brought forth by valid injunctions. (p. 84)

Thus, to gain access to any of these valid modes of knowing, the person needs to be adequate to the injunction. By this Wilber means that they need to be able to use the tools of the paradigm. It is important to use these tools otherwise the results cannot be confirmed within the communion of confirmation. Wilber emphasises this point with regard to contemplation and knowing mysticism. Hence experience can only be adequately apprehended by the person experiencing her or his own being. Understanding and learning through lived experience would fit into the subjective-individual quadrant. Experience cannot be observed. Wilber notes:

'the only way you and I can get at each other's interiors is by dialogue and interpretation. And yet when you report to me your inner status you might be lying. Moreover, you might be lying to yourself.' (p. 14)

Knowing self being and becoming can only be adequately represented in a reflexive narrative form. Other eyes of knowing may be manifest within the narrative yet integrated within it according to their various tools and rules of injunction. The narrative integrates the strands of experience, whether body, mind and soul, into a coherent whole. As such, the narrative cannot satisfactorily be validated from any one paradigm because the rules of each are necessarily different, focusing as they do within their own forms of injunction.

A valid narrative would seek to reveal truthfulness. However, I am conscious that what practitioners say they did may not correspond with what they actually did, and that people may distort their reality. Indeed, reflection has been questioned in the light of a psychological theory which suggests that people do not recall accurately (Newell 1992). However, the issue is not one of accuracy of recall but of the meaning of events for people. People reflect on events in the present. If practitioners distort events, they do so for reasons which are part of their reality, or to deliberately create a false impression. As Albright (1994) notes:

> 'How much of our remembered self is carefully, scrupulously edited in order to conform to some vision of how we would like our self to appear? If we speak of a remembered self, we should also speak of an editorial self that consciously or unconsciously selects the memories that wrap us around with the sense of our dignity, our erotic power, our nonchalance, our good will toward mankind, all those pleasures that our self-consideration craves.' (pp. 32–3)

The very nature of reflection is to surface and explore contradiction and to reveal self to self, if it is significant in becoming an effective practitioner. Just as the developmental process is rooted in revealing and working towards resolving contradiction, so it is within the guided reflection relationship itself. Are the 'horizons' of the supervisor and the practitioner continuously woven in co-creating meaning, transcending each perspective? Is the dialogue conducted in an interactive, dialogic manner, where meaning is negotiated through 'free and open dialogue' (Elliott 1989) so that agreement as to what would count as a more truthful description of work-life can be reached (Kushner & Norris 1980–81; Lather 1986a)? From this perspective validity is properly concerned with processes of engagement and dialogue, and an emergent reflexive sense of what's important, rather than on outcomes.

The guide and practitioner must reflect on their relationship in ways that allow 'living contradictions' (Whitehead 2000) to be revealed and worked towards resolving. In other words, a particular focus of guided reflection is a mutual reflexive self-consciousness on the guided reflection relationship itself.

We do not live in a perfect world with perfect answers to situations. As such, failure of correspondence between 'what I say' and 'what I do' remains a potential yet acceptable flaw. The ability to recall more accurately and penetrate self-distortion is enhanced by using models of reflection that give the more novice reflective practitioner access to reflection in a systematic way. The use of such models gives confidence to the reader that reflection is not merely haphazard and dismissed as anecdotal in its most pejorative sense.

'Validity' themes

Lather (1986a, b), in searching for more adequate ways to fit *validity* to new paradigm research, identified three key validity criteria: catalytic validity, face validity, and construct validity. Lather (1993) did not claim these criteria in a prescriptive sense. She felt these criteria best 'fitted' empowering type research, 'openly committed to a more just social order' (p. 66). The explicit focus of guided reflection on shared vision, collegial working, working with patients and families, and creating and sustaining conditions where being available is possible, all point towards a more just social order with its focus on liberating practitioners from oppressive conditions in order to realise desirable work.

Face validity

One test of the truth of critical theory is the considered reaction by those for whom it is supposed to be emancipatory (Fay 1987). Reason and Rowan (1981) note:

> 'Good research at the non-alienating end of the spectrum ... goes back to the subject with the tentative results, and refines them in the light of the subject's reactions.' (p. 248)

The 'results' are co-created as they unfold within the reflexive process. As such the conditions for face validity are implicit within the research process. Hall and Stevens (1991) note that the active voice of participants is enhanced:

> 'by using their language to describe phenomenon and create theory, and by presenting their verbatim stories to illustrate analytical arguments.' (p. 26)

As such, the use of dialogue to construct narrative enables the practitioner's voice to be heard and enables my interpretations of dialogue to be transparent and open to competing discourses.

Construct validity

Construct validity focuses the researcher on ensuring that emergent insights (or tentative theory) are grounded within a wider community of knowledge. This condition is met through theoretical framing in which the researcher/practitioner frames emerging insights within extent theory as a dialogic process. The truth is not 'out there' as some objective reality that the personal notion of truth must be judged against to qualify as the truth. Neither is it simply subjective, because people are not isolated. They exist in communities where some common understanding of what counts as truth is adhered to; a constant interplay between knowing as revealed through reflection and extant theories towards co-creating meaning that is always unfolding and evolving within the reflexive spiral of being and becoming.

Catalytic validity

Catalytic validity is concerned with illuminating the way practitioners come to see themselves reflexively (Agar & Hobbs 1982). This requires the narrative to represent adequately what took place without textual distortion. As Steele (1986) notes:

> 'All narratives leave out people, events, or ideas which if included would cast doubt on the truth of the theory being expounded or the story being told. Textual distortion by omission of relevant data is difficult to see when reading a work because there are only often obscure signs in the text that point to what is missing from it.' (p. 262)

Steele notes that 'textual distortion' is difficult for the reader to perceive and perhaps can only be challenged through a reflective scepticism. Are the 'results' well founded in and consistent with the dialogue? Are the results systematically connected within a coherent sense of the whole? Where research intends to be empowering, then clearly the construction of the narrative that represents the practitioners' experiences must have been negotiated as a continuous process, not just at the end, when the account has largely been formulated.

Rhizomatic validity

Madden (2001) develops a view on validity from a feminist perspective that picks up Lather's concerns with 'validity'. She writes:

> 'Lather (1993) advocates an anarchistic view of the growth of knowledge that denies the idea of a smooth, orderly progression from ignorance to knowing; she argues that "there is no trunk, no emergence from a single root, but rather arbitrary branchings off and temporal frontiers which can only be mapped, not blueprinted" (p. 680).
>
> Any consensus of what it is that we know is, for Lather, a "temporal contract". Her notion of validity, rhizomatic validity, is both post-modern and feminist in that it refuses to fragment the narrative into forced codes and categories. Rhizomatic validity refers to new knowledge that "taps underground", and in so doing creates new locally determined norms of understanding. It is based not on criteria of permanency and rationality, but on its power to open up new discourses, and subvert taken-for-granted ways of interpreting the world. Irigaray (1987) adds that women need to pay special attention to the language of science, stressing how such language forbids the first person, the subjective, as a way of masking the agents through whom it is propagated. Thus the political effects of the discourse are blurred behind a screen of neutrality. If one accepts these arguments, at least in part, then the notion of "validity" within research (even our notions of what "research" is and is not) loses a certain degree of power. It can itself be viewed as an oppressive technology, as it serves to downgrade the personal, the subjective, the untidy story within each of us. The crucial distinction that marks feminist research from other forms, is that it is carried out for women, that it is self-consciously partial. Admitting the impossibility of impartiality and neutrality, it seeks instead to own its political core. Acker *et al.* (1983) reconstruct validity in terms of "worthwhileness". This worthwhileness is judged by the emancipatory qualities of the research, using three criteria:
>
> (1) whether the voices of participants are heard in research reports
> (2) whether the role of the investigator is theorised as well as those of the investigated, and

(3)   whether the analysis reveals the social relations that lie behind the lives of those being studied.

How are these criteria represented here?

(1)   *Participants' voices* – The stories of women relayed by my diary
(2)   *Role of investigator* – Exploration of my pre-understandings, influences, or fore-structures
(3)   *Social relations* – Exploration of the discourses inherent in the listening role of the visits – the nature of the clinical intervention.

The rejection of the traditional concepts of validity within research, those built around ideas of objectivity, impartiality and rationality, opens the door to a different frame of meaning – one that accords with the greater eclecticism of much feminist research (Webb 1993). For Weir (1995), those different frames of meaning are to do with self-identity, and the ways in which it is constructed. Weir looks to a concept of self-identity that sees women as active participants in the social world, and central to this understanding of identity is the capacity to sustain, and resolve, multiple and often conflicting identities. To do this we need cognitive and practical capacities for self-knowledge, self-realisation and self-direction. Combining the critical theory of Habermas (to visualise the interested nature of knowledge), and Kristeva's emphasis on the power of affective relationships (to facilitate feelings of participation in the world), Weir (1995) talks of a responsibility "to problematize and define one's own meaning (and identity) (which) is both the burden and the privilege of modern society – as a subject who is relatively free to determine, through my own practices, who I am and who I am going to be. The flip side of this is the burden of self-definition – every action, every decision becomes self-defining – every position is open to question".' (pp. 26–9])

Madden illuminates that validity for guided reflection research cannot, because of its very nature, be pinned down within rigid rules or set criteria. This is pertinent because Madden's work was presented as a master's dissertation and achieved an excellent mark. You might argue she beguiled her markers but I do not think so. One reason for her success was her debate around validity; i.e. she addressed validity in a reflective way and justified her position. Jane Groom presented her work as an undergraduate dissertation and was sharply criticised for failure to adhere to set criteria and because one of her examiners had his own rigid understanding of what validity meant. Yvonne Latchford similarly presented her narrative as part of her undergraduate dissertation and was awarded the highest mark. The risk is that this concern with validity detracts from the merit of the narrative itself. I feel I am a guardian eagle swooping low to protect this work within the academy.

Reader validity

'The story writer does one half of the work, but the reader does the other. The reader's mind becomes the screen, the place, the era. To a large extent readers create the world from words, they invent the reality they read. Reading, therefore, is a co-production between writer and reader.' (Okri 1997, p. 41)

Readers may relate to the narrative simply because they share common meanings and experience similar situations. As such, narratives have enormous value to inform other practitioners. Relating to narratives is made accessible because they are subjective and contextualised. The reader knows where the other person is coming from. Meaning does not have to be interpreted from generalisations. The text offers examples based on concrete experience rather than rules to be followed. As Read (1983) asserted, people relate more easily to examples, particularly within complex situations, than following a set of rules. It doesn't matter which characteristics are unique and which are general within the reflective perspective. Generalisation is never an intention of empowering research.

As such, the ultimate test of coherence lies with the reader – the extent to which the reader relates to the text. The art of reading texts, or hermeneutics, is dialogue – the engagement between text and reader, other and self, in coming to a mutual understanding or clarifying disagreement. Readers (as interpreters) will approach these narratives with their own horizons, and whilst they may not share my interpretations, they should be able to make sense of it. Gadamer (1975) expressed the hermeneutic belief that the reader projects, in advance, a sense of the whole as soon as an initial sense appears. This is because the reader brings to this text a viewpoint on what to expect from the text, i.e. his or her own meanings and experiences with the world. This position assumes:

> 'The audience is not composed of isolated, passive consumers of social spectacle but is in a position to use this work as a resource, critically appropriating aspects of it to help them to clarify the basis of everyday life and the possibilities for its transformation.' (Simon & Dippo, 1986, p. 199)

The reader is the final arbiter of truth and is invited to close the hermeneutic circle. The responsibility of the story-writer is to write the story in such a way that the reader is able to make sense of it; the writer establishes a system of signs to guide and provoke the reader. Narrative must find the balance between communicating the meaning of the text and opening a door for others to find meaning. This may not be easy because stories are in themselves contradictory and complex, reflecting the nature of clinical practice. A well-written narrative will point out the scratches, the deep etches, the flaws that flow across the polished surface of life, even as nurses endeavour to put on a polished face to the world. The fragility of our competence lies just below the surface waiting to be revealed. We must become open to ourselves in authentic ways to move beyond ourselves towards self-realisation. The stories do this beautifully. This is their magic. And at the end of it all, the reader will be closer to themselves, will have become more open to their own experience and will know themselves better. They will be touched by the wonder and terrors within the stories. They will feel their compassion tingle and flow more freely as they reveal themselves to themselves, lifting the masks that have clouded their vision as they reconnect to the essence of caring. They will identify the factors in their own practices that constrain realising desirable practice and understand the way these factors work and are formed, and ways these factors might be swept away. In doing so they will continue the flow of their own experiences yet more consciously, more reflectively, more knowingly, and so begin to change the tradition's trajectory. The reader may even pick up a pen and begin to reflect or more formally undertake such research as advocated in the book. Reading the stories is to participate in research because it triggers powerful reflectors within each reader. That is why such stories are such powerful learning opportunities for all levels of practitioners.

I shall let Okri (1997) nearly have the last word:

'It suggests that, at bottom, and never wanting to admit it we really want to face the minotaur within, we want the drains unblocked within, we want the frozen river of our blood and compassion to flow again, we want the pain so that we can be free.' (pp. 65–6)

As a hermeneutic reader, surface and suspend your own concerns as you engage the text and relate to it in terms of your own experience.

References

Acker, J., Barry, K. & Esseveld, J. (1983) Objectivity and truth: problems in doing feminist research. *Women Studies International Forum*, 6(4) 423–35.

Agar, M. & Hobbs, J. (1982) Interpreting discourse: coherence and the analysis of ethnographic interviews. *Discourse Processes*, 5, 1–32.

Albright, D. (1994) Literary and psychological models of the self. In *The Remembering Self: construction and accuracy in the self-narrative* (eds Neisser U. & Fivush R.), pp. 19–40. Cambridge University Press, Cambridge.

Argyris, C. & Schön, D. (1974) *Theory in Practice: increasing professional effectiveness.* Jossey-Bass, San Francisco.

Borbasi, S. (1995) To be or not to be? Nurse? Researcher? Or both? *Nursing Inquiry*, 1, 57.

Bruner, J. (1994) The 'remembered' self. In *The Remembering Self: construction and accuracy in the self-narrative* (eds Neisser U. and Fivush R.), pp. 41–54. Cambridge University Press, Cambridge.

Chenail, R. & Maione, P. (1997) Sensemaking in Clinical Qualitative Research. *The Qualitative Report* 3(1) at http://www.nova.edu/ssss/QR/QR3-1/sense.html

Cochran, L. & Laub, J. (1994) *Becoming an Agent: patterns and dynamics for shaping your life.* State University of New York Press, Albany.

De Francisco, V. (1997) Gender, power and practice: or putting your money (and your research) where your mouth is. In *Gender and Discourse* (ed. R. Wodak). Sage, California.

Dewey, J. (1933) *How We Think.* J.C. Heath, Boston.

Doran, F. & Cameron, C. (1998) Hearing nurses' voices through reflection in women's studies. *Nurse Education Today*, 18, 64–71.

Elliott, J. (1989) Knowledge, power and teacher appraisal. In *Quality in Teaching* (ed. W. Carr). Falmer Press, London.

Fay, B. (1987) *Critical Social Science.* Polity Press, Cambridge.

Gadamer, H-G. (1975) *Truth & Method* (Trans. Barden G. & Cumming J.). Seabury Press, New York.

Gergen, K. & Gergen, M. (1986) Narrative form and the construction of psychological science. In *Narrative Psychology: the storied nature of human conduct* (ed. T. Sarbin). Praeger, New York.

Gergen, K. & Gergen, M. (1991) Toward reflexive methodologies. In *Research and Reflexivity* (ed. F. Steier). Sage Publications, London.

Giorgi, A. (1985) Phemenological psychology of learning and the verbal learning tradition. In *Phemenology and Psychological Research* (ed. A. Giorgi). Duquesne University Press, Pittsburgh.

Hall, J. & Stevens, P. (1991) Rigor in feminist research. *Advances in Nursing Science*, 13(3) 16–29.

Irigaray, L. (1987) Is the subject of science sacred? (Trans. C. Mastrangelo) *Hypatia*, 3(3) (Fall), 66. Cited in Tong, R. (1989) *Feminist Thought: A Comprehensive Introduction*. Routledge, London.

Johns, C. (1998) *Becoming an effective practitioner through guided reflection*. PhD thesis, The Open University.

Johns, C. (2000) *Becoming a Reflective Practitioner*. Blackwell Science, Oxford.

Jones, Blackwolf & Jones, G. (1998) *Earth Dance Drum*, p. 54. Commune-a-Key Publishing, Salt Lake City.

Kieffer, C. (1984) Citizen empowerment: a developmental perspective. *Prevention in Human Services*, **84**(3) 9–36.

Kushner, S. & Norris, N. (1980–81) Interpretation, negotiation, and validity in naturalistic research. *Interchange*, **11**(4) 26–36.

Lather, P. (1986a) Research as praxis. *Harvard Educational Review*, **56**(3) 257–77.

Lather, P. (1986b) Issues of validity in open ideological research: between a rock and a soft place. *Interchange*, **17**(4) 63–84.

Lather, P. (1993) Fertile obsession: validity after post-structuralism. *The Sociological Quarterly*, **34**(4) 673–93.

Lawler, J. (1998) Phenomenologies as research methodologies for nursing: from philosophy to research practice. *Nursing Inquiry*, **5**(2) 104–11.

Madden, B. (2001) *Working with women following traumatic child birth*. MSc dissertation, University of Luton.

Martin, M. (1998) Emerging innovations: caring in action. A fragment of love from practice. *International Journal for Human Caring*, **3**(2) 16–27.

Mattingly, C. (1994) The concept of therapeutic 'emplotment'. *Social Sciences and Medicine*, **38**(6) 811–22.

May, C. & Fleming, C. (1997) The professional imagination: narrative and symbolic boundaries between medicine and nursing. *Journal of Advanced Nursing*, 25, 1094–1100.

Miller, T. (2000) Losing the plot: narrative construction and longitudinal childbirth research. *Qualitative Health Research*, **10**(3) 309–23.

Newell, M. (1992) Anxiety, accuracy, and reflection: the limits of professional development. *Journal of Advanced Nursing*, 17, 1326–33.

Okri, B. (1997) *A Way of Being Free*. Phoenix House, London.

Paget, M. (1983) Experience and knowledge. *Human Studies*, **6**(2) 67–90.

Polkinghorne, D.E. (1996) Transformative narratives: from victimic to agentic life plots. *The American Journal of Occupational Therapy*, **50**(4) 299–305.

Read, S.J. (1983) Once is enough: causal reasoning from a single instance. *Journal of Personality & Social Psychology*, **45**(2) 323–34.

Reason, P. & Rowan, J. (1981) Issues of validity in new paradigm research. In *Human Inquiry* (eds P. Reason & J. Rowan). John Wiley, Chichester.

Robinson, J. & Hawpe, L. (1986) Narrative thinking as a heuristic proces. In *Narrative Psychology: the storied nature of human conduct* (ed. T. Sarbin) pp. 111–25. Praeger, New York.

Simon, R. & Dippo, D. (1986) On critical ethnographic work. *Anthropology and Education Quarterly*, 17, 195–202.

Spence, D.P. (1982) *Narrative Truth and Historical Truth: meaning and interpretation in psycho-analysis*. WW Norton & Co., New York.

Steele, R. (1986) Deconstructing histories: toward a systematic criticism of psychological naratives. In *Narrative Psychology: the storied nature of human conduct* (ed. T. Sarbin). Praeger, New York.

Thorne, S. (1997) Phenomenological positivism and other problematic trends in health science research. *Qualitative Health Research*, 7, 287–93.

Van Manen, M. (1990) *Researching Lived Experience*. State University of New York Press, New York.

Wagner, L. (2000) Connecting to nurse-self through reflective poetic story. *International Journal for Human Caring*, 4(2) 7–12.

Wainwright, S. (1997) A new paradigm for nursing: the potential of realism. *Journal of Advanced Nursing*, 26, 1262–71.

Webb, C. (1993) Feminist research: definitions, methodology, methods and evaluation. *Journal of Advanced Nursing*, 18, 416–23.

Weir, A. (1995) Toward a model of self-identity: Habermas and Kristeva. In *Feminists read Habermas: gendering the subject of discourse* (ed. J. Meehan). Routledge, London.

Whitehead, J. (2000) How do I improve my practice? Creating and legiimating an epistemology of practice. *Reflective Practice*, 1, 91–104, 105–12 (reply).

Wilber, K. (1998) *The Eye of Spirit: an integral vision for a world gone slightly mad.* Shambhala, Boston.

Part 2

Narratives

Chapter 4
Awakenings

Introduction

Aileen Joiner is a psychiatric nurse. Her narrative unfolds the 'reality shock' of reflection as she came to confront and work towards resolving the forces that diminished her. It is a powerful drama that reveals the way intelligent nurses can become disempowered within health care systems. Aileen's narrative is constructed from the three assignments she wrote while undertaking the English National Board for Nursing, Health Visiting and Midwifery (ENB) A29 course – 'Becoming a reflective and effective practitioner'. This four module course is offered (at level 3) within a BA Health Care Studies degree for post-registered health care practitioners. On this course, students work in small guided reflection groups (maximum of eight) to reflexively learn through the stories of everyday practice that they bring to the group. Aileen was guided by myself and by Cheryl Watson, my colleague at the University of Luton, who worked with me as co-supervisor on this course. The students' first assignment asks them to write up a reflection they shared within their guided reflection group. The second assignment asks them to construct a personal theory of reflection. For their third assignment the practitioner constructs a reflexive account of personal development around an area of practice. Each assignment has been designed to plot the practitioner's development through the course.

Narrative

'I have been and still am a seeker,
But I have ceased to question stars and books;
I have begun to listen to the teachings my blood whispers to me'

Herman Hess – prologue to Damian (cited in Dossey 1989)

This is my story of my journey whilst a student on ENB A29 – 'Becoming a reflective and effective practitioner'. The course spans eight months. This narrative has been pieced together and edited by Christopher Johns from the first and third assignments I wrote during the course.

My first assignment

People live in crisis that ripples across their beings, rippling below the surface of conscious thought. Such crisis can be observed by paying attention to the signs, yet most people live in a state of partial visibility as if wrapped up in themselves, perhaps to keep self from exploding. Reflection is a trigger to release this tension.

Johns and Freshwater (1998) state that reflection 'gives us wings to soar as we emerge from our cocoons' (p. x). I certainly feel that I am at the stage of wanting to burst from my own cocoon and I want to use my fledgling attempts to ensure that I do soar professionally and personally.

Reflection is the personal opportunity for me to look through my own window, which Johns (1998) describes as 'a window to look inside, to know who I am as I strive towards understanding and realising the meaning of desirable work in my everyday practice' (p. 9). This definition seems useful to me as it provides the image of a personal space . . . I am beginning to associate reflection with personal time out . . . *permission* to break from 'performing' in order to consider the 'performance' and the need to plan future 'performances'.

I have always kept a diary and have been encouraged to reflect in my journal through the course. Much of the course is delivered in small guided reflection groups. After our first session I wrote in my journal:

'I sat in a room full of strangers stating I had left nursing in the 1970s because I didn't like it. With that came the realisation that after all the studying, all the work, I still felt the same way! It washed over me, a strange experience, a flooding sensation from foot to finger tips. Physical but deeply emotional. I tried to explain in a later session of clinical supervision with my ward manager . . . "but you're a good nurse Aileen, very professional, everyone says so, etc." . . . Yes, but is the professionalism the armour I use to keep self together through a multitude of experiences I find exhausting, stressful, distasteful and frustrating? Nursing is far from my expectation, my personal practice is not what I want, it is confined by so many limitations. All my idealism forced to the recesses of my mind, never perhaps to be realised. To change the face of something so massive at what cost to myself? At what worth to others? Chris Johns has spoken of people being marginalised. I have always had the capacity to marginalise myself, never good at conforming to satisfy others. What am I doing? Onwards with studying. Why? Will this provide some key to unlock disappointment, or will it be a balm to bring about acceptance of what is, and where I'm at? Reflection so far seems to raise more questions, but can I answer some? I am unable to separate myself from my practice. So much of nursing is personal, the professional may separate the personal side, but the personal fragility provides much of the human touch. There is not much opportunity to personalise the rigid practices of the ward routine. Much verbal encouragement is given, but little happens. The routine continues, the relentless routine. Probably there is safety in the routine, and a workforce of long serving nursing assistants who pride themselves on maintaining the routine, continue the past and reduce the future; although I work with people who would reshape what we do. I need to reshape what I do, because it swallows me like a whale. This all seems negative, but I feel more positive in expressing my doubts. I am aware of my feelings within myself daily. I am always aware of my impact individually, I am not complacent about the issues that affect my feelings about my job, but maybe I am worn down . . .'

It seems to me that this piece of reflection has enabled a much needed cathartic therapy for myself. Heron (1975) felt that catharsis enabled the dissolving of scars from emotional vulnerability. Valentine (1995) said that nurses and women were nurturing, caring, loving kinds of people – the antithesis of confrontation. This does not allow for the integration of assertiveness as a personal trait. I believe that many women like myself, are skilled at being assertive, but consciously choose to use alternative traits to deal with certain issues, to reduce exposure of vulnerability. By this I mean I can reflect on several ways of dealing with my dislike of my current situation, but know that I will not act alone, or completely independently choosing just for myself, since the consequences affect far more people than myself. Bendelow (1983) found that by avoiding conflict it was turned inwards and experienced as stress, a feeling I relate to, knowing stress and frustration are constantly with me at work.

My reflective account shows a lack of energy throughout. Peers [from the group] described feelings of sadness, hopelessness and profoundness. I reveal some of myself and my conflict within to weigh what I would like to change personally against the reality of what I work with daily.

I felt that this group of people saw me then as helpless and hopeless. Yet this is wrong. People who know me well would laugh at that suggestion. Yet honesty causes me to acknowledge my restrictive upbringing, strong on conforming (though I do not always do this), doing what is right, not challenging, with little meaningful communication. All this leads me to feel I have long fought to be different and yet fundamentally remain the same. Graham (1998) cited in Johns and Freshwater (1998) talks about a sense of humanness and personal identity belonging to the patient. I would argue that the nurse too, has that right of personal identity, especially during reflection and essentially during practice. Social groups (such as our reflective group) are very important in maintaining a sense of humanness. I think this ties in well with the fragility I talked about. I know I am fragile; that makes me sensitive to myself and others. Humanness allows us to remember that fragility is part of being human.

My second assignment

It occurs to me that at the point of narrating my journal I had viewed my professional manner as armour to hold myself together, but with reflection I review my original feelings and now wonder if this was also a valuable tool to prove to others my sense of capability, sense of responsibility, etc. With the unfolding of my reflection, I can begin to see how my own notes illuminate and transmit meaning to theory. My personal learning curve is increased as I start to see beyond myself and understand, liberating the tight rein on my emotions.

On reflection, clearly I am incongruent in my beliefs and have been guilty of holding back, to my own cost. Although I hold strong beliefs related to equality of opportunity, personal rights, etc., I have been confused by the complex world of the struggling nurse where there is no automatic right and I lost sight in my attempts to be submissive, in order to conform and be accepted. This perception, I now feel, is distorted and I struggle to make sense of my feelings.

Miller (1977) cited in Oakley (1984) identified characteristics that develop from belonging to a dominant or subordinate group, which helps me underpin my difficulty in changing my situation, while nurses continue in the subordinate group of submissiveness, and the culture in my own environment is managed, based on submissiveness and ever coping!

My recent experience would have been less stressful had I been myself from the onset and unafraid, but I was brought up to practice self-sacrifice – 'you can't always have what you want...', and I have transferred my upbringing to my career, fearing I could not make wrong right and I should sacrifice my own values to be employed.

There is now within me a recognition to change. I have highlighted fundamental problems and surfaced my tension. I can see how important my need is to bring to the surface the underlying value systems from my past which are valued as of crucial importance to change. Johns (1998) was so right about being unable to cleanse ourselves from our histories.

Even within my own reflective group where I am the junior grade listening to others' reflections, I am reminded that I am merely an E grade! Especially when I listen to reflections by others that highlight attempts of managerial grades to rule over others with patriarchal supremacy. I do believe Newman (1994) when she says that 'who people are' can be read as a pattern rippling across the surface of their being, and just as I read my own ripple (guided by my supervisor), I can read those patterns in my group and I vary in response. I am ambivalent, frightened and bloody-minded all at once in sharing my thoughts with theirs. I feel I began as a qualified nurse after a difficult training period, where there were definite and known attempts by the college where I trained to make life more difficult when I 'fought' them on several issues that I felt strongly affected my values. In this way I felt at first hand their power over me and the effect it wielded over my future, and I currently consider whether that experience so affected me that I lost my autonomy to express my opinion without fear of punishment. This view has been further supported by experience within the team where I work. The reality of the situation means I must work with what is, yet I carry some bitterness, a useless emotion, which always adds to through life's path and saps me of energy to grow. I can see some fluttering that is within me to grow, and this may encourage me to seek a new job in due course.

When I shared my reflection within the group I was offered the visual image of a jungle; to cut space in the undergrowth using a machete, to sit in the trees dropping anger into the space below. I am amazed at how effective this visualisation has been. I have added my own pattern – dropping coconuts on people I feel anger towards. It is surprising how many coconuts I have dropped! This has made me aware that I do hold on to anger, not only towards myself, but to others, especially to those I cherish and value. I think I am very self critical and know I can be caustic and hostile and so have avoided the confrontation and need to utilise 'pricking the bubble' in order to reduce the anger I hang onto.

I can see that the questions will continue in my reflection because, although one can consider the contradictions and debate ways forward, there is then the need to make choices. I stand in front of a bridge I must cross. That is, making the choice. For me, I think it is essential that I do make the correct one as much of my personal well-being will depend on it. It seems I must repair some confidence along the way.

Johns (1995) found that reflective practitioners always interpreted extant knowledge for its relevance to their practice. Watson (1998) states that it is necessary to use theory as a lens for reflective seeing, which helps bring the mountain and the marsh together, the mountain being Schön's high hard ground of technical rationality, whereas the marsh is Schön's enduring metaphor for the messy indeterminate nature of professional practice (Schön 1987). I feel I have inhabited the depths of the marsh and can now see and find meaning in the mountains and their relationship with the marsh in the wider landscape, and in doing so I am understanding more of how my feelings are impacting so strongly on my practice. But this is not an automatic process, rather an extremely complicated one, a long therapeutic journey where I will look back on this analysis as crude and unskilled as I become more proficient. I have acknowledged my own discomfort but surfaced some strengths in my abilities too. I have shown a pattern in my life. There is much truth that learning through experience is arduous work (Johns 1995).

My *third assignment*

I pick up my journey through the third assignment some four months later.

During this course a lecturer commented on her awareness while reading my work, of tentative steps occurring in becoming more positive and affirmative of myself as both a person and practitioner. This is true – I am aware of subtle and real changes taking place within myself and my work. One major change has been the acquisition of a new role with promotion. This was a result of exposing and surfacing tension in [my previous role] where I began to realise I was totally frustrated, unable to meet my practice potential or any personal satisfaction.

Guided reflection gave me the opportunity to allow myself time and space to 'spring clean' emotions long held onto, deep within emotional depths. The theme of these emotions has been ever present in my reflective work. Now my reflective practice feels like a new dawn, a new horizon of opportunity towards realising nursing therapeutic potential (Johns 1998).

> Reflect the actions and the words
> The good times soar on wings of birds
> The sad times tear my soul apart
> And cause my heart, my life to chart
> I look within myself so deep
> My thoughts remain within my sleep
> They stay aside my waking day
> Over and over, in encased depths they lay.
>
> Reflect the care, the love, the act
> The need to show an emotional pact
> Between what I am, what I do, why I care
> Was it just, was it right, was it fair?
>
> And if I can reflect who I am
> Will you challenge me if you can?
> And if I reflect that I care
> Will things change? Do they dare!

I wrote this poem when I began to reflect on the meaning that reflective practice had for me. In the poem I express some inspiration for improvement in my life as a whole. I now realise how central the many emotions I carried within me were to the nurse I was becoming. I was inspired by Johns' comment (1998) that reflection gives us wings to soar, as we emerge from our cocoons, but this was balanced alongside many arduous years of being many things to many people where I arrived exhausted from the emotional labour of dealing with other people's feelings and regulating my own emotions, what James (1989) has termed emotional labour.

Over time I have been able to create the time and space to recover from emotional entanglement, having come to recognise that nursing is almost parasitic in the way it takes psychological reservoirs of one's personality and that one needs a strong sense of self to recharge our batteries. When evaluating emotional work, what we say depends on who we are talking to, what shared knowledge may be assumed, and what kinds of reaction are anticipated (Frith & Kitzinger 1998). My own emotional work has been influenced by many complicated personal and practice events. Initially, as a newly qualified nurse, I found the stress of coping with adults attempting behaviours such as self mutilation and attempted suicide, draining and isolating since there was little opportunity to explore feeling, especially in a unit where such behaviours were an almost daily occurrence. One positive aspect of listening to others reflecting is to realise my stresses are shared by others. At the same time I was nursing my mother who died of cancer and my son left home to go to university, and I changed jobs and my batteries went flat. Emotions are fruitfully seen as embodied existential modes of being. Work commitments and a busy lifestyle contributed to me carrying my emotions as baggage – picking them up and dumping them as time allowed, but not exploring them, letting them go or renewing them. Work spent considering this now is charging my batteries. I have come to recognise how dangerous my lack of self-interest in sorting them may have been, and if I am honest, I can see how I reduced myself as a practitioner by 'capping' my true feelings as this extract from my journal illustrates:

'Don't hold my hand, please don't hold my hand. I cannot hold yours. You are dying and you know it. I know it too – I see it in your eyes. I know you are frightened. Your fear is not within the layers where most people hold onto theirs, when they are well. No, it is on the surface, covering you. It is beyond your skin all around you in the room. I feel it. I know it and I must cope with it.

I do everything to make Margaret comfortable. The position, the pillows, the light , the warmth. All are considered. A sip of water, a fumble with the charts, take the blood pressure, keep the oxygen nearby. Soothe the relatives, say the right things. Are you watching me? I'm good, you can tell I've done this before. They think I'm an expert and unaffected. There are no experts in this and the effects mix with my own bereavement.

Her hand is so fragile, small and like a bird shaking as life flows away. How large my hand seems. Ugly next to Margaret's. Every time I approach the bed she attempts to grab my hand – she is seeking reassurance. I know I must hold her hand and show reassurance in my eyes. I say something soothing but I'm not there. I think now as I write of all the hands I've held and wonder if anyone will be there to hold mine. When you think about how many people we love in our lives that hold onto our hands, parents, partners, children, no wonder Margaret wants hers held now as she dies...'

As a nurse I have held many people's hands during times of pain and stress. It is never easy to do. To me it connects you so physically with them. I think I am exposing more of my shadow self but I'm cautious since there isn't enough guided reflection space to deal with it all and like others this year I worry about the impact of coping with newly surfaced emotions.

Zerwekh (1995) wrote that it is always a turning point when nurses can find and celebrate humanity and competence that at first may be hidden by suffering and degradation. She says nurses search for ways to validate people who have lost faith in themselves or no longer believe in their own power. I'm searching in my practice for their humanity and mine. If I must find it to be considered an effective practitioner I may fail, but if I work amongst people who can see how elusive this achievement is, I can relax in being human and frail... my recurring theme. Possibly I am becoming a more effective practitioner because I accept fragility. I have learnt that while I can create a therapeutic environment for others to release their emotions, I am not a machine and must therefore find appropriate expression of my own, in order to be available to others. I use the being available template (Johns 1998) as a mirror to see myself. Do I like the reflection? I like it more. I recognise now that I am very strong, have coped with much and those aspects of me that show fragility are warm, human and okay. Life experiences force me to be more honest about who I am and what and why I contribute towards others as I do. Having previously looked in some depth at the gender issues and prevailing attitudes between doctor and nurses, I concur that there is a definite set of constraints as to what nurses are able to do for patients and themselves.

It seems realistic to say that some of my reflective patterns have been painful and I have had to think about managing myself during reflection. If I am hard on myself, does it follow that I am hard on my patients? I have discussed being less hard on myself and know the kindness I extend to others can be extended within, but the barrier is not altogether down. Chapman (1983) concluded from Menzies-Lyth's work (1988) on the ritualistic practices utilised by nurses to protect them from anxieties, that individual behaviour attempts to defend one from the primitive anxieties evoked by death, dirty tasks and intimacy. I have found myself attempting that protection, yet overtly steering myself from ritualistic practice in the hope of achieving more holistic care; being much more comfortable with a strong belief that patients are people with minds and soul and feelings and not object bodies given up to medical domination.

However, my delivery of effective care is variable since my reflection about Margaret shows a gap between the performance to meet the need as I interpret it and the deeper levels of myself as I reveal them. Cultural patterns of avoidance, the forbidden topic of death govern interactions around dying patients in hospitals (Glasser & Strauss 1965, cited in Chapman 1983). This must surely contribute little support for the nurse who cares for these patients, attempting somehow to support patients, relatives and others, while managing their own emotions throughout.

Fortunately, I find myself thinking about many issues in a different way, attempting to step free of ingrained cultural and socialisation limitations. Now I am beginning to see how restricted I have been in myself.

Watson (1998) said that reflective caring practice helps us to stop and think, to pause in the midst of action. I have certainly done much of that. Watson felt this resulted in us being more aware, more mindful, authentically present, allowing a redirection. She likened it to being a simple shifting of one's consciousness from being harried, hurried or rushed, to being still, to finding one's quiet centre. When I think of this I am inspired to be calm, yet the days are often so hectic. I was known to say to those who knew me well that I want peace in my life, but the reflection I have *laboured at* this year makes me think that the peace I seek is here in the quiet centre of myself; and if I had the courage to exorcise my shadow self I would find more peace. In response Chris Johns said: 'The shadow self does not need exorcising, it needs embracing because it tells us important things about ourselves'. Through reflection I come to acknowledge and value my shadow self and integrate my shadow self with myself. Perhaps on this level we most need the challenge and support of guidance.

During my first assignment I realised I was at a bridge that I must cross successfully to maintain my own mental health. Now I view myself crossing that bridge and reflect on Johns' (1998) words: 'Assure your bridge is strong with a well defined plan'.

Truthful reflection has helped me focus my plan and I begin to see what the future could hold and more importantly, there is now a time for me to be kinder to myself.

I have changed my job. I was not prepared to continue in a restrictive routine that didn't recognise individual patients' needs. I've grown by becoming more self-determining, by choosing my own values and ideals, grounded in my own experience (Mayeroff 1971, cited in Johns 1996). This shows a personal right to become whole (if that is fully achievable) through choice and based on experience. It fills me with confidence that the person I am, while unique, is okay and in that I feel less isolated from other practitioners, but also some independence which shows progress in itself since I previously commented on feelings of isolation and lack of harmony.

I have explored relationships amongst work colleagues and I am finally realising some of the effects these relationships have had on my well-being. I was seen as a confidant and was lent on for support, yet needed much support myself . . . more than I admitted to openly, whereas now I look for support. I was seen as capable, yet often questioned that of myself, feeling that my integrity and logic opposed others. While I am guilty of using others in the workplace I too was used and exploited by friends and superiors and when it was overt at times I tolerated it even when I recognised it, but that perspective is changing. Johns (1992) states that nurses must develop new ways to effectively support each other in their mutual roles.

I wrote in my journal:

> 'my time on the unit has been fraught with frustration and I have seen myself wanting to be more involved, often part of a routine I disliked, in events that I wanted to challenge, and part of a team whose support varied . . . yet again nothing is certain, I cannot be sure my choice of job will be better . . . I often ask myself why do I put myself through so much?'

Already I see events repeating themselves, yet I do see them and work towards responding differently even as the less than welcoming reception has left me guarded and confused, wondering about the psychological cost. My sensitivity re-emerging, depleting my batteries again. Yet the opportunity to reshape something is not lost on me and I am able to utilise new reflective coping strategies, ensuring not to absorb too much. Let them keep their problems and prejudices which are not mine.

Reflection has equipped me with so many intrapersonal and interpersonal skills, but it is there for the reader to see that there is great turmoil between what I am and what I do:

> It's not that I am black or blue
> Nor any shade that's blurred from view
> It's just that when I want to care
> to show for you that I am there
> The nurse I am just doesn't dare!

But there is a new and changing me
A person grown who now can see
The callous cruelty of what was done,
The right to care, but live, have fun.
And in doing that change the job for which I trained
So there's more of me and less that's drained.

I'm not where I want to be
I want more, I want to be free
To give to others better choice to start
To practise life and work from their heart
A sense of self in all they do,
That's not dependent on hierarchy such as you!

The ghosts I have carried from my experiences as a student nurse are not laid to rest. I am trying but still they are not exorcised – 'the callous cruelty of what was done'. 'The right to care, but live and have fun', is my hope that nurses will drop this need for devotion and sacrifice and come to understand the best ones have a life as well and all have the right to one. The final verse of the above poem shows a desire to have a role in shaping the experience of other beginners in nursing so that ultimately more will be able to challenge the hierarchical structures and professional dominance that restrict us from realising our therapeutic potential and destiny. Then the mountain and the marsh may well come together.

References

Bendelow, M. (1983) *Managerial women's approaches to organisational conflict: a qualitative study*. Unpublished doctoral dissertation. University of Colorado, Denver.

Chapman, G. (1983) Ritual and rational action in hospitals. *Journal of Advanced Nursing*, 8, 13–30.

Dossey, L. (1989) *Recovering the soul: a scientific and spiritual search*. Bantam Science, New York.

Frith, H. & Kitzinger, C. (1998) 'Emotional work' as a participant recourse: A feminist analysis of young women's talk-in-interaction. *Sociology*, 32(2) 299–320.

Glasser, B. & Strauss, A. (1965) *Awareness of Dying*. Aldine, Chicago.

Graham, I. (1998) Understanding the nature of nursing through reflection. In *Transforming Nursing through Reflective Practice* (eds Johns C. & Freshwater D.) pp. 119–33. Blackwell Science, Oxford.

Heron, J. (1975) *Six category intervention analysis*. Human potential Research Project. University of Surrey.

James, N. (1989) Emotional labour: skill and work in the social regulation of feelings. *The Sociological Review*, 37(1) 15–42.

Johns, C. (1992) Ownership and the harmonious team: barriers to developing the therapeutic team in primary nursing. *Journal of Clinical Nursing*, 1, 89–94.

Johns, C. (1995) Time to care? Time for reflection. *International Journal of Nursing Practice*, 1, 37–42.

Johns, C. (1996) Visualising and realising caring in practice through guided reflection. *Journal of Advanced Nursing*, 24, 1135–43.

Johns, C. (1998) Opening the doors of perception. In *Transforming Nursing through Reflective Practice* (eds Johns C. & Freshwater D.) pp. 1–20. Blackwell Science, Oxford.

Johns, C. & Freshwater, D. (1998) Preface. *Transforming Nursing through Reflective Practice*. Blackwell Science, Oxford.

Mayeroff, M. (1971) *On Caring*. Harper, New York.

Menzies-Lyth, I. (1988) A case study in the functioning of social systems as a defence against anxiety. In *Containing Anxiety in Institutions: selected essays*. Free Association Books, London.

Miller, J. (1977) *Towards a New Psychology of Women*. Beacon Press, Boston.

Oakley, A. (1984) The importance of being a nurse. *Nursing Times*, 83(50) 24–7.

Newman, M. (1994) *Health as Expanded Consciousness*. National League for Nursing, New York.

Schön, D. (1987) *Educating the Reflective Practitioner*. Jossey-Bass, San Francisco.

Valentine, P. (1995) Management of conflict: do nurses/women handle it differently? *Journal of Advanced Nursing*, 22, 142–9.

Watson, J. (1998) A meta-reflection on reflective practice and caring theory. In *Transforming Nursing through Reflective Practice* (eds Johns C. & Freshwater D.) pp. 214–20. Blackwell Science, Oxford.

Zerwekh, J. (1995) Making the connection during home visits; narratives of expert nurses. *The Hospice Journal*, 10, 27–44.

Chapter 5

Striving to Realise Clinical Leadership

Introduction

Tessa's narrative was one of 14 narratives that I constructed as part of a research project – 'Clinical supervision as a model for clinical leadership'. As the project title suggests, I worked with 14 nurses of varying leadership grades (F–H) in guided reflection relationships with the explicit aim of guiding them to become more effective as clinical leaders. Each relationship was constructed as an individual narrative using the clinical leadership template as a developmental marker. When Tessa commenced her guided reflection relationship with me she was a junior sister (F grade) on Lavender ward, a care of the elderly assessment ward. She accepted my invitation to participate in a guided reflection relationship with the explicit intent of developing her clinical leadership role. We contracted for one year during which time we met on 11 occasions.

The narrative offers a powerful and disturbing insight into the pressures of being a modern ward sister struggling with the everyday pressures and the challenge of the leadership agenda.

Narrative

Clarifying the clinical leadership role

In our first session Tessa reflected on the nature of her clinical leadership role using the clinical leadership template (Fig. 5.1). I had constructed this template by reflecting on and interpreting my own role as a clinical leader at Brackley and Burford Community Hospitals. Tessa considered that the leadership template reflected her leadership role and she felt it would be an appropriate template to frame her own experiences and mark the growth of her leadership ability. In using the template, I suggested we would test and revise the framework as necessary rather than view the template as a rigid model that was definitive of the clinical leadership role.

With regard to a vision for practice, Tessa believed practice should be holistic, concerned with working with patients and families towards meeting their health needs. Almost as if she was preparing herself to be unmasked, she confessed that she knew that many respects of practice did not match her holistic vision. However she was positive about this and agreed that the ward needed to develop a strong vision of nursing to guide and direct practice, roles and practice development. I suggested her initial reflections were likely to be triggered by uncomfortable feelings about some-

- To facilitate a vision for practice.
- To facilitate the growth of staff into appropriate role responsibility.
- To maintain 'expert' clinical credibility.
- To facilitate the development and support of staff competence within defined roles.
- To facilitate the development of clinical practice.
- To ensure the overall quality of care.
- To manage the unit effectively by:
  - appointing personnel
  - managing resources
  - meeting and influencing organisational objectives
  - co-ordinating activity and ensuring effective communication systems
  - establishing effective working relationships.
- To ensure self-development and support.

Fig. 5.1 Clinical leadership template.

thing. Tessa responded: 'You mean like the irritation I felt today? Three staff were late coming on-duty this morning. I'm especially irritated with Jane, a nursing auxiliary who is often late.'

Tessa explored her need to confront Jane yet in ways that emphasised Jane's responsibility as a member of the ward team. We also discussed the potential for developing clinical practice, notably preceptorship, developing the existing team nursing, and developing standards of care and learning resources.

Reflection

I felt enthusiastic about working with Tessa. She was very interested in developing her role and had responded positively to the challenge before her. However, I was also conscious of my enthusiasm pushing her too quickly towards change. The focus on her role had exposed many aspects of the leadership role that were not being fulfilled by her senior sister who was also in the research project. As such, I needed to be sensitive to the ward hierarchy and patterns of relating between Tessa and Delia.

Nurturing responsibility

In session two Tessa reflected on the session notes: 'I spoke to the nurse who was constantly late. She was late again – she walked in at 07.25! So I asked her nicely to see me and then confronted her. She blamed the buses. I suggested she started later – say 07.30 – and pointed out the impact of her lateness on others, that it wasn't fair and that she was getting a reputation, although people didn't observe the fact that she was often left late. She thought that was a great idea. We both felt good.'

I drew a transactional analysis map to help Tessa see the pattern of communication between herself and Jane in the way she had confronted Jane in adult to adult mode in a non-threatening way (Fig. 5.2).

Tessa could see that if she had responded as a critical mother she would most likely have prompted Jane to respond as a child and that may have reinforced Jane's irresponsibility and made her defensive.

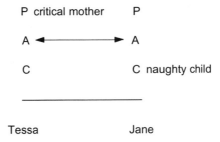

P critical mother   P

A ◄──────────► A

C   C naughty child

Tessa   Jane

Fig. 5.2 Transactional analysis pattern between Tessa and nurse.

Tessa exclaimed: 'That's how I felt! I felt like a critical mother wanting to tell her off!'
Chris: 'Yes but you managed to control that feeling.'

Tessa acknowledged the need to reinforce a ward culture based on supportive responsibility that cut across the prevailing conflict-avoidance culture.

Tessa noted: 'I don't like conflict. I feel quite anxious confronting these staff.'
Chris: 'But you did it with a good result. You asserted your role responsibility. In doing so, you have established a new pattern for dealing with such problems in the future. A key feature of clinical leadership is to positively manage situations of conflict.'

Enabling responsibility

Tessa linked the experience with Jane to another situation:

Tessa: 'This is related to a staff nurse. I had delegated her a small task. The task involved completing a monthly form to monitor the time between referral to community care and actual discharge. This time gap has become an increasing problem within the Trust. I had previously allocated the task to everybody as a collaborative effort. It was everyone's responsibility but it was not happening. I wanted the task done better. I felt that one person responsible should ensure that it would be done. It was a failure of the ward that it hadn't been done. It reflected badly on me as ward sister. I felt guilty about that.'
Chris: 'Because of the potential of negative feedback from managers?'
Tessa: 'They picked up it hadn't been done in December. I had done November but now it's not been done halfway through January. I felt cross at staff . . . well perhaps not cross, more disappointed.'
Chris: 'Because of their lack of responsibility?'
Tessa: 'They weren't aware it was something to be done. They work hard all day then it is time to go home. They have no motivation to stay and do that one thing.'
Chris: 'Is that a pattern – that tasks like this get stacked up to do at the end of the day?'
Tessa: 'They won't accept the fact that you are too busy. I understand the pressure of workload. I don't know if I expect that little bit extra from them to do this. I think I do but another bit of me says I shouldn't expect it.'
Chris: 'Have you shared this ambivalence with them? If they knew they could understand and support you more?'
Tessa linked this to Delia: 'She never asked me to help her with any of her duties.'
Chris: 'Do you think she should have?'

Tessa: 'I have gone out of my way to help her, things that needed to be done. I was willing to help and she was always grateful. She's always shown appreciation of this, but I don't think anyone else on the ward makes the effort to find out or offer help. I feel they should all take some interest. This form was pinned to the board asking for offers to help.'

Chris: 'You might need to invite them to do this?'

Tessa: 'Yes, they might not know. They might think I am happy with their busy work. They may see this as something that Delia and I get up to. One thing I will try to encourage if I become ward manager.'

Chris: 'How did you delegate this to the staff nurse?'

Tessa: 'I explained exactly what was expected of her and checked her understanding "if she didn't mind".'

Chris: 'Did she have the choice?'

Tessa: 'She did.'

Chris: 'But did she *really* have this choice? Can she easily refuse sister's request?'

Tessa: 'I hope she could if that's what she was feeling.'

Chris: 'Did you choose this nurse for any particular reason?'

Tessa: 'No – I just picked her . . . no explicit reason. She is a relatively junior staff nurse. I felt it was something she could be successful and reliable at. She was apprehensive at first, unsure what was expected of her. She felt it would be time consuming, tedious. She couldn't understand the relevance of doing it. I could tell by her facial expression she was negative about doing it. How did I feel? – In control, relieved that I had confronted her. I felt I had lifted the responsibility off me. I was pleased with myself.'

Chris: 'You felt relieved as if confronting staff was something difficult to do?'

Tessa: 'Yes . . . my actions were matched by my beliefs. I was calm, pleasant, thankful, appreciative. She now does it in a few minutes. That makes me feel relieved I suppose. The evidence is that she is doing it well. I shall see that it lasts by discussing and supporting her regularly. It's the way of the future, to involve other staff, focus on career development/roles – generally staff are keen to help if approached. There is not enough emphasis on the ward for development, probably no time with the emphasis on workload.'

Chris: 'Can you turn that round?'

Tessa: 'Yeah – this has made me more aware, to ask them what they want to achieve, what they want to do.'

Chris: 'How does this link with the last experience?'

Tessa: 'I acted from adult ↔ adult mode to confront my colleague. She initially resisted this approach because it was a management task and because such work has been viewed as the business of the sisters.'

Chris: 'You felt a tension between managing your own concerns – to get these management tasks done and facilitating the growth of responsibility within junior staff to accept this responsibility. The tension is apparent within your concern about putting staff under pressure – the "protective mother" posture? Yet support for the staff nurse is reflected in her improved performance.'

Tessa: 'Yeah, it's difficult because the organisation are not interested in this pressure, simply that the task had to be done.'

Chris: 'I felt this pressure in your comment "It reflected badly on me as a ward sister. I felt guilty about that" . . . as if you have internalised this pressure and fear criticism. It's significant the way this fear prompts you to transmit this fear into staff by being "critical" and yet you feel guilty about that and become "protective" as if you are caught in a protective-critical mother trap, and yet in both experiences you acted to reinforce responsibility. Do you think you have learned anything through this experience, either writing it out or sharing it with me?'

Tessa: 'It has made me think more. I would not have seen it in all these aspects.'
Tessa noted her anxiety with her forthcoming shift in role as Delia had decided to take early retirement: 'I'm going to act-up into the G grade role, and apply for the G grade post. I have begun to organise the ward in the light of taking over the ward leadership role from Delia.'

Reflection

Tessa reveals a culture where junior staff were not involved in *management work*. The delegation of management work is passively resisted by junior staff. With this insight Tessa can plan to enable staff growth of responsibility into management work, particularly as she wants to spend more time on the ward with patients and families.

Perhaps Tessa is also passively resisting the monitoring initiative as simply another time-consuming task to do irrespective of its value. The task is complied with because of power relations that insist it should be done. Tessa fears sanction if it is not done. As such she becomes anxious and transmits her anxiety into her staff – 'I felt cross at staff'. She begins to respond to staff as she imagines hierarchy will respond to her. Tessa's usual response to staff is both the critical and protective mother – telling them off for being naughty and protecting them from pressure. She oscillates between the two roles, yet both act to reinforce dependency rather than foster responsibility.

Preparing for interview

In session three Tessa rehearsed with me her G grade interview. I projected Tessa forward into the interview and explored the sorts of issues that she may be asked about, in particular her plans for ward development, things such as preceptorship and supervision. Tessa said that recent staff nurse interviewees asked about preceptorship and that this would be offered to them. We talked through the nature of preceptorship and key issues that would be on her 'preceptorship programme'.

Tessa: 'It's difficult to focus on anything with the interview coming up and with keeping the ward "ticking over" with Delia gone. They expect everything to carry on regardless, as if Delia's post had been dissolved. The impression of coping is important for the interview. There are so many issues to deal with – The King's Fund Organisational Audit self-assessment forms, a new nurse management system. I've done them all but it has been an enormous effort.'
Chris: 'The modern G grade post?'
Tessa: 'All staff are now expected to stay behind in their own time – the expectation of a 10 hour day – the day doesn't finish at 3.30 PM anymore. I can't expect staff to stay in their own time, especially if they have been on since early morning. Sometimes they don't even get to breaks or only get 15 minutes for lunch.'
Chris: 'How can you best manage that?'
Tessa: 'People watch what I do!'
Chris: 'The significance of role modelling.'
Tessa: 'What about time?'
Chris: 'Are we slaves to time or do we control time? We know the real world is tough – diminishing resources where managing resources best is vital. The challenge – does Lavender ward use time well? Can you prioritise the best use of time? For example, the delegation of management tasks to junior staff that we discussed last session.'

Tessa acknowledged this: 'There is this rush to get things done in the morning it's true, but it does create time to get other things done in the afternoon.'

I supported this by noting: 'I expect patients prefer to have a wash in the morning?'

Tessa: 'Usually by 08.30! And relatives want to see their patient looking as if they have been cared for! I get little opportunity to do everyday care. My work is focused more on changes in treatment, dealing with social services, relatives, discharge arrangements and doctors' rounds, besides management tasks.'

Chris: 'Aren't these roles for team leaders and named nurses?'

Tessa: 'To be truthful, the team nursing concept in practice is an illusion. In reality there was a nurse in charge who dealt with these issues because of the trained staff ratio – we do not have that continuity. Where possible I try to maintain continuity of nurse with patients if on for a number of shifts.'

Chris' commentary   I noted how our dialogue had revealed a number of cultural norms interacting and reinforcing each other – hierarchy, tasks, shifts, lack of time, being busy, staff are stressed, no vision, no culture of development – all potent barriers to developing change. Tessa saw that initiatives such as the named nurse were illusions. Despite her obvious discomfort with such contradiction she felt committed and motivated to resolve them.

Chris: 'I know it's tough for you at the moment and I don't want to increase this pressure by forcing these ward development issues or by getting you to focus on patient care experiences.'

Tessa paused: 'It doesn't threaten me – I know what I need to do!'

Reflection

Although Tessa's mind was full of her forthcoming interview for the G grade sister's post, I was able to pick up issues from the last session and challenge Tessa with managing time and prioritising work. Tessa was able to pull away the illusion of the 'named nurse' and 'team nursing' and in doing so cleared the ground so new ideas can be sown and watered. The dialogue also illuminates the significance of commitment in order to face up to things that are tough to deal with.

Changing gear

I commenced session four by congratulating Tessa on becoming a G grade.

Tessa responded: 'My thoughts about the new role have affected my sleep. I keep thinking of all the things I want to do … of silly little things.'

Chris: 'Such as?'

Tessa: 'What I want to do! I see myself as a perfectionist, but I want everybody else to be like this besides myself. I want staff to know this but I don't want to throw my weight around straight away. I don't want to be negative with staff but I want things to change. The first ward meeting is on Saturday. I am developing an agenda for this. I expect things to be taken on board as I expect things from myself.'

I shared with Tessa my work with another ward sister within the project who had been focusing on values, roles and relationships as the context for knowing and developing effective practice. I suggested that Tessa might need to focus on these issues so staff know the boundaries of their responsibility. Tessa noted this but felt it was the 'little things' rather than 'major role things' that she needed to focus on – the impressionable things like a patient being able to reach a glass of water whilst sitting out of bed: 'Things you would expect from senior staff, and not just junior staff to do.' I asserted my point about putting such 'small things' into a sense of caring context and role responsibility: 'My advice – if I were you at my first ward meeting I might articulate my vision of the ward and invite staff to discuss this and jump on board.'

I sensed a tension between Tessa's 'horizon' to focus on 'little things' and my 'horizon' to focus on 'major things'. Tessa's focus was to 'make good' things that were not done well enough, reflecting her anxiety that the ward, and hence she, would be seen as imperfect. I felt anxious that her agenda would be to manage her anxiety rather than continue her previous work of staff becoming empowered to develop role responsibility within a vision of holistic practice.

Managing caring or managing complaint?

Tessa continued: 'I'm still finding it difficult to find experiences to reflect on. I have been so preoccupied, but I have brought an experience for today. I've written it down. It's related to a patient and his relatives – something that wound me up. The patient was not particularly sick but the relatives were phoning every half-hour asking the same questions from different relatives. Then the distressed wife and neighbour came in. I spent a long time with them – about three-quarters of an hour, that impacted on other things I needed to do. The wife was very anxious if the husband was going to die. She had two sons who lived abroad. She was debating whether to contact these sons. She wanted me to tell the neighbour, who was going to contact them, whether she should ask them to come over? We talked it through and then the neighbour asked me to talk it through again so he could write it down. And then later, early evening, a third son came in and wanted me to go through it all again! He said that he was going to contact his brothers. At the time I was putting up some blood plus trying to do the 6 PM drugs and we had three admissions that evening. The son was following me around into the clinical room. At first I might have seemed dismissive – telling him that I was doing this and that, the ward was busy – and then immediately I felt guilty for being like that.'
Chris: 'Were you off-hand?"'
Tessa: 'I don't think so. I would never do that. He could see that I was busy. He just stopped me and I stopped what I was doing and invited him into the office.'
Tessa paused: 'Is this was the sort of stuff you want me to share?'
Chris: 'Yes. You stopped what you were doing?'
Tessa: 'Yes. I finished what I was doing just then. I had told him in the clinical room that I had spoken with his mother and neighbour but he asked "will you tell me?" I felt sorry for him. He looked upset about his dad – I felt what he was going through. To me his dad was just another patient – one of 23. I gave him all the time he needed. In myself I calmed down, got my priorities right, and went through it all again – not rushed.'
Chris: 'How long did you spend with him?'
Tessa: 'Twenty minutes. It made me feel better afterwards and I'm sure I made him feel better.'
Chris: 'You could tell that by the way he responded to you?'
Tessa: 'Yes. He was quite young, late twenties. My age – unusual on the ward where most

relatives are themselves in their fifties. It made me relate to him more, especially with him being so upset.'

Chris: 'It brought your sympathy out?'

Chris' commentary   I noted the concept of affinity where perhaps we are more attracted to patients and relatives who are like us. I linked this to a recent experience shared by another practitioner where the practitioner illustrated her 'attractiveness' to the patient because he was very similar to her in lifestyle, and to the literature on unpopular/good-bad/difficult patients. I said I would send her these papers (Stockwell 1972; Kelly & May 1982).

Tessa: 'I'm developing resource files that I can put this information in.'

Chris: 'How ill was this man?'

Tessa: 'They wanted me to make the decision. Whether to ask these two brothers to come over. I didn't want to do that – not my job to do that. I gave it back to them – gave them the facts to let them make the decision, but I do "weight" advice in some cases. I said that if that was my dad I would want to be there.'

Chris: 'You actually said that?'

Tessa: 'Yes.'

Chris: 'But you also said that you don't want the responsibility of making the decision for them?'

Tessa: 'The decision to come over or not is the sons'.'

Chris: 'Yes – however it is also a question of emphasis to influence this decision to come over. Your decision had other implications, for example – how you used your time, and was giving this time the best use of time considering other priorities? And also how this decision was primarily based on your guilt – that you at first didn't respond to his needs.'

Tessa: 'I can see the time I spent with the neighbour was a waste of time, having to go through it all again. I felt a real sense of frustration with this family and then with the son who made me react like this. I was also conscious of complaints – would this have been a consequence of not acting – to get a complaint? On reflection I know I can't ever be rude and that I always need to calm potential complaint situations down.'

Chris: 'The need to avoid complaints reflects the reality of the real world and how this influences decision making, but it may also mask the most appropriate decision. Another way of responding might have been to acknowledge the son's feelings – "I can see this is tough for you", or, in other words, to show him you care and are concerned for him and his dad. Then assert your action with the neighbour – suggest the neighbour will help him contact the sons?'

Tessa: 'The son might have gone away with a strong message that "the sister" didn't care very much. This caring image is important for me. I need to be perceived this way. I didn't know the wife had a third son!'

Chris: 'It would have helped to know this. Was it in the notes?'

Tessa: 'I should have asked if there was another son although many families don't communicate well. This family was "difficult" – they communicated as such between the nurses. I did reflect on what could have happened within that 20 minutes. I could be at fault because of that, although the place didn't fall apart in this time.'

Chris: 'You're giving yourself feedback that your actions had no obvious impact on other patients? Perhaps you do need to be tougher on the issues, otherwise you'll lose control of time in the face of such requests by relatives. Your judgement will always be based on compassion rather than sound judgement of priorities.'

Tessa: 'Caring is the prime focus for my actions. I felt good afterwards. It's what I'm here for ... it's what I do and do well.'

Chris: 'Acting like this, you role modelled caring for others – the way you prioritised time to be available to this distressed son cut through perceiving the family as difficult and reinforced caring values to the observer. Could you share this experience with your staff? You can do that in a casual way such as – "oh you know that family? well yesterday it went like this" – as a way of emphasising caring values. It may help them think and confront their own attitudes whilst reinforcing your caring expectations.'

Tessa said she liked best: 'That I had brought something to talk about and the points you have made – "try these" – I can weigh them up in future situations – happening all the time. I especially liked the idea of sharing the experience with staff.'

Reflection

Tessa acknowledged that the ethical dilemma confronting her was stark, whether to continue her 'tasks' or to stop and respond to the person seeking help. Tessa's dilemma exemplified the cultural shift between being 'task' focused and being 'person' focused. Within the immediacy of getting through the work on a busy ward, the ability to stop the task and respond to the person is a true realisation of caring. However, there is a 'twist' to this experience – the extent that Tessa was motivated to respond to the son because of her fear of complaint. This is particular apposite with Tessa because of her concern with her image – she was a perfectionist and needed to be seen as a perfectionist. In the real world of competing priorities, being a perfectionist rather than being a pragmatist was difficult for her. Hence her concern for caring was matched by her concern to be seen as caring. On reflection she felt she had responded appropriately and in doing so she had reinforced the primacy of caring and realising the satisfaction that caring brings.

This experience was the first experience that really exposed herself as a caring person. It was unlike her earlier experiences which resembled problems to be solved. Tessa wanted me to affirm that her response to the son was 'caring', and to resolve her sense of unease that she had wanted to brush the son aside. My response was to help her see the underlying norms of practice that prompted her anxiety. Yet I also had one eye on the clinical leadership framework, helping Tessa to see how this experience fits into her leadership role: role modelling, de-briefing, managing priorities, expert self, clarifying caring values, managing self, ensuring quality of care, responding to the organisational agenda of managing complaints, and responding positively to situations of potential conflict with carers.

Yet, perhaps underlying all these factors is the issue of developing the powerful self, so such situations can be controlled within a deep understanding of what is trying to be achieved and role responsibility, and within a deep understanding of self.

Establishing vision and collaboration

In session five, Tessa reflected on her first staff meeting:

Tessa: 'I told people what I expected of them – the "small things" I will be monitoring and setting some ground-rules. It was also an opportunity for people to say things.'

Chris: 'Did you ask people what they expected of you – the other side of the coin?'
Tessa: 'I didn't say that … it wasn't that deep. It was very basic things although people could say what they wanted to say. For example, Annette mentioned appraisal. I was able to give feedback from our team briefing – the approach to introducing appraisal.'
Chris: 'She wanted to be appraised?'
Tessa: 'Yes. She has objectives. I would like to see everybody in time, especially the junior staff nurses. I want them to know I am concerned about them, that I value them, more than just numbers. With the dawning of PREPP [Post-Registration Education and Practice Project] they will have to keep a record of study days, etc. It would also be nice to know what people want to do.'
Chris: 'How do you develop responsibility and commitment in staff?'
Tessa: 'Take the "language difficulty survey" – at the staff meeting I said to the staff nurse I had asked to do this, that it had not been forthcoming. I had a peep to see how she was getting on – there was no record made so far in April. I asked myself – What should I do about it? Do I leave it a bit longer or do I confront her? I feel I should inquire how the staff nurse was progressing otherwise I'll become increasingly anxious.'
Chris: 'Your dilemma relived from session 2! The challenge – are you the critical mother responding to the naughty child or can you confront her irresponsibility in ways to enable her growth of responsibility? Are you reluctant to confront her because you don't want to upset her?'
Tessa paused and smiled: 'A case of déjà vu. Can I apply this theory in practice?'

Peering out from the medical shadow

Tessa continued: 'This is about two recent experiences where I was told what I should do. I wasn't told off exactly but I did feel I couldn't say anything. I was doing the ward round with the consultant. Each patient has a named nurse and consultant slot on each bed. This patient had the wrong consultant's name. The consultant took it out and threw it on the bed towards me with a sarcastic comment – "it's not working is it?" This was in front of the patient and four other doctors. I picked it up. I felt angry with him and felt angry with staff who put me in this situation. I could explain why this happened, the patient had changed consultants. Afterwards I had a moan about him to other staff – I closed the door to make sure he couldn't hear!'
Chris: 'Is he normally like that?'
Tessa: 'Yes.'
Chris: 'Why do you think he responds like that?'
Tessa: 'He thinks that because he's a consultant he can talk to nurses like that. I felt humiliated. It was awful for the patients as well.'
Chris: 'I can sense your outrage at his behaviour.'

Chris' commentary   I framed this in terms of humiliation techniques that doctors use to keep nurses in their place, maintaining the status quo of medical domination. I noted a paper by Chapman (1983) to help Tessa understand this as a socialised form of oppression rather than a personal attack.

I reflected: 'You've projected some anger into your staff for putting you into this situation. Could you have redirected this anger by confronting him?'
Tessa: 'He moved on.'
Chris: 'Could you have seen him after the round?'

Tessa: 'Yes.'

Chris: 'So why didn't you?'

Tessa: 'He's busy. I know – I'm just making excuses ... yeah.'

Chris: 'Could you arrange to see him – give him feedback that you didn't appreciate this behaviour?'

Tessa: 'It' a bit late now.'

Chris: 'I know it's tough – it's a difficult barrier to overcome ... something for you to think about in future experiences?'

Tessa: 'He says obvious things like asking if we are doing pressure area care for an immobile patient and with a patient "nil by mouth" – "are you doing mouth care?".'

Chris: 'You could always be ironic – "Gosh that's a great idea – I would never have thought about that" – reflect his comments back to him?'

Tessa: 'Can you do that? ... He'll always find something wrong with someone somewhere.'

Chris: 'If you feel oppressed by him then you have to learn to give it back – not just in terms of the type of professional relationships you want, but also in terms of respect as a person. Your staff watch the way you respond – you risk role-modelling subordinate behaviour. Before we meet next time – maybe read Ann Dickson's (1982) rights of women in terms of being assertive? I always keep this book in my "supervision kit-bag" for moments like this – let's talk through these rights:

- I have the right to state my own needs and set my own priorities as a person independent of any roles that I may assume in life
- I have the right to be treated with respect as an intelligent, capable and equal human being
- I have the right to express my feelings
- I have the right to express my opinions and values
- I have the right to say "yes" or "no" for myself
- I have the right to make mistakes
- I have the right to change my mind
- I have the right to say I don't understand
- I have the right to ask for what I want
- I have the right to decline responsibility for other people
- I have the right to deal with others without being dependent on them for approval.'

Tessa felt she didn't score too highly with these statements. Chris continued: 'I feel your self-esteem has been flattened at a time when you need to be respected by the consultants in the context of your new status. Are you okay about this?'

Tessa: 'I am ... this is a real challenge – to become assertive and demand respect from him.

Chris: 'It's crucial to your sense of being a powerful and effective leader. But it's also important not to judge yourself harshly if you cannot assert yourself with him. We have embodied normal ways of relating that are not necessarily easy to shift quickly. At least you are now sensitive to the dynamics between you.'

Frustration at management attitude

Tessa: 'The second experience, a senior nurse gave me feedback regarding my off-duty. The business manager had noted how much weekend and nights I was doing and had said that he would prefer me to work Monday–Friday, preferably 9–5. I felt cross it was a secondhand message – what do you do about that?! I could see it made sense what he said – it was just the way it was said. I wanted to be treated with respect – it made me defensive. I felt it was being suggested that I had been doing this for my own benefit – creating negative impressions! Why didn't he give me this feedback directly when we met earlier?'

Chris suggested: 'Perhaps he's a conflict avoider? Whose responsibility is it?'
Tessa: 'The senior nurse's.'
Chris: 'Perhaps he was telling her do her job properly? Perhaps she's avoiding conflict with you by telling you that he had said it?'

Chris' commentary   We reflected on the significance of these two experiences. Tessa felt undermined at a time when she was vulnerable. The experience exposed a *blame and shame* culture and a management culture that saw issues essentially from its budget consequences rather than from its caring consequences. Tessa drew links with the consultant experience, the way she absorbed this anxiety rather than giving it back. Tessa's leadership task was to respond to others assertively in terms of challenging oppressive ways in which others related to nursing staff, and to overcome her fear of sanction.

Tessa said she liked best: 'I thought I didn't have anything to talk about – you got that out of me. The first part at least. I liked least how I feel a bit inadequate. It highlighted my weak points. I felt before that I was strong and assertive.'
Chris: 'You felt uncomfortable?'
Tessa: 'I feel what have I let myself in for! If only someone had taught me things before I got the job!'

Reflection

The themes within the narrative become clearer. Tessa shared another experience concerned with staff responsibility and considered her ideal response within a collaborative rather than parental-hierarchical framework. I surface her concern with upsetting her staff, what I describe as 'misplaced concern' whereby practitioners are soft on the issues and soft on the staff rather than tough on the issues/soft on the staff. Challenging the protective parent. The situations of conflict with the consultant and her managers reflect the difficult terrain Tessa had to journey in order to create patterns of relating that were congruent with her clinical leadership role. Her first task was to develop her assertive self whereby these people could not disempower her. Tessa was stressed by these situations. She carried them around in a metaphorical rucksack that weighed her down. She had no-one within her everyday practice to help her deal with them. I almost literally had to wrest her free from consultant domination and begin to help her see herself as a person who demands respect. I also confronted the projection of her anxiety into her junior staff in an effort to break a cycle of transmitting anxiety rather than direct the anxiety at its cause. Projecting it into a softer target, one where some blame may be legitimately attributed, was another reflection of the 'critical mother' scolded by the angry dominant father. It was not easy because Tessa wanted to be valued by the consultant and by her managers. Her self-esteem was linked to such feedback. If she broke out of this mould she was likely to attract further criticism or 'hell to pay' for not playing the subordinate/loyal wife game (Stein 1978). Such games or norms ripple just below the surface of all experience and are easily read.

Yet Tessa struggled with guided reflection – '*I like least how I feel inadequate. It highlighted my weak points. I felt before that I was strong and assertive*'. Tessa pulled away her own mask to reveal herself. It was uncomfortable as her self perception and normal mechanisms for managing anxiety were being exposed as inadequate, leaving her vulnerable. My supportive role was vital to help sustain Tessa through this crisis transition.

Drowning in staff conflict

In session six Tessa reflected on appointing Annette to the F grade post, and her response to Sylvia's reaction (the other E grade nurse who had applied for this post):

Tessa: 'Sylvia accused me of having made my mind up prior to the interview. I knew Annette would interview better. It was a horrible day as was Sylvia's backlash over the following days! I saw Sylvia after the interview with the personnel officer and informed her of the appointment decision. She took it badly – shouting, storming out. I discussed it with her the following day and she did ring Annette to congratulate her. I was off next day, but I was bothered by this. So I phoned Sylvia. She was furious the off-duty had been changed so she could avoid Annette. I decided to go in. Sylvia was very angry at me. I tried to be sensitive but she accused me of not knowing how to interview. She demanded staff development for future F grade posts.'

Chris' commentary   Tessa was very upset sharing this. I acknowledged how tough this was for her. We tried to pick up some ward organisational issues but Tessa was too distressed and my probing was not helping her, although she acknowledged the need to sort them out prior to moving ward location on 1 June. We agreed to involve Annette to seek some practical answers to the idea of team nursing.

Chris: 'You can see the way people blowing their top is so destructive, reflecting a culture where difficult feelings are suppressed. So when they are expressed you feel uncomfortable, even intimidated. Perhaps Sylvia had been given some false expectations and was genuinely grieved that she had been disadvantaged in some way? How could you have responded to her more appropriately?'
Tessa: 'I don't know … it was so awful.'
Chris: 'Perhaps a cathartic response would have acknowledged Sylvia's distress. For example – "I can see you are upset and angry by this". This type of response creates an opportunity to support her. On the other hand she may need time to come to terms with her sense of being rejected and hence, nothing you do will help her. Rather like an angry child having a tantrum against her unfair mother.'

Reflection

To be an effective clinical leader, Tessa needed to learn to create an emotional space between her and her staff so that she could see these issues for what they were and to stop herself from becoming entangled. She must come to terms with the fact that she is no longer 'one of the girls'. Tessa has absorbed Sylvia's distress as her own and, as a conflict avoider, she feels uncomfortable with the ensuing conflict. Although she responded appropriately within the situation she feels she hasn't because Sylvia's anger has not been appeased. Tessa must see that this is Sylvia's problem and must not accept responsibility for Sylvia's hurt.

Planning change

Annette joined us for session seven. Tessa acknowledged a tension between staff lacking responsibility and senior nurses responding to them as if they were irresponsible. Did staff expect senior nurses to make decisions? Was it easier for the senior staff to do it themselves in contrast with flogging 'dead horses'? Tessa felt she needed to know everything – a sense that she can't leave it for anybody else. She and Annette felt that staff were often not happy with managing the same group of patients – a factor against introducing primary nursing.

I guided them to view managing change from a 'bottom-up approach'(Ottaway 1976) that helped Tessa's dilemma with imposing change from a hierarchical perspective. I challenged them to review the existing ward philosophy which had little meaning for either of them, and was an inadequate representation of the ward's nursing practice. We felt it had been a productive meeting. Annette and Tessa could spend time together to consider areas of development, challenged yet supported by my technical and philosophical input. Tessa and Annette wanted to develop clinical practice quickly. Indeed their enthusiasm was evident, but at every turn they saw barriers, either within themselves or in terms of ward resources. I was left with a strong feeling of 'taking things slowly' – to minimise resistance and conflict.

Reflection

Tessa now has a supportive colleague working with her on the ward. She is not so isolated within everyday practice. Annette is her primary change adopter and enables Tessa to review more formally the possibilities for developing clinical practice. However I felt they had an over-concern with 'taking things slowly' because they wanted to avoid resistance and conflict, the barometers for managing change. Of course, these sensations cannot be avoided but they can be best managed within the change process. There was no culture of being proactive with practice development. As such, it seems an alien world to proceed with extreme caution. The session had confronted Tessa's natural passivity towards developing practice. She begins to embrace this aspect of her role responsibility.

Chasing up Tessa

Between sessions seven and eight I visited Tessa on Lavender ward after its relocation. I noted how tired she looked. She smiled knowingly. Tessa had cancelled our previously arranged sessions and I had made the decision to let her contact me if she wanted another appointment. She hadn't done this. I asked her: 'Do you want supervision?'. She didn't know but she made a new appointment.

Caring for self

By session eight we hadn't met for four months. I confronted Tessa that she had not had a break since becoming the senior ward sister six months ago and that she had even been working her holidays! In response, she felt she needed to be there but that she had become very tired. She agreed she needed to 'let go' and create some space between herself and the ward. She was like a new mother with a baby anxious about letting the baby out of sight. As a consequence Tessa was becoming overwhelmed.

Tackling staff sickness

Tessa wanted to use the time today to talk about how she can reduce sickness levels on the ward. These levels were not acceptable from the hospital's viewpoint. She had been told to do something about it by the directorate management.

> *Tessa:* 'What can I do? One of my objectives when I was interviewed was to reduce sickness levels. They have always been very high and now it's my problem. If anything sickness has increased. I haven't achieved this reduction – it is one of my IPR [individual performance review] objectives.'
> *Chris:* 'What are your options? What makes people sick?'
> *Tessa:* 'People have been off for long spells, back injuries, diarrhoea.'
> *Chris:* 'The first thing to deal with a problem is to understand its nature – can you see patterns within people's sickness histories? Take back injuries? Is it caused by poor lifting?'

Chris' commentary   We explored the nature of the staff sickness and ways Tessa could respond. Focusing on making the issues a ward issue rather than just a Tessa issue.

> *Chris suggested:* 'You could raise staff sickness as a group concern – "We have this problem", to make it a ward issue rather than just a Tessa issue. We need to break into a vicious cycle of stress → sick → increased stress → increased sickness, etc. Hence the need to make this cycle visible and everybody's concern. Help people to consider that the consequence of their sickness is increased stress for everybody else – prick people's consciences. Whereas now, going off sick may be normative – "everybody else does it so why not me?". Could you use the ward meeting for this agenda?'
> *Tessa:* 'We now have monthly ward meetings and we do set an agenda, yet there is often only four people there, who are those on duty at that time. So, another problem – how to increase attendance at ward meetings?!'

Chris' commentary   Another problem to solve. Tessa despaired of knowing how to reduce her staff sickness in the face of organisational expectation that this would be achieved and yet management did not support her adequately to resolve the problem. Tessa's pressure is visible as a time-bomb counting down. She is already reluctant to be in supervision because it confronted her with these issues and she felt she didn't have time to be in supervision. An irony considering her need for support. Yet, the session had been positive. Tessa had regained a sense of control over this particular problem. Tessa had been guided to understand the problem, explore ways of tackling the problem, and support towards taking action. I had been quite directive, but I felt Tessa needed this 'firm hand' to focus her options.

Reflection

Tessa and I had spent the whole session exploring the nature of the problem of staff sickness and ways in which Tessa might reduce it. The problem arose because she had been confronted by her manager that the level of staff sickness was unacceptable. Tessa was anxious because she felt this problem put her in a bad light and she desperately wanted to be valued by the organisation. One of the disadvantages Tessa faced within the ward hierarchy, is that responsibility is pushed upwards, whereas the solution to such problems is found in a mutual responsibility – that the problem belongs to all the staff and not just Tessa. However, she had not yet created this type of collaborative team and perceived the problem as her responsibility.

Acting on staff sickness insights

I had written to Tessa in the session notes – 'A sense of you struggling with this problem without adequate support from management'. In session nine Tessa said she had read the last session notes but she didn't comment specifically on my note. She unfolded her business plan that addressed as one of its objectives to reduce sickness levels.

> *Tessa:* 'I discussed the problem at the ward meeting – the same staff turned up but more than usual as more were on-duty at that time. The plan didn't go down too well, received with silence.'
>
> *The look of resignation on Tessa's face was all too evident. She continued:* 'I wrote a bulletin to all staff which outlined the problem and making it everybody's problem. I've tightened the rules for reporting sickness to make it less of an easy thing to do. I've discussed the issue with my senior nurse and plan to pick up the three main culprits and refer them to Occupational Health.'
>
> *Chris:* 'That feels good to involve the senior nurse, challenging her to support you, that is her role? Taking this action illustrates that you're breaking down the barrier of needing to be seen as coping.'
>
> *Tessa:* 'I'm putting pressure on the culprits. One, an E grade on night duty, has a chronic back injury, had just returned to work from her latest bout of sickness, even though her GP wanted her to stay off work longer. I asked to see her and showed my concern for her. We talked through the issues. She acknowledged my perspective – we talked about the future, our options. I hadn't done this before. I was surprised and relieved it went well. I'm helping her to look for a new post. She said she had been looking for some time. She realised she needed a lighter job but also how she can't afford not to work. It may be possible for her to take early retirement. We are arranging an Occupational Health appointment. There's still a division between night and day staff which made this chat more difficult, but overall I'm pleased with myself. I did "love" them a bit extra as you suggested – they thanked me for that. There were more smiles around.'

Chris' commentary   Tessa smiled. I sensed how important it was for her to work in a warm caring environment, not just for her own needs but to reflect caring for patients and families. If staff did not feel cared for, could they care for others?

> *Chris responded:* 'I feel this will lead to more mutual support – you need to continue being more "loving" to staff. If I was a staff nurse and you made a point of "loving" me I would feel pretty good about that.'
>
> *Tessa:* 'I put a suggestion box to encourage staff ideas. I'm now booking up to establishment – 7 and 5s when previously only booking up to 6 and 4s [staffing numbers for early/late shift].'

Chris: 'Blow the budget – an example when you need support from management as that opens you up to criticism if you overspend despite your rationale for this action. However, you seem much less stressed than last session?'

Tessa: 'Last time I was very stressed.'

Chris: 'I predict a significant fall in sickness statistics within six months. Your work highlights the essential need for dialogue in resolving "team" problems and creating a "new team" based on shared values and responsibility.'

Tessa: 'I don't know about that but I do now feel in control of this situation.'

Reflection

Tessa felt in control of the staff sickness problem by being tough on the issues and soft on the people. She had converted much of her negative energy into positive energy for taking action. Significantly she had sought organisational support for the problem, highlighting the way the effective leader seeks support at appropriate times rather than try and cope (and fail).

Managing risk

Tessa continued: 'The night staff were handing over to the day staff – there was only one A grade nurse on the ward when we heard a crash. A woman getting off the commode had fallen on her face. The nurse was there with her and had helped her back onto the bed. The patient had nasty bruises. I completed an accident form when her daughter arrived. She comes in every morning – we allow that – she is a school teacher. She helps her mum a bit. I knew she was coming in so I anticipated meeting her to warn and inform her of what had happened. She was concerned but I felt I managed to reassure her. She accepted it. Then she went to see her mother who gave her a completely different story. She came back to me and confronted me and said her mother was very upset. I took her into the office. She said her mother had told her that the nurse had let her fall to the ground. I explained that the nurse had been on the other side of the bed doing the draw-sheet. The nurse had said the woman had stood up from the commode and had then fallen. She said: "My mother said there had been two nurses behind the screen". I knew that was wrong and told her as such. However the daughter retorted her mother was "not silly". She confronted me whether only one person on duty was enough? Should her mother be left like that? I tried to explain the circumstances at the time with the staff handover.'

Chris: 'The complaint is a serious allegation. It does challenge you to consider whether just one nurse was adequate at this time?'

Tessa: 'I got the nurse to come into the office to explain with the daughter present. I was trying to defuse the situation. I could sense the daughter was ready to complain. I offered to let her see the doctor again.'

Chris: 'The nurse – do you trust her?'

Tessa (with a knowing look): 'She was moved from Cowslip [ward] for personal reasons. She has been all right with me but she doesn't come across as the most caring when she talks with patients.'

Chris: 'How heavy was this woman? Perhaps the nurse let her fall deliberately because she couldn't manage by herself?'

Tessa: 'I would have been there at the woman's side as the woman is quite unwell, helping her, not on the other side of the bed.'

Chris: 'Imagine I am the investigating officer – we can see what her line of questioning would be like – the nurse probably made an error of judgement?'

Tessa: 'Yes – I can see that. I was wondering if I made the right decision to bring the A grade into the office. The daughter backed down in the end yet, just half an hour later, her husband telephoned me and asked for her to be moved to the private wing. However, the consultant thought that she was too unwell to go the private clinic. So she stayed with us.'

Chris: 'She obviously felt she wouldn't get anywhere with you so she went home and raged at her husband. His call was a reaction to that emotion. What was the relationship like between the daughter and mother?'

Tessa: 'The daughter was not the carer – her mother had a husband.'

Chris: 'I just wondered, knowing how carers often feel guilty with admission into hospital, are they more ready complain as a reaction to their guilt?'

Chris' commentary   I noted some research to support this view (Dawson 1987; Nolan & Grant 1989) that I would send her.

Tessa: 'I felt I had a good relationship with both the mother and her husband. We have had several chats since the fall. I've paid this family more attention since the fall.'

Chris: 'That sounds as if this is a compensatory gesture to "keep them sweet"?'

Tessa: 'I was sensitive about a possible complaint. The biggest source of complaint from relatives is lack of information. Neither is her mother getting any better – she has pleural effusions secondary to heart failure. I want to be there for the relatives.'

Chris: 'I don't doubt your sincerity and caring. Your previous experiences have illustrated this, most notably the experience with the son, where the same issues between caring and managing a possible complaint was evident. How do you intend to respond with the A grade? Would it be useful to de-brief with her?'

Tessa: 'Can I do that?! It was two weeks ago.'

Chris: 'That's a judgement you need to make. You still feel concerned about this situation. Perhaps link it with your other observations of her lack of caring?'

Tessa: 'Perhaps I am avoiding that. It reminds me of the night–day culture. I didn't want to inflame that. I overheard this A grade talking to a relative today and how unsatisfactory that had been. I need to deal with that otherwise she will give the ward a bad name. I've got to get her to consider the consequences of her actions, to reflect on how the relative had felt being spoken to like that.'

Chris: 'Let's reflect back. Your reaction was to defend against the relative's "attack". You realised that bringing the A grade into the office heightened the confrontation and had been an error of judgement. Despite her performance, you have avoided confronting her and indeed, rationalised the A grade's behaviour as typical of her reputation, reinforced by overhearing the interaction between the A grade and another relative. So, without me being judgemental, what should you do?'

Tessa: 'Speak with her.'

Chris: 'Avoiding dealing with conflict means issues are not adequately resolved. You feel very negative yet you can use that energy in positive ways to tackle the issue and role model being tough on issues yet in ways that reinforce responsibility rather than as the critical mother we've discussed in the past. The culture of the harmonious team (Johns 1992) suggests that avoiding conflict is a cultural norm within nursing. Within this theory, you avoid conflict because you would be blamed for being disloyal to the staff member irrespective of the care consequences. You may also avoid conflict as a way to "hide" such complaint from becoming visible to the organisation, where you might be "blamed" for the poor practice? Perhaps your ambivalence of response is influenced by a need to "protect" the team and yourself from organisational backlash?'

Tessa answered my question in an oblique way: 'It's true what you say about my need not to upset people. I need friends not enemies! This type of situation has never been confronted before. I know I avoid conflict and yes, I guess I would like to be more assertive and more collaborative but how to get there!?'

Chris: 'We can reflect more on this in subsequent experiences you share with me. How do you feel now?'

Tessa smiled: 'Exhausted.'

Reflection

Tessa was again confronted with her ability to deal positively with conflict. The experience revealed the culture of the harmonious team whereby Tessa was in a dilemma whether to be loyal to her own team rather than advocate for the patient/family. As Tessa reflected, she needed friends not enemies, fearing that if she took the relatives' side then staff would be hostile towards her for 'breaking the rules'. Tessa was entangled with these politics as previously revealed within Sylvia's outburst. Tessa has to learn to disentangle herself from these politics to take responsible action – being 'tough on the issue/soft on the people'. By being soft on the issue, Tessa felt guilty that the patient had fallen and the relative had become angry. She felt angry at the nurse for causing the fall, and was subsequently anxious that the organisation would view her negatively. It hurt and Tessa suffered. Neither was it easy for her to see what she needed to do.

Growing frustration

In session ten Tessa felt sickness rates were no better.

Tessa: 'I was advised by Colin [business manager] not to send out the memo to staff. He felt this was not the best thing to hand out at this moment. I accepted that. These other problems; some staff are complaining about me! Therefore I didn't want to wind the staff up even more! This was not what I want to talk about today – this was just going on. I'm hoping to address these issues at the ward meeting on 3 December. I've put up the agenda late as I've been on holiday. I left spaces for staff to fill in extra agenda items – somebody wrote "Staff morale – lack of "! I'm distressed with the ward atmosphere. I don't know what more I can do! I tell myself there's nothing more I can do. It's soul destroying. All I've done is implement things from above. All I'm told is how rude I am by certain staff, and that I've got to earn respect from them! I do respect people. I am nice to people. I make a fuss of people, I respond to their requests etc., but even then I've been accused of favouritism when I do respond to people's need! I can't win! I wrote on the agenda – "bring along good suggestions to deal with agenda items".'

Chris: 'Who's giving you the tough time?'

Tessa: 'It's only a couple of people who are really giving me a tough time, undermining me. A lot of staff are saying they have had enough of this, even these two staff are not faulting my care!'

Chris: 'That's the most important part of your esteem. Perhaps you need to confront them?'

Tessa: 'Colin said that. I had one of them in. That was when she said that I had to earn her respect. What could I say? I ended up praising her! My comment about wanting friends and not enemies was ringing in my ears! I haven't had the courage to see the other one. Both are nice to my face and then, the other night she was moaning about me to other staff. I confronted the E grade who put the "low morale" on the agenda. She said she had put that on as staff were generally moaning about everything. She gave an example when Annette had arranged five staff for a late duty, in spite of senior nurse's criticism about the budget implications. I defended this in light of staff sickness and low morale at the present time. This staff nurse didn't feel we needed five on late as we had a reduced number of patients. It caused bad feelings between this staff nurse and Annette, even though Annette and myself were trying to help. That's now resolved. I confronted other staff who were late or who had social difficulties due to children – I'm always trying to accommodate people but also being tough on the issues when I needed to be, helping people adjust their work times to make their lives easier. However this was often interpreted as "favouritism" by the complainers, always looking for an excuse to turn the knife.'

Chris: 'Is it a reflection of the culture shift from Delia to you? The shift from a parental-hierarchy to a team based on responsibility? I feel you caught in a trap between the critical and protective mother.'

Tessa: 'I confronted one of them that she would not have spoken to Delia like that – when she told me she had changed the off-duty. I had accepted this. In fact I thanked her for informing me. Although I was angry, I remained calm on the outside, and then later she confronted me when I was giving an IV drug to a patient – she asked me if I had a "problem" with what she had done, suggesting that I had spoken to her in a "rude way". An A grade phoned me at home today saying how distressed she was with listening to how these nurses were talking about me ... how you couldn't walk into the canteen without people noting "that sister" on that ward.'

Chris: 'Perhaps you need to seek appropriate support. How about personnel?'

Tessa balked at this idea.

I picked up Tessa's distress cue: 'I'm not getting at you.'

Tessa: 'I thought perhaps you were.'

Chris: 'Look at your options – you can back away from it as you are doing, hoping that it would go away? Your other choice – you can take tough action even though the situation may get worse and reach a crisis! It's important to try and understand why these nurses were behaving like this?'

Tessa: 'I'm committed to change and yet I can't understand why they act like this. The holiday was just in time [Tessa had spent two weeks in the USA], I was at the end of my tether. I now feel differently about things but I can't go home and stop worrying about it. Colin suggested that!'

Reading Tessa's pattern or thoughts, I felt she needed me to tell her what to do: 'Try talking to personnel and talk through this problem and your options. My advice is to see these two nurses separately. Confront them and assert:

- it is no longer acceptable to get feedback that undermines your authority;
- you expect these two nurses to co-operate with change and contribute positively to the nursing team;
- you expect that no recrimination will be taken against those nurses who gave you feedback;
- that if these conditions are broken, then you will proceed with an informal disciplinary.'

Chris' commentary   Tessa listened, nodded but was subdued. She said she hadn't talked about what she was going to share. I noted that this issue was 'on top' and had to be dealt with *even* though it was tough to face up to. I noted that she had spent the whole session talking about her despair concerned with the way these two staff nurses were responding to her. Tessa had taken their 'resistance' personally reflecting how entangled she had become, and like an entangled fly caught in a web she felt helpless. Tessa's manager gave her confusing and contradictory messages. He suggested that she shouldn't wind the staff up, yet he also suggested she should confront these two staff nurses. He tells her she shouldn't worry about it at home! There is no real concern, his concern is for organisational smoothness. I had absorbed some of Tessa's despair.

Reflection

Despite her good holiday I feel Tessa is arching towards crisis. She feels isolated, attacked, unsupported, and yet she feels she has acted in everyone's best interests. The criticism, even from just two members of staff, is destructive, highlighting the way change resisters champion the status quo and undermine Tessa's confidence. I sensed she needed to hang on tight and ride out the storm rather than assert her change agenda. Her clinical leadership work was to establish a ward team based on mutual responsibility. Yet before she could do this, she needed to disentangle herself from these destructive forces. Whilst Tessa can gain insight it doesn't help her to act differently because these ways of relating are so embodied within her. Yet her actions around staff sickness were positive and self-affirming. Yet she is so vulnerable and easily knocked back.

Wiping the tears

We next met for session eleven 44 days later. A new year. I noted how tough the last session had been.

> *Tessa responded:* 'Things don't get any easier I'm afraid. I did go to Lorna in Personnel. She said that I needed to see these staff – but she wouldn't see me with them. I felt very anxious about doing this because it would cause me more problems.'
> *Chris:* 'So all these people – Colin, personnel, Vera [senior nurse] – all ostensibly "available" to support you, fail you in this support role?'
> *Tessa looked down and away, clearly upset. She said:* 'Is it worth coming? It's not what clinical supervision is about is it? I come here and moan a lot … it's no better today.'
> *Chris asked:* 'What should supervision be?'
> *Tessa:* 'To bring some experience along to share … more about patient care … more positive things!'
> *Chris:* 'It's natural for you to share things that concern you most. Patient care issues are not where your head is at right now.'
> *Tessa:* 'I don't know what it was but when I come here, I seem to end up crying.'

Chris' commentary   Tessa was clearly uncomfortable about crying. I tried to reassure her that it was good to let out these emotions, to express her distress. She was like a bottle filled up, waiting to burst with all this distress, yet leaking around the seams. I noted my perception that it was important for Tessa to be seen to be coping within her everyday practice, and how she strained to maintain this facade.

Tessa responded: 'I'm not sleeping. I'm getting up at 5.30 AM for early shifts and not getting off work until 11 PM on late shifts. I've tried to share it with my husband. He's sympathetic but he really doesn't understand.'

Tessa talked about the ward: 'I feel the fundamental issue is a shortage of staff. The ward had both high dependency and a high turnover, usually six admissions and discharges each day. The bed manager is always ringing, up to six times a day – "is the bed ready yet?" It's hurting me. I'm going home knowing I haven't looked after patients as I know I want to. Feedback from relatives confirms this, things like knowing that mouth care has not been done more than twice during the day. It's amazing there have been no formal complaints. And seeing staff distressed. This D grade nurse, she is committed, she's in tears as she goes off duty each day, and then having to fill in these forms – ANSOS, Peggy [nursing information systems] . . . I can't even do "Peggy" properly because staff don't fill in activity during the day – they're too busy and so the senior nurse has to do this at the end of the day. You know what has generally happened but not the detail.'

Chris: 'Can you use "Peggy" figures to illustrate the short-fall of staff?'

Tessa: 'No-one pays any attention to them. I have the same staffing as other wards with 23 patients – we've got 32 patients! Other sisters seem to cope. The other day I went to Daisy ward, a medical ward, and the staff were just standing around. Sister was in the office doing her bank nurse/agency nurse figures. Maybe it's just me? Supervision with Annette has dropped off. I am the D grade's preceptor but when do I get the chance to spend time with her? I cannot ask her to stay at the end of the shift – she is like us, already giving so much more of her time. And staff sickness – that's no better. In fact it's even worse! The staff are under so much pressure – it's not a patch we are going through. This is the norm now, unremitting, relentless. The staff are exhausted so any slight complaint they go off sick. What motivation can they have? We drag ourselves in. Vera [senior nurse] insists that "we" go to her Wednesday meetings – if we don't then she said she wouldn't tell us what Colin had passed to her. Others don't go. It's a joke. They expect me to send nurses on all these courses linked with reduction in doctors' hours/technicians – ECGs, cannulation, etc. I don't want these things to happen! I did stand up for myself when Vera tried to put an E grade onto me. This nurse had ophthalmic experience in London. She had applied for Buttercup ward. I clearly felt that Vera was thinking: "Tessa has a vacancy – she will do for her". I did agree to try her as a bank nurse, but she was hopeless. It was the same with an A grade. I had gone along with that, but this person had not turned up for ward today, again "given" to me by Vera. I'm going to choose my own staff. I put an advertisement in the bulletin.'

Chris' commentary   Tessa explored her options to grab some control back into her work life by managing her time. I suggested writing memos, apologising but explaining the reasons for non-attendance to meetings, for example Vera's meeting. I noted that this takes time to do, but it also serves the purpose of making visible the issues. I strongly urged Tessa to keep a diary of risk practice, fulfil her responsibility for recording and reporting unsatisfactory care. This 'evidence' would also be useful to anticipate management's response to her – where is your evidence? I asked Tessa if she felt she could shout *How I'm feeling* at Colin's and at Vera's meetings. We also explored other forms of support – I asked: 'Can you go to the new chief nurse?'

Tessa: 'I couldn't face going to see the chief nurse. I've got to try and cope, to be seen as someone who can manage. I don't want to be labelled a "failure" – I fear that more than anything.'

Tessa then said: 'Will you visit me in hospital?'
Chris said: 'I'll bring you flowers and a poem.'

Reflection

It was a most tragic session. Tessa cried throughout. On the one hand Tessa was out of control, and on the other hand she was hanging on at all costs. Her need to be seen as coping handicapped her ability to take effective action – she will always try and paper over the cracks until the cracks get so big they will swallow her – but she has to try – she has no real choices. That is why supervision was tough for her because it was the time when she cried and could say she couldn't cope. She needed to cope, yet she also needed comforting and support, to be helped to look at things positively. She had no-one to support her. This could be understood in terms that the management expected people to cope, wanted the cracks papered over and relied on Tessa to do that. Hence, the organisation was always shoving 'responsibility' into Tessa's face. Where was her 'management training'? Why did the organisation allow this most talented and caring person to be so distressed? The reason was that the organisation itself tried to cope, it looked inwards at itself and its own survival. It couldn't afford to acknowledge Tessa's experience as valid. Tessa was just a replaceable victim in a system that did not acknowledge individuals.

She did not make another appointment – an ironic twist that at the time she most needed support she shunned it because it was too painful. Ironically, I noted that perhaps we should increase our supervision to increase her support. I felt battered by the session and very conscious of wanting to 'fix-it' for Tessa – to make it okay for her. Hence I said I would ring her in two weeks to see how she was. In fact I didn't contact her – believing that I was available to her but that she must take responsibility for her supervision. She didn't contact me.

Tessa was full of hope and expectation in becoming a G grade. It is the realisation of her ambition. The experiences she shared illustrated her difficulty in developing her clinical leadership role under the specific circumstances of this ward. She knew from Delia's regime how difficult it was to focus staff on positive action towards change, a consequence of Delia's management and leadership. Delia had created a passive hierarchy where things drifted along smoothly enough, at least on the surface. Tessa had been part of this way of things but wanted change quickly at a time when resources had become more compromised. The consequence was failed strategy, and conflict resulting in a spiralling pattern of stress for Tessa. Her shared experiences indicate that the content of her supervision was focused on management issues concerned with managing conflict with staff and ward organisational issues. Although Tessa was motivated to develop clinical practice, this effort floundered in practice. The conditions were not fertile enough for change to flourish. Tessa had to spend time on cultivating the soil for later harvests. Tessa was committed to practice but was not empowered, or enabled to become empowered by the organisation, to shift existing unhelpful norms towards new norms congruent with realising her vision of caring and support within practice. In the end, supervision could not sustain her.

Consider each of the clinical leadership roles set out in Fig. 5.1. To what extent did Tessa develop? Perhaps she became more enlightened as to her predicament but did that actually benefit her? Supervision increased the pressure on Tessa because it made her confront issues and look positively at change. The reality could not match this. I don't feel this was an error of my judgement as her supervisor. I feel this was largely due to her own hopes and expectations within an environment she was neither prepared for nor supported within.

Tessa and I met in May 1996 and agreed the narrative even though she said it was painful for her to read.

References

Chapman, G. (1983) Ritual and rational action in hospitals. *Journal of Advanced Nursing*, 8, 13–20.

Dawson, J. (1987) Evaluation of a community-based night sitter service. In *Research in Nursing Care of Elderly People* (ed. P. Fielding). John Wiley, Chichester.

Dickson, A. (1982) *A Woman in Your Own Right*. Quartet Books, London.

Johns, C. (1992) Ownership and the harmonious team: barriers to developing the therapeutic nursing team in primary nursing. *Journal of Clinical Nursing*, 1, 89–94.

Kelly, P. & May, D. (1982) Good and bad patients: a review of the literature and a theoretical critique. *Journal of Advanced Nursing*, 7, 147–56.

Nolan, M. & Grant, G. (1989) Addressing the needs of informal carers: a neglected area of nursing practice. *Journal of Advanced Nursing*, 14, 950–61.

Ottaway, R. (1976) A change strategy to implement new norms, new styles, and new environment in the work organisation. *Personnel Review*, 5(1) 131–38.

Stein, L. (1978) The doctor-nurse game. In *Readings in the Sociology of Nursing* (eds R. Dingwall & J. McIntosh). Churchill Livingstone, London.

Stockwell, F. (1972) *The Unpopular Patient*. RCN Research Monograph, London.

Chapter 6

Becoming Available within the Hustle of a Medical Ward

Introduction

Caitlin is a team leader on Sunflower ward, a typical medical ward within a large district general hospital. Caitlin and I worked together in a guided reflection relationship for 12 months, spanning 10 sessions. The narrative reveals her struggle to realise holistic practice on a very busy medical ward, steeped as it was in a medical model approach to patient management. I suggested to Caitlin that we used the being available template (see Fig. 3.1) to frame her reflexive development of effective practice. She agreed, although it's worth noting I did not offer her an alternative. I am conscious of a contradiction of imposing dominant frameworks and yet I genuinely believe the being available framework is the most adequate framework available. I am conscious of a criticism – 'well you would say that wouldn't you because you constructed it?' Two reasons for using the framework to frame Caitlin's development are its empirical roots in framing practitioners' development towards realising holistic practice through guided reflection, and the lack of viable alternatives.

Narrative

Asserting self

In our first session we contracted our relationship and talked generally about 'holistic' values and to what extent such values were realised within practice. In doing so, we set the plot for our work together. In our second session Caitlin felt she was a softy because she had failed to tell Debbie, a junior colleague, to do a ward round with the consultant.

> *Caitlin:* 'The consultant was asking me questions he could have asked the patient, which I then had to do, questions that Debbie could have answered. I felt uncomfortable, so I asked Debbie to take over from me when she had finished hand-over. She offered but was reluctant. She said she didn't know the patients particularly well and was anxious about this. So I didn't insist. I got home at 4.40 PM. Debbie got home at 3.40! I asked myself "Why did I do that?" Why didn't I insist when she asked – "Do you want me to do the ward round?"'
> *Chris:* 'So why didn't you insist?'

Caitlin: 'A number of reasons really. Debbie has personal difficulties right now and I was conscious that the consultant likes "sister" to do the rounds. He plays to the audience. He makes little jibes to keep nurses in their place.'

Chris: 'His humiliation tactics. Chapman (1983) has noted how these tactics keep nurses "in their place". You suggest he's a stickler for tradition, likes "his" ward sister buzzing around him, a focal point for his humiliating "wit".'

Caitlin: 'I felt guilty expecting Debbie to do the ward round but also angry at myself! I feel I am a softy. If anybody is doing the giving in – I feel it's going to be me! I feel I am telling tales! Is that usual?'

Chris: 'It does seem to be a cultural norm, part of a climate that discourages conflict and seeks to protect people against external threat! You're not telling tales. You're not attacking Debbie in any way. Neither is being a "softy" a weakness – it shows how much you care about people, wanting to make it all right for people, but a consequence for you is to take this all on board when this responsibility belongs to others. Consider – who would have benefited if you had "insisted" that Debbie did the ward round?'

Caitlin: 'The consultant would have got a better deal. I wouldn't have had this frustration. For patients probably better care? For Debbie – to help her accept responsibility and grow in her role. Before "team nursing" the most senior nurse would take the ward round.'

Chris: 'Perhaps Debbie still saw it that way – that you were the senior nurse and that she felt uneasy doing the ward round? Because the structure of the ward organisation has changed doesn't automatically mean that people's expectations and behaviour change so quickly? Why not de-brief this experience with Debbie to help her learn through this?'

Caitlin felt this would be difficult to do although she should: 'I don't like conflict and try to avoid it. Perhaps that's why I'm a softy?'

Chris: 'How do you feel about this situation now?'

Caitlin: 'Right now – recognising I am a softy, I feel better! – immediate off-loading . . . given the same situation I would act differently . . . I would phrase this as a question to Debbie. Something like – "are you going to do Dr Grouch's ward round?"'

Chris: 'But why give her the choice? If there is no choice – you want her to do the round and you feel this is legitimate – then tell her: "Please do the round Debbie". If you give her choice you also allow her to say "no" – then what do you do? You can either accept it and experience internal conflict as you have done within this experience, or confront her and risk inter-personal conflict with her. I think your concern for Debbie is "misplaced" because it was essentially about avoiding conflict rather than right practice. We need to develop open and honest relationships where we can tell people what we really think rather than avoid dealing with difficult feelings.'

Reflection

On reflection Caitlin could see that she had not asssserted that Debbie join the ward round. She could see that this was not the best decision. She explored those factors that constrained her ability to assert herself. She had been confronted with rationalising herself as a 'softy' and helped to see her role responsibility within this situation. We had explored ways she could assert herself if a similar situation occurred.

When we next met in session 3, Caitlin said 'I've been saying to people "don't give people a choice if there isn't one" and it doesn't make me think that I'm not nice to people.'

Caitlin disclosed the way she had tested her assertive ability in relation to giving a 'difficult' student some uncomfortable feedback about her personal mannerisms that had alienated her from the ward staff. She reiterated how difficult these situations with Debbie and the student had been because she was so anxious of upsetting people and causing conflict. She felt that adopting the mind-set of 'being tough on the issues, soft on the people' had really helped to move her beyond viewing these situations as personal. She felt that refocusing the issues in terms of her role responsibility had helped her to be tough by seeing that her concern not to upset her colleagues was misplaced. She felt this had not diminished her concern for them, rather it had enhanced it because it had enabled her to deal with an underlying sense of frustration with these people.

Managing resistance

In session 4, Caitlin related her difficulty with giving the student feedback to her 'difficult' relationship with Mrs Driver, the wife of one of the patients.

> *Caitlin:* 'There's a relative I feel negative towards – Mrs Driver.'
> *Chris:* 'Do you know why you feel that way?'
> *Caitlin:* 'How do I put this into words? I think she is being critical of how we care for her husband in indirect ways. She says something like: "My husband is meant to have three 'fortisips' a day – how do you expect him to pierce the top himself!?" I responded that earlier he didn't want it and so we didn't pierce the top to keep it fresh. She drives me onto the defensive.'
> *Chris:* 'Why do you think she's being critical?'
> *Caitlin:* 'Because she cares … she is his main carer at home.'
> *Chris:* 'So how does that influence the way she comes across?'
> *Caitlin:* 'I don't know … maybe she thinks we don't care as much?'
> *Chris:* 'There are theories that suggest it's tough for carers to give up the caring role to the nurse. They may feel they can care better. Dawson (1987) noted that spouses, in particular, may perceive giving up caring as failure, equating the failure to care with failure of marriage role with consequent guilt. Spouses may project this guilt into you through complaining about little things that are not good enough. Nolan and Grant's survey (1989) identified that "professionals" failed to identify and respond to carer needs within the care setting, in particular recognising and responding to the carers' emotional needs. Your experience highlights the need to see the whole family rather than just a patient in a hospital bed, especially elderly people who are likely to be discharged back into the community. You've perceived this wife as a nuisance, rather than empathise with her. You've only seen a crabby woman giving you an unfair hard time. Her criticism is a projection of her anxiety. As a consequence you want to avoid her. Hawker's research (1982) illustrated the way acute ward nurses responded to relatives as essentially a nuisance to be managed because they interfere with the smooth running of the patient's management. Ask yourself – what support does Mrs Driver need?
> *Chris paused:* 'Does that feel like a lecture?'
> *Caitlin smiled:* 'A bit … but it's useful. I can relate to what you're saying. It fits the picture.'
> *Chris:* 'So what could be your tactic for dealing with this?'
> *Caitlin:* 'I could involve her more in care, acknowledging her role, sympathising how tough it must be for her?'
> *We talked this through. I then challenged Caitlin:* 'Try it out – is she in today?'
> *Caitlin:* 'Yes she will be. Okay. It feels good.'

Reflection

Caitlin had felt anxious because she resisted Mrs Driver's demands. The consequence was Caitlin was unable to establish a caring relationship with this woman or respond to her needs in any meaningful way. On reflection, Caitlin explored her resistance to Mrs Driver, to put aside her own concerns in order to see Mrs Driver in terms of her experience rather than the abrupt and aggressive signs she presented. Caitlin had taken these signs as a personal affront that clouded the way she perceived Mrs Driver. Caitlin had become entangled in her emotions as if caught in an emotional trap. Worse, she felt guilty because she knew that she was failing Mrs Driver.

In the reactive busyness of the medical ward it was easy for Caitlin to see the way adversarial relationships with relatives were established and resulted in conflict and uncaring practice. That when Mrs Driver needed understanding and love, she received an uncaring glance.

Managing conflict

Caitlin continued by disclosing another situation of conflict with Claudia, a newly qualified staff nurse.

Caitlin: 'I was on an early shift. I had been off for a couple of days. I noted all the ill patients were in the top half of the ward [team A] much more than in the bottom half of the ward [team B]. I decided to balance the load by moving a terminally ill patient to Team B. I discussed this with Claudia in Team B – she was okay about this. I said I would discuss it with his family. They were fine about it as well, in fact they were happy for him to have a single room. Later, one of the patient's relatives came to me and said that the patient was wet – could we come and help him? I went with Beth, who was taking the bottom half of the ward after hand-over. We were appalled at his condition. He had a bottle between his legs that had filled and spilled. It made me think he had been neglected. We washed and shaved him, did his pressure area care. These were much worse than I had seen them before. The crease of the sheet was clearly indented on his hip even though he was on a "Nimbus" bed. I immediately felt guilty with moving him.'

Chris: 'But you didn't feel guilty earlier when you moved him?'

Caitlin: 'No ... but he should have got a better deal. I felt I had dumped him! Beth said to me that I needed to speak to Claudia about this, so I asked her who was allocated to care for Mr Smith that morning. Claudia responded that "we all mucked in". She was defensive, she denied my accusations. She said the family were going to wash him that afternoon and that he had been turned.'

Chris: 'Did the family normally wash him?'

Caitlin: 'No. They help him shave.'

Chris: 'So her comment probably wasn't true. Is one of the dangers of "Nimbus" type beds that nurses think they can leave patients?'

Caitlin: 'But not when they're wet!'

Chris: 'Do you think your hand-over to Claudia was adequate?'

Caitlin: 'Perhaps it wasn't, although Claudia had the same hand-over as I had from the night staff. I assumed she would know what to do.'

Chris: 'Consider Claudia's response. I take it you were unhappy about that?'

Caitlin: 'She was defensive which irritated me.'

Chris: 'Can you use transactional analysis to reflect on your pattern of communication with her.'

Chris' commentary   I talked through transactional analysis theory and drew the characteristic Parent – Adult – Child pattern on some paper for Caitlin to consider (see Fig. 6.1). Caitlin drew a line between her critical parent and Claudia's naughty child.

> *Caitlin:* 'I can see how I became anxious about the relative's complaint and went into "critical parent" mode. It must have made her feel like a "naughty child" and squirm to escape responsibility. I need to encourage Claudia to accept responsibility for her actions without fear she was being told off. I can clearly see how I fit into that pattern, that's really enlightening!'
>
> *Chris:* 'Perhaps Claudia does need support to prioritise care. Perhaps she lacks experience at this. Maybe you need to spend a few minutes after morning hand-over helping her prioritise care? She may not feel competent; it is important for newly qualified staff to be seen as competent (Cherniss 1980) – this might constrain her asking for support because it would expose her lack of competence. Does she have preceptorship?'
>
> *Caitlin:* 'No. I feel I have got off on the wrong foot with her.'
>
> *Chris:* 'I sense you have three barriers to being positive about Claudia; you are angry at her because of this incident; you are angry at her because of her defensive response; and you don't like her very much.'
>
> *Caitlin:* 'Andrea, the other new staff nurse, does not have preceptorship either. She's in my team. I will set that up with her.'
>
> *Chris:* 'One option might be to arrange a formal appointment to de-brief with Claudia about this situation?'
>
> *Caitlin:* 'Go on.'
>
> *I continued:* 'You could role model being *big* about admitting mistakes, something like "I should have handed over to you better. I should have helped you prioritise care. I should have arranged preceptorship for you." Help her to learn that its okay to drop any façade of competence, that there is "no need to be defensive with me".'
>
> *Caitlin:* 'I know I need to deal with it but not how to go about it. I just thought "I've pointed it out and she's denied it. Where do I go from here?".'
>
> *Chris:* 'Consider your role responsibility to protect patient care and support staff. The experience highlights the way new staff nurses are expected to be competent. Failure to acknowledge need and to provide support leads to poor care and defensiveness when care is challenged as inadequate. This fits a cultural norm of only being spoken to when something is wrong. Feedback might make you feel more positive towards Claudia?'

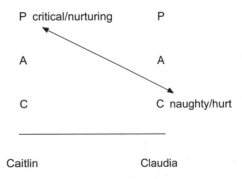

Fig. 6.1 Transactional analysis pattern between Caitlin and Claudia.

Caitlin: 'I like being open and honest about these issues but it's difficult to contemplate tackling Claudia. As you know with Debra, I shy away from conflict with staff although I know I need to deal with these issues more positively. Such care really wasn't good enough and neither was Claudia's response.'

Reflection

As Caitlin's earlier experiences had shown, her learning was to assert her role responsibility so difficult feelings could be explored and resolved without blame and shame, and ensure newly qualified staff were adequately supported. Yet there is no culture for this type of work, illuminating the prevailing culture of the harmonious team where difficult feelings are not disclosed and conflict is brushed under the carpet (Johns 1992). Because Caitlin had embodied non-assertiveness and avoidance as a way of responding to conflict, it was not easy for her to respond in new ways. I felt it was important for Caitlin to realise this in case she judged herself as failing to respond differently, emphasising the significance of my guidance role to both challenge and support Caitlin as she moved along this transformatory trajectory. Transactional analysis assisted Caitlin to perceive and explore her pattern of communications with Claudia, and to consider what pattern would have been more desirable and to explore ways that might be achieved.

Reasserting self

As if to prove the point, when we next met in session five:

> *Caitlin:* 'I re-read the notes this morning. I felt very bad not speaking to Claudia. I decided not to bring up old issues with her but as time went on I felt I should have done that because another situation cropped up. It brought it back into my mind. I felt as if I had opted out because she is not in my team – why me dealing with it? The ward was very busy after that over the bank holiday weekend. When I came on duty they said how awful it had been, including Claudia. She was already stressed – I felt I would I be adding to her stress. I need to be assertive but I see myself as a softy.'
>
> *Chris:* 'We've talked about this before. The culture of conflict avoidance is very powerful so you mustn't give yourself a hard time over this. We can understand the culture and the need to change, and we can chip away at this as you are doing.'
>
> *Caitlin:* 'Maybe I mix up assertion with aggression but when I think about it I can be assertive. There is a situation I'm thinking of where I challenged the medical decision. The patient, Elsie, was clearly dying. She had a PEG tube [feeding tube] inserted but since the tube was inserted she had been having excess secretion following her feeds. I felt it was inappropriate to feed her. However, the consultant, Dr Pierce, said it was his duty to feed her. We are excluded from this type of decision ... so we need to assert our right to be involved ... to have a voice.'
>
> *Chris:* 'Let's use "ethical mapping" [see Fig. 1.5] to reflect on this situation from the different perspectives of the nurses, doctors, the patient and family, and the organisation, and then consider the ethics in terms of the "best" decision, and how the decision was actually made. The dilemma is whether Elsie should be fed?'
>
> *Caitlin:* 'Elsie had expressed her wish to George that if she ever got like this to "let her go". George was distressed at Elsie's "bubbling" – asking can't we deal with it? I am sitting here thinking how am I going to assert no-feeding with Dr Pierce?'

Chris: 'He intimidates you?'

Caitlin: 'In the past when his domination was threatened his response was to threaten to inform managers.'

Chris: 'Like a "bully-boy" using coercive/positional power to get his own way. But this power is weak when challenged because it was not grounded in the "right" decision. You hold the moral high ground.'

Reflection

Caitlin felt she could assert her voice with doctors although they did not necessarily listen. Her experience with Dr Pierce revealed the norms embodied within the nurse-doctor relationship. Understanding where different people were coming from and the ethics of the situation enabled Caitlin to feel more powerful and less intimidated, and to assert her position more knowingly by taking the moral high ground. In doing so, she shifted the conditions of practice to be more available to the patient and her husband.

On reflection Caitlin could frame herself in terms of her role responsibility, that her responsibility lay with the patient and her husband, rather than passively accepting the medical decision. I asked Caitlin why she felt it easier to assert herself with the registrar than with her nursing colleagues.

Caitlin: 'It's because I work with them every day, it does seem more personal.'

Positive feedback!

Caitlin then picked-up Mrs Driver: 'We have become the best of friends! I did go to her the next day and chatted with Reg and then asked how she was/how were things? She just opened up and shared her fears. She talked about the empty house. I "invited" her in to care for Reg. It was really easy!'

Chris: 'What have you learnt from this?'

Caitlin: 'Give someone's carer acknowledgement and build relationships. It's happened a lot since then. A patient's 'stroppy" daughter was talking at me ... agitated, tutting. I acknowledged how she must be feeling. She just stopped and started talking about her anxieties.'

Chris: 'Like bursting the bubble – you enabled her to express her fears and feelings.'

Caitlin: 'It is much easier to talk about difficult things within a relationship. For example, making a decision whether to resuscitate a patient at the weekend. I could talk to the daughter about it as the locum doctor didn't know the patient. I could make the decision with her.'

Chris: 'It shows how working with the family makes such decisions easier.'

Caitlin: 'I now feel much better. When Mrs Driver visits she always asks for me now! I shared it with a staff nurse who commented how well I was getting on with the wife.'

Chris: 'This has taken some stress out of your life?'

Caitlin: 'It has. Before, I had this risk of becoming involved. I linked it to controlling work time. But this was all done in ten minutes. The results were well worth it and on reflection I can see how this can save time in the long run ... it brought us a long way. The only trouble is that they all want to talk to me now! The "she listens, she'll understand" syndrome.'

Chris: 'Such irony! It shows how available you have become to them. Imagine before – all that distress and unmet need without nurses being available to respond?'

Reflection

Caitlin had realised her caring self. I felt this was very significant because it was the first positive experience Caitlin had shared with me. Mrs Driver now felt understood and cared for. I had a strong sense that the experiences concerned with conflict had battered Caitlin. As Caitlin said 'I now feel much better'. And so did I. The realisation of caring in others is very sustaining and exemplifies the significance of this type of research. Yet, reflecting on why I felt better, I realised how I had unwittingly absorbed much of Caitlin's tension.

Asserting ethical action

In session six, Caitlin picked up Elsie's care:

> *Caitlin:* 'We reduced Elsie's feed because she was so "chesty" but ten days later she was still alive against all predictions! Dr Pierce wanted her feed re-commenced – well ... "all hell broke loose". He discussed it with us. He was reasonable with us but he cited the Tony Bland case, noting the court ruling that the case was not to be set as a precedent and therefore each case had to be judged on its own facts. He said his "hands were tied", and hence we had to resume feeding her. He left it to me to tell the family. Well, I was not happy with that, so I informed the family to come in and arranged for them to see the doctor. The family didn't want it – it was difficult for George, Elsie's husband. He was influenced by the daughter-in-law who was also a nurse. The family responded by threatening to cut the tube. They asked if another consultant would take over her care so she could go to the hospice. Dr Pierce wanted the feed continued the next day so it was arranged for her to go to the hospice that night. Dr Pierce was not happy with this in case she died in the ambulance. Elsie died the day after. This was a real predicament for me. I really cared for Elsie and George. George was being pulled in all different directions and he had to sign that she agreed to take her own discharge. George was tortured seeing her groaning. He wanted her to live as the old Elsie – not this Elsie. He hoped she would wake up and be her old self.'

Being available

Caitlin enabled the family to assert their views and arrange transfer to a hospice. Caitlin illuminates her being available to this family, prepared to challenge the consultant's decision making fuelled by her deep sense of concern for this family. In knowing the family's perspectives she is more in tune with them and works with them to ensure best decisions and appropriate action is taken. Yet, because she is so concerned, she has a sense of moral outrage at the consultant's actions, yet is able to convert this energy into positive action. She does not set out to compete. Indeed she seeks to collaborate with the consultant, yet is also able to take the moral high ground exposing the inhumanity in the feeding regime, the relatives' distress, and the inadequate analgesic response. She moves outside the shadow of medical domination, changing the conditions of practice where she and her staff can become more available to work with their patients and families. It is profound.

Understanding collaboration

In session seven, Caitlin basked in a sense of achievement with her work with Elsie and her family:

> *Caitlin:* 'It felt really good to talk about Elsie's care. It made me much more aware of the ethical issues involved. Dr Pierce listens to me more now than before. I can highlight that. We have a 62 year old man, Ray, who has a terminal meningioma which has been controlled by steroids. He was last admitted in a coma because of steroid omission. This time, we will keep him in hospital until he dies. We've stopped his steroids – this has been agreed with his wife Lucy. She wasn't coping well with him at home.'
>
> *Chris:* 'How does Ray feel about the steroids being withdrawn?'
>
> *Caitlin:* 'He was not involved in this discussion.'
>
> *Chris:* 'Okay, that might be something you want to reflect on. Tell me – why is his wife not coping? Can she be helped to cope better? Might dying at home be Ray's preferred option? Has anybody talked to him about his forthcoming death? Is he lying there wondering why his drugs have been stopped?'
>
> *Caitlin paused before this battery of questions fired at her:* 'Ray's talk is "confused" which limits conversations with him.'
>
> *Chris:* 'Is this the rationale for not involving him in his own death management? Callanan and Kelley (1993) consider that dying people are often labelled confused without adequate assessment. They challenge us to be more open and listen carefully so we can understand their messages. They claim that the dying person's messages are usually attempts to describe what they are experiencing, or requests for something they need for a peaceful death, for example reassurance that the other person can cope. What do you think?'
>
> *Caitlin:* 'I'll listen to him again with "new ears"... I'm uncomfortable with this idea of collusion with Lucy and excluding Ray from the decision of withdrawing his steroids because I hadn't seen it and felt this was a good example of managing death ... yet, if Lucy's coping should I challenge this? It would surface a potential conflict of interests between her needs and Ray's needs.'
>
> *Chris:* 'What are Ray's rights, needs? Did we know these? Is his humanness diminished by becoming an object within others' decision making process? We seem to have opened up a number of issues. What do you need to do?'

Chris' commentary We explored how Heron's (1975) cathartic and catalytic interventions might help Lucy to express and talk through her feelings, and perhaps to create the opportunity for Ray to respond and explore to what was happening to him if he desired.

> *Chris:* 'Is she on the ward now?'
>
> *Caitlin:* 'Yes she is. Perhaps I could do this tomorrow. I'm off at 3 PM today.'
>
> *Chris:* 'Why not just spend five minutes with her now and ask her how she is and maybe suggest you have a long chat tomorrow?'
>
> *Caitlin:* 'Yes, I'll do that. I feel good about that although I'm left feeling ineffective.'
>
> *Chris:* 'Be more positive, draw an analogy with shutters – I have helped you lift some shutters that limited how you saw this situation.'

In session eight Caitlin picked up the story:

'I went back to the ward. Lucy was in the dayroom with Ray's brother Len. Ray was being turned at this time. I said: "Hello, how are you coping?". Lucy became tearful. I thought: "Oh lord I've delved into it now!". She said: "When I'm here it's all right, I don't cry". She was trying to keep a stiff upper lip coping at the hospital. I realised this but challenged her: "Is it important that you don't cry in front of Ray?" and then "What would Ray think if he knew the steroids had been withdrawn?". They both jumped in. Lucy said that Ray had always buried his head in the sand! I don't know if I told you last time but Ray's operation was open and closed. They never said to Ray that the tumour was still there. He was told the operation had gone well, that he could get on with the rest of his life. I further confronted her: "Had Ray got an inkling because he had deteriorated so much?". She said: "Oh no". She was getting upset again. She said: "Please don't ask me about it Caitlin, it makes me cry and I don't want to cry". I respected this.

The next day I was on an early shift. Lucy didn't come in the afternoon and therefore I didn't see her for some days. I kept thinking about it over the weekend, that Lucy didn't want to tell him but I felt she should. When I next saw Ray I asked him how he was feeling – was he feeling rough? He could barely whisper to me. He indicated that he was feeling very rough. I said: "Do you realise the steroids are stopped now?". He said something to me but I couldn't tell what it was. I got some help to sit him up and gave him some sips of water, and then asked him again but I still couldn't make it out – you know how that is. I said something like: "You must be feeling very sad". I sat with him and held his hand. I asked myself: "Have I left it too late?". Had I created turmoil inside him? . . . I was really frustrated! That evening Lucy was there with him by herself. She was crying. I went in there and sat down with the two of them. She said she was sorry, wiping her tears away. I said: "No – it's okay. Ray knows how you are feeling. I am sure you have had some very good times". Lucy then reminisced about their times together. He knew what we were talking about. He opened his eyes but he did seem just sad really . . . that air about him.'

Chris: 'How do you think Lucy responded to you?'

Caitlin: 'Initially she didn't want me to see her crying but once I was in there I could see she was animated in talking about their life, going through it all. It was a different kind of chat we had. I felt I got to know her much better. She came especially to see me when she went home and thanked me for the chat. Len had encouraged the suppression of feelings for her protection. She was too vulnerable on her own.'

Chris: 'You were there for her now – you were not available to her before – you had not really shown her how concerned you were for her before.'

Caitlin: 'I can accept that. I shared it with the staff as you suggested. They were very responsive. They were saying: "How do you start a conversation like that?". Susan [staff nurse] came up to me later – she said: "I thought about what you shared with us. I didn't know what to do!". She had obviously picked up that we hadn't responded to this situation. She cared, she wanted to be available but hadn't known how.'

Chris: 'And therefore she avoided it?'

Caitlin: 'I felt a lot better. Ray died the next morning at 7 AM. Lucy came in later for the death certificate, etc. We had time to sit down – she was really pleased she had had that chance to be with him and myself at the end.'

Chris: 'So it made a difference?'

Caitlin: 'It probably did, but I wondered if it was enough. Lucy had often helped Ray – shaving, washing him but not sharing this with him.'

Chris: 'We can see two levels of involvement – one on a physical level, helping him but using this level as a way of avoiding dealing with the emotional level but fulfilling her need to feel useful. The cost of the collusion was that she hadn't said goodbye – or enabled him to say goodbye. You facilitated that, that must feel very good.'

Caitlin: 'I felt as if I had climbed a mountain. The good thing was that all the pretence had gone. It's been really good to go through that. I have been feeling very negative. It has given me a real lift.'
Chris: 'Why so negative?'

Chris' commentary Caitlin painted a picture of a really busy ward all summer, problems with instigating nine hour night shifts and the impact on day staff; how work was disorganised, things not being done, patients not happy. Caitlin had challenged this situation with management:

Caitlin: 'I was shouted down at a meeting when I expressed these concerns. I was so frustrated I went home and cried. I felt like a moaning minnie.'
Chris: 'As if somehow you are to blame for feeling like this? Once again we can see the significance of creating an environment to nurture and support our caring effort. It sounds as if you have battle fatigue.'
Caitlin: 'Yes, that's it – battle fatigue! I'm going on holiday for a week so what I like best is feeling less battle fatigued!'

Reflection

Reviewing the being available template, Caitlin felt she had truly been available to Ray and Lucy at this momentous time. By sharing her experience with colleagues Caitlin felt she had begun to shift the ward culture into a more reflective mode where people could talk more openly about their feelings rather than pretend to cope or bottle feelings deep inside. Not only that, Caitlin felt that sharing her story with Ray and Lucy enabled caring to become more visible within the medical model, that caring was significant and did make a difference to people's lives. Caitlin said she did feel more empowered to care and that was what nursing was all about. Yet the shadow of 'battle fatigue' was a dark shadow that threatened to obliterate the light of caring. As caring became more significant for Caitlin, her frustration was growing that the environment always seemed to stifle rather than promote caring as a lived reality.

Applying insights

In session nine, Caitlin related Ray's confused talk to a new patient.

Caitlin: 'I met him on the Saturday. He said: "I'm dying – I saw an angel – I'm dying". I immediately identified that with what I had been reading. I confronted other staff that he might not necessarily be confused. People were saying: "why is he so confused?". The doctors are open to what we have to say – we have a good team at the moment, but as time went on he actually thought he was dead and as time went on it did develop into confusion. Doctors were saying: "He's no more likely to die than us!". Later he couldn't remember a thing, except that he did remember my name!'
Being conscious of Caitlin's sense of 'battle fatigue' Chris asked: 'How are you?'
Caitlin: 'I feel disillusioned just now. The plans to extend the staff nurse role to include reduction in doctors' hours, no extra cover and plans to take away the blood ladies and the dawning of nine hour night shifts! We try so very hard and we don't get listened to. They ask us for our comments and these just get filed away!'

Chris: 'How is this affecting you?'
Caitlin: 'I care so much for my patients and colleagues. I care nothing for management!'

Reflection

Caitlin reflected her increased sensitivity to confused people and a greater willingness to know them through their apparently confused haze. Again I feel and fear the clouds of despair shadow Caitlin.

Dark clouds

Before we met for session ten I had sent Caitlin a note asking her to contact me, which she hadn't done. So I phoned her on the ward to make this appointment. She had seemed reluctant to do this, saying how fed up she was with everything.

> *When we met I said:* 'You sounded desperate on the phone? Reading the notes I can see how you felt when we last met.'
> *Caitlin:* 'It's been going on for a long time really. It does help just to feel listened to. I just want out now. The major thing is the lack of nurses on the ward.'
> *Chris:* 'So how does that impact on how you feel?'

Tim

> *Caitlin:* 'Let me tell you about Tim, then you can better understand my frustration. The other shift I was finishing the 6 PM drug round at 8.15 PM when a man started talking to me about his cancer. I had a million other things to do before the night staff come on, and that was wrong because I needed to sit down and talk with him when he was ready to talk.'
> *Chris:* 'So what did you do?'
> *Caitlin:* 'I stayed and talked with him for five to ten minutes.'
> *Chris:* 'You finished the drugs afterwards – therefore the last people to get their 6 PM drugs got them at 8.30 PM?'
> *Caitlin:* 'Yes, and then I did the 6 PM IVs.'
> *Chris:* 'What were your options to get round this?'
> *Caitlin:* 'There is no other support available on the ward or from other wards ... wards are struggling with sickness just now. The doctors could not be approached to do the IVs. They would refuse.'
> *Chris:* 'Did the patient appreciate the five to ten minutes?'
> *Caitlin:* 'I say he did ... yeah.'
> *Chris:* 'He knew you were busy?'
> *Caitlin:* 'I'm not sure because he was in a side room being reverse barrier nursed. He has "neutropenia". He's away from the hustle and bustle. Our talk came to a lull so I said: "Tim, I have left the drug trolley outside. I must go and finish these".'
> *Chris:* 'And he understood?'
> *Caitlin:* 'Yes. He had been on the main ward and would have seen how we work.'
> *Chris:* 'What was his fear?'
> *Caitlin:* 'He was expressing how he felt in general ... how he had worked hard all of his life ... never smoked, only drank a little, his wife had left him and how he had cancer.'
> *Chris:* 'The "why me?" feeling ... and he's going to die?'

Caitlin: 'Yes, and he has this pain which is not well controlled. I tried to explore that with him. He won't take the pain killers – he has this fear of becoming addicted to morphine.'

Chris: 'You must see a lot of people who are dying and yet afraid of addiction?'

Caitlin: 'Yes. It was the first time that he had shared this with someone.'

Chris: 'That's important – does he have any family?'

Caitlin: 'None – he feels quite alone.'

Chris: 'I was just thinking of Ray and Lucy – when you said "Oh lord, I've delved into it now" – here you are under pressure of time and you open up this at this time. Did you feel guilty when you left because of time or feel good that you had spent that time with him?'

Caitlin: 'Good initially. I recognised that sitting down and talking with him at this moment was more important than finishing the drugs, but by 8.30 PM the 6 PM drugs became more pressing!'

Chris: 'So did you feel OK about leaving him then?'

Caitlin: 'I felt bad about leaving him because it was the first time he had shared that. He had been in denial. He said: "This tumour, this cancer … whatever this damn thing is … why me?".'

Chris: 'Could you have made contact with the Macmillan support nurse? Bring her in to support him?'

Caitlin: 'She's already involved, but I have no confidence in her – she doesn't deal with these issues well. He felt the tumour was caged in his body limiting the way he moved his trunk. He only ever had pain killers when he was in agony. I explained to him the pain killers would loosen him up – enable him to move more easily. He then said he was worried about the addiction. Because he was in denial – he couldn't see that he was going to die. I confronted him with this fear of addiction. I knew he needed to be given this information and to think about it for a while, so I left him to think about it. The next day I saw him – he said he had thought about it but rejected the pain killers because of the risk of addiction. I put some leading questions to him – "How was he feeling today?" – but he just answered these as either yes or no.'

Chris: 'He was putting up his barriers again.'

Chris' commentary   We explored his reasons for doing that, speculating that he may have felt too vulnerable admitting to the tumour at this time.

Chris: 'Perhaps there were ways that you could have continued the work – for example, reminding him of the words he had used last night and confronting his return to denial? A question of judgement?'

Chris' commentary   Caitlin acknowledged this. I clarified the situation – Caitlin had recognised this man's need at that moment and judged her priorities.

Chris: 'Would most staff have done that?'

Caitlin: 'No, and most staff would think me a fool for doing so. It illustrates my problem of having time to be with patients like this – there is no time.'

Chris: 'I can see you're hurting with this and struggling to cope.'

Caitlin: 'Going part-time and being on the ward every other week will help. I'll have time to recover each time although I won't know the patients so well. I'm disappointed with myself. I saw myself climbing the ladder – becoming a ward sister – but not under these conditions.'

Chris: 'And the future of supervision?'

Chris' commentary   Caitlin gave me a knowing look. We left it for Caitlin to contact me if she wished to continue supervision.

Reflection

Caitlin was frustrated and pessimistic about caring within the context of responding to a dying patient's request to talk whilst doing the drugs two hours late. Caitlin weighed competing priorities against each other. She illustrated that all decisions are essentially ethical decisions, yet she had made a choice she felt that her colleagues would not have even recognised, and even if they did they would not have made the same choice. To spend time with this patient impacted on the care of others. The experience continued a pattern of Caitlin coming to know caring. She strove to be available to this patient but felt battered by circumstance and guilty at having not done enough. I mused with Caitlin how quickly the glow of working with Ray and Lucy had faded. I felt that caring needed to be sustained on a daily basis not simply in peak experiences, as much as these were in themselves sustaining and empowering.

Footnote

Caitlin never did contact me. She went part-time, working part-time in her own nursing home venture she had set up with two colleagues. The narrative is a gathering crisis towards this climax of despair. And yet the narrative is also full of realisation of self as a holistic practitioner. Consider the extent to which Caitlin had become more available to her patients and families. She had strengthened and clarified her beliefs about holistic practice. She had nurtured her concern for her patients. She had developed profound insights into the patients' and families' experience. She could respond with more effective action, especially to meet patient and relative needs. She knew herself better within relationship. And yet, overall, her despair at the system proved to be overwhelming. She was unable to create and sustain an environment whereby she could be available to her patients.

In the busyness of the medical ward this is perhaps not surprising. Her experiences give glimmers of caring possibility within such environments. Yet they are only glimmers. Her concern was nourished and nurtured yet it only exposed her to the contradictions that her beliefs could not be realised. Perhaps it is better to live in a dark cave if we are to survive the maelstrom of failed caring. As it was, Caitlin was no longer prepared to suffer the conflict of contradiction between what she desired and the realities of her everyday practice. The narrative can be viewed as pulling away masks of self-distortion that had limited Caitlin's perception of her reality. Yet pulling away masks, whilst unleashing her caring potential, also exposed her vulnerability. When we touch the essence of caring, nothing else can ever be good enough again.

Working with Caitlin was a profound experience for me. It touched the core of my own being, enabling me to reflect on 'who I am' and my work as a teacher and researcher, and illuminating the way guided reflection is a mutual process of growth as our horizons were fused and transformed in co-creating meaning.

References

Callanan, M. & Kelley, P. (1993) *Final Gifts: Understanding the special awareness, needs and communication of the dying*. Bantam Books, New York.

Chapman, G. (1983) Ritual and rational action in hospitals. *Journal of Advanced Nursing*, 8, 13–20.

Cherniss, G. (1980) *Professional Burn-out in Human Service Organisations*. Praeger, New York.

Dawson, J. (1987) Evaluation of a community-based night sitter service. In *Research in Nursing Care of Elderly People* (ed. P. Fielding). John Wiley, Chichester.

Hawker, R. (1982) *The interaction between nurses and patients' relatives*. Unpublished doctoral thesis. University of Exeter.

Heron, J. (1975) *Six Category Intervention Analysis*. Human Potential Resource Group, University of Surrey, Guildford.

Johns, C. (1992) Ownership and the harmonious team: barriers to creating the therapeutic team in primary nursing. *Journal of Clinical Nursing*, 1, 89–94.

Nolan, M. & Grant, G. (1989) Addressing the needs of informal carers: a neglected area of nursing practice. *Journal of Advanced Nursing*, 14, 950–61.

Chapter 7

Realising the Therapeutic Relationship with Head and Neck Cancer Patients and Families

This narrative tells the story of my work with Alexia within our guided reflection relationship. We met for nine sessions between July 1998 and April 1999. Each session lasted approximately one hour. Our relationship was discontinued by Alexia's maternity leave.

I met Alexia when she was a student on the clinical supervision module which I teach at the University of Luton. We agreed to enter into an individual guided reflection relationship. At that time she was the ward manager and clinical nurse specialist for a regional head and neck unit. She had commenced this post about six months previously.

Developing the therapeutic relationship

In our first session we contracted that we would monitor the impact of guided reflection in enabling Alexia to become a more effective practitioner, whatever that might mean. I suggested I would take detailed notes of our dialogue and construct a narrative to unfold our experience of working together in guided reflection in ways that illuminated Alexia's growth (or non-growth) of realising desirable practice. We agreed to meet at four-weekly intervals for one hour. After formally contracting our guided reflection relationship Alexia disclosed the following.

> *Alexia:* 'Three weeks ago I was upset about a situation. I unwittingly took it home with me and it impacted on my home life. I didn't know what the reason was at first. I also know it will happen again. It's about the amount of support patients need. This patient, Paul, he had had a malignant melanoma removed from his ear in the past. His neck had become swollen and he required a 13 hour operation – a radical neck dissection that involved pulling muscle up from his chest. Body image was a problem for him. I knew it would be. I didn't admit him. An E grade did this but I wish I had done. I would have been better prepared to respond to his needs. He was very British – "chop the bugger out and I'll be fine" attitude. I challenged him then: "And what happens if it's not fine?". He discarded this. I felt the family dynamics were "odd". His wife only visited at visiting times although relatives of patients who have such surgery have open visiting. This made it difficult for me to talk with them as a couple. Then on Sunday afternoon the ward was very quiet and I could chat to him without guilt! I felt I

had a good rapport with him. He was going to Addenbrooke's on the Monday for radio-therapy. That made a good opener to the conversation: "How was he feeling about that?". I chatted about myself, I think that's important so they get to know something about you.'

Chris stated: 'The significance of using self disclosure in developing therapeutic relation-ships.'

Alexia responded: 'I asked him about his children – he said his son had committed suicide a year ago. He said that matter of factly. I acknowledged my shock at this news and how difficult that must have been when we expect our children to bury their parents not the other way round. This had happened when he and his wife were on holiday – he was angry at his daughters for letting this happen. The son had been depressed. I noted the coincidence that it happened when he was on holiday, that the son would have done it if he was determined to. He said his son's death had coincided with the Princess of Wales' death and how angry he felt when people were grieving for someone they didn't know – when he was grieving for his son. I noted I found the family dynamic strained. He admitted this – that he had never shed a tear. I also fedback my perception that his wife didn't seem to know. He agreed – that he didn't want her to know … didn't want to bother her with it. I then picked up the "what if" question – linking it to Addenbrooke's. He said: "It won't happen to me".'

Drawing on Bolen's work (1996) Chris noted: 'Patients tend to respond to imminent death in three ways: to deny it; to be stoic about it; or to fight it; which as Bolen suggests often leads to the best outcomes. Does that fit?'

Alexia acknowledged the fit: 'He's a bit of denial and a bit stoic. I challenged his denial of events – going out on a limb, prodding him to respond … to get him to show some emotion. I felt guilty about doing that. He just said: "I don't want to talk about that". He was going next day! That's why I wanted to talk to him about it. He just went back to talking about his son. He felt that somehow his stress about his son had caused the recurrence of his mela-noma. Then his family came in – he didn't want to talk in front of his family. At hand-over I raised the need to enable Paul to talk about his feelings. The next day, Monday, we had two hours before he left to go to Addenbrooke's at 9 AM. It was really busy. I couldn't create the opportunity to be with him. And then the transport arrived – he was about to go and he burst into tears and gave me a hug, thanking me. I asked the ambulance men to have some tea for 15 minutes so I could spend some time with him. They agreed. It was all they could spare. We went into the office. He was distraught. He's coming back in one week but I felt I hadn't done my job. I felt bereft. Sad for him and sad for me. I was thrown back into my job. At hand-over the staff asked me how it had gone with him. I didn't handle that well. They said: "We knew he would crack at some time, but when!"

I rang Addenbrooke's each day to see how he was. He was isolated in a side room which made it impossible to speak with him. My husband picked up the vibe and suggested I visit him … that put me into the dilemma of whether I should visit him or not – where to draw the line of taking work home and becoming involved with patients and families. I do have some regret about not visiting.'

Chris picked up Alexia's sense of self-doubt: 'Reinforcing your sense of being over-involved? And yet you are only human and need to accept that sometimes you become drawn into the other's suffering. That's a consequence of your holistic beliefs and a part of your daily work life … perhaps you need to accept that's okay rather than punish yourself?'

Alexia simply said: 'I know … but that doesn't necessarily make it any easier.'

Chris' commentary   I used the being available template to guide Alexia to reflect on her involvement with Paul and the type of relationships she desired with her patients. Being available is the non-reducible core of therapeutic practice, working with the patient and family to help them find meaning in their experience and make best decisions and take subsequent actions to meet their health/life needs. Alexia and I viewed the forces that influence the extent she could be available:

- Knowing what is desirable
- Being concerned
- Knowing the person
- Responding with appropriate and effective action to meet patient need
- Knowing self and managing involvement of self
- Creating and sustaining an environment where being available is possible.

> *Alexia felt that knowing Paul was paramount – 'who is this man?' She asked herself:* 'What were his feelings and thoughts? What meaning did he give to this health event?' It was significant tuning into what was significant for him … it might have been assumed that his melanoma was the most significant issue for Paul and yet his unresolved feelings about his son most occupied his mind.'

Chris' commentary   I linked this to an experience a surgical ward sister shared with me about a woman with breast cancer whose greatest concern was being made redundant from her job.

> *Chris asked:* 'Does your assessment tool enable knowing patients/family well enough?'
> *Alexia paused to consider this challenge:* 'I don't know … I'm very perceptive but other staff? I need to consider this. I feel very attached to Paul. It's important to understand his sense of loss and unresolved sorrow … to understand where he is coming from.'

Chris' commentary   I linked this feeling to some theory on chronic sorrow (Eakes *et al.* 1998) and said I would send Alexia this paper for her to reflect further on Paul.

> *Alexia:* 'Now I do feel I responded appropriately to Paul, although having discussed it with you maybe I did absorb Paul's distress and had become distressed myself.'
> *Chris smiled:* 'You ask me this question? It wasn't easy to manage your work priorities differently, yet you did create the space to be with him and your concern for him enabled him to cry and communicate his distress. It's good to become more sensitive to these processes.'
> *Alexia responded:* 'I desperately wanted Paul to respond. I can see now that this had to some extent become my need and that when he couldn't respond except at the very end I felt I had failed. When faced with such family turmoil, I did become entangled. I had wanted to fix it for Paul.'
> *Chris confronted this:* 'Whether he responded was his responsibility not yours – we can't force people to make use of ourselves. I am going to assume that when you talk about a holistic philosophy you acknowledge that the nursing role is to facilitate Paul and his family to find meaning in the experience in order to make good decisions about his life/health?'
> *Alexia accepted this perspective:* 'Working with such cancer patients and families that is important. The emotional, psychological, social, spiritual aspects of care are really important. Since I have been on the ward we are moving towards embracing this approach rather than the medical model which had prevailed. I think we are getting to know our patients well over time.'
> *Chris clarified:* 'In other words you nurture involved relationships with patients even if some of them like Paul initially resist you in their efforts to cope?'

Alexia agreed.
Chris continued: 'Hence it becomes imperative that nurses learn to manage themselves within such relationships. As your experience has highlighted, nurses are at risk of absorbing the patient's distress as their own. Nurses are well prepared for this type of relationship.'

Chris' commentary I then challenged Alexia's role in working with the family, asking her a battery of questions. Did she support the wife/daughters enough? Was she overly influenced by Paul's request not to tell his wife what was happening to him? Could she have made an appointment to speak with the wife? Could she have mitigated between competing and conflicting needs within the family to bring the family together, even to the extent of confronting Paul's attitude towards secrecy with his own family? Did saying that she didn't have an opportunity to speak with the wife reflect a reactive rather than proactive stance to relatives? If so, does this reflect a culture on the unit where the focus on care is more on the patient than the family needs? Did she take over care of this man because she felt the named nurse could not respond adequately? Did Alexia feel that the patient would have got a less good deal if the staff nurse had had these conversations with him? Such questions, but gently asked like peeling back the leaves of a lettuce to reveal its heart.

> *Alexia:* 'It's true, I hadn't perceived the named nurse's role. I simply responded as I felt able. However she could see the value of de-briefing and the way the staff's comments reflected their anxiety with Paul. I think that generally we are good with relatives... I was in a dilemma about Paul's response. I can see that perhaps I should have confronted that. I don't know.'

Chris' commentary I guided Alexia through ethical mapping (see Fig. 1.5) to reflect on this dilemma. The dilemma hinged around the extent to which Alexia should respect Paul's autonomy and her empathy with the needs of Paul's wife. Alexia felt the 'solution' was to help Paul express his deeper fears and to confront him if his 'best' decision was his stoic attempt to protect his wife from facing up to this issue. Perhaps he was protecting himself from his own anticipated discomfort, or he viewed his role of man within the family as to protect his wife, or indeed perhaps his decision was a reaction to his son's death. His wife was quite passive yet she may need to explore with Paul her fears and their future together.

> *Chris asked:* 'What has been significant about sharing this experience?'
> *Alexia thoughtfully:* 'I suppose recognising my sense of failure and guilt ... thinking that I should be there for my patient at all times.'

Chris' commentary In response to Alexia's lingering feeling of failure and distress I guided Alexia to imagine a space outside herself where she could stand back and look at these feelings for what they are:

> *Chris:* 'Ask yourself how do we come to feel these things? Turn them over and have a good look at them. Why are nurses so riddled with guilt? It is as if we take on responsibility for everything and blame ourselves harshly if things go wrong. Dickson (1982) calls this the

"compassion trap", as if we are trapped by our caring ethic. You've absorbed his pain as your own, and suffer. You know it is not your pain but can't easily break free from it. Your work is to balance your sense of concern and involvement without diminishing your concern. So let's stamp on this guilt now ... let go of this pain.'

Chris' commentary   I stood up and stamped on it. Alexia laughed.

> *Chris:* 'Through understanding and focusing our actions to future situations, much of this negative energy can be converted.'
> *Alexia exclaimed:* 'I do feel as if I've unloaded my rucksack. I do feel better by discussing it.'
> *Chris said:* 'Linking your own feelings and supporting your staff, maybe you might have used staff more for support?'
> *Alexia was uncertain:* 'In this situation I felt I needed to be "professional", to be strong which meant appearing to cope.'
> *Chris challenged:* 'So, tell me, what does "being professional" mean? Does it mean that good nurses cope? That good nurses don't burden their colleagues? Put that into context of the type of team you want.'
> *Alexia:* 'I want a team that can support each other ...'
> *She broke off and immediately saw how she had been led into this contradiction:* 'I am trying to let go, to trust the staff. I can link this back to previous experience where this had not happened ... I had needed to appear to be tough, to win respect and trust ...'
> *Chris:* 'Yet the price you paid for this was perhaps role modelling that good nurses cope. Might it be useful to de-brief your feelings with your staff?'
> *Alexia was hesitant:* 'I don't know if I could do that.'

Chris' commentary   I took the *Tibetan Book of Living and Dying* (Rinpoche 1992) from my briefcase and turned to a well worn page, 316, and read:

> 'Suffering ... gives you such an opportunity of working through and transforming it. The times you are suffering can be those when you are most open, and where you are extremely vulnerable can be where your greatest strength really lies. Say to yourself then: "I am not going to run away from this suffering. I want to use it in the best and richest way I can, so that I can become more compassionate and more helpful to others". So whatever you do, don't shut off your pain; accept your pain and remain vulnerable. And don't we know only too well, that protection from pain doesn't work, and that when we try to defend ourselves from suffering, we only suffer more and don't learn what we can from the experience?'

For Alexia these words were a revelation. She had responded with an openness and passion, able to look at herself in the mirror I held for her. She said she would de-brief with her staff and see what happened.

Reflection

I utilised the being available template to frame Alexia's development of effective practice:

Knowing what is desirable	Alexia had reflected on and clarified her beliefs about her practice. As a consequence she had a stronger sense of purpose.
Being concerned	Alexia's concern for her practice is very strong. However by the end of the session it has been nurtured, she has gained strength, and has become more focused.
Knowing the person	Alexia's sense of knowing Paul and his family has gained new dimensions by reflecting on the way she 'tunes' into and rides Paul's wavelength, and in understanding the way he responds to his illness.
Responding with appropriate and effective action	Alexia explores new ways of working with Paul based on understanding his needs and the unspoken conflicts within the family. Her confidence is strengthened.
Knowing self and managing involvement of self	Alexia is able to view herself in relation to Paul and understand her own fears and emotional responses. She is able to view herself within the resistance–reciprocation continuum as she contemplates riding with Paul on his shifting wavelength. As she does, so she begins to understand and work towards shifting the weight of negative emotions, such as guilt and failure, that bore heavily in her experience with Paul.
Creating and sustaining an environment where being available is possible	Alexia is able to place her work with Paul within the wider organisational and cultural context and the way forces interact to create the caring moment. She feels more in control and able to influence the environment.

Knowing and managing self

In session two Alexia related her experience with Paul to another patient who had aroused strong emotions within staff:

Alexia: 'He's a 42 year old Asian man who had throat and tongue cancer. This is attributed to the Bangladeshi habit of berry nut chewing and smoking. I brought nurses together to de-brief strong feelings aroused by this man's attitude ... sharing my own feelings of frustration and anger at this man, which I felt enabled other nurses to share similar feelings ... feelings which had been bottled up. One nurse had been having nightmares about this man, which stopped after she had been able to release the tension.'

Chris: 'How nurses bottle up feelings ... reflecting the prevailing culture whereby good nurses cope.'

Alexia: 'I felt I acted as a significant role model by enabling and empowering staff to share their feelings. We agreed we must spend more time in this way. I told them we will spend 20 minutes, the patients can wait.'

Chris: 'We can frame this release of tension within the metaphor of the water-butt theory of stress (Johns 2000). In this metaphor, stress, like rainwater filling a water-butt, fills up the body until it reaches the point where the practitioner feels she is drowning. By then it's too late to relieve it except by "blowing your top" which makes a mess everywhere and this distracts people from the issues that caused the mess. People hurry around to mop up the mess. We need to become sensitive to the stress filling up. Now water-butts have a drainage tap which enable the gardener to draw off water at appropriate times to water the plants and help them grow and bloom. In a similar way the practitioner can draw off stressful energy and use this energy positively to grow and bloom. You might say that my guide's role is to help you do this. That's what you did, you helped staff to open their taps and use their stress in positive ways to care.'

Alexia related this back to Paul: 'I was reluctant to disclose myself with my staff because I felt I needed to be seen as strong. Now I feel confident about this, about letting go of this need ... I can see how this worked to bring the team together, a team that could become mutually supportive acknowledging the tough work it did and that we are only human – and suffer from human vulnerability.'

Chris acknowledged the significance of what Alexia had said and asked: 'How did this man feel about what was happening to him?'

Alexia: 'He had rejected radical surgery that would have seriously disfigured him whilst only adding months to his life. This had raised ethical issues about such surgery. The surgeon had discouraged the man's acceptance of the surgery option – but nevertheless he had offered the patient the choice. I doubt whether he would accept the offer of radiotherapy – although palliatively this would increase his comfort. He had refused a gastrostomy tube (he was in fact booked into theatre next week to have a tube inserted). He had also taken out a long peripheral line for total parenteral nutrition (TPN). This type of line was now used more and more instead of central lines. He had Asian food brought in – the smell filtered across the ward.'

Chris: 'How do you feel about the smell?'

Before Alexia could answer Chris joked: 'The food must have deodorised the smell from his tumour.'

Alexia laughed: 'It didn't – the two don't mingle well!'

Chris' commentary   I imagined the tumour smell and commented how awful the smell must be for the man and his family. Alexia agreed.

Alexia: 'His wife looks about 12 – she doesn't speak English. He dominates her. The nurses haven't been able to respond to her in terms of her needs.'

Chris: 'How much is this an issue?'

Alexia: 'He has a 15 year old son who acted as his interpreter although he could speak English. He had rejected an official interpreter. One came up but was dismissed by him. He wanted everything said through his son. It was his son who had to tell his father his prognosis. I'm concerned about the son being expected to do this – the son had been in tears.'

Alexia laughed in anticipation of my next question: 'Yes, I do feel maternal ... to protect the son.'

Chris: 'Indeed the son may have been in tears anyway. At least the son telling his father enabled the son and father to share this moment ... that such feelings have been openly expressed. I assume the son will take over the mantle of the father in the household.'

Chris' commentary   Alexia (using the being available template) reflected on who this man was and why he responded in this apparent off-hand manner. Alexia acknowledged the risk of taking his behaviour as a personal affront and labelling him negatively, with the uncaring consequence of avoiding him.

Alexia: 'I can identify the cultural issues and can make sense of the man's attitude to women and that being a white woman and nurse made little difference. The man was quite happy for a nurse to do "menial chores" – like take his urinal bottles away. He had been unco-operative with his tracheostomy tube changing. I had to confront him sternly about the need for her to do it. He had ceased to talk to her after that. A nurse who spoke his language had, off her own back, tried to create the opportunity for him to talk about his illness, but he rejected this approach and ceased to have anything to do with her as a consequence.'

Chris challenged: 'Does all this explain why the staff had felt so angry at this man? Do we expect him to be "nice" whilst he struggled to come to terms with his cancer and forthcoming death? What are his deeper needs? Maybe he responds as he does in his effort to control his environment – a proud man brought to his knees?'

Alexia picked up this cue: 'He had been a school teacher in Bangladesh – now he's a cook. Perhaps that has eroded his pride? He wasn't receptive to the tales of my Indian travels. Perhaps he had hang-ups about the colonial past, or perhaps it made him reflect on his death – and that was too painful?'

Chris: 'You highlight how easy it is to assume "who he is". Perhaps his needs are not to be prised open and talk about his feelings, but to shut them up in his pride – a man who must cope for his own and his family's sake. Maybe the time will come when this facade falls apart and he needs spiritual and emotional support? Linking this back to Paul's experience, do we impose this need to talk and be co-operative because he and the family are suffering – seeing our role is to ease their pain? And when the approach is rejected, and rejected in a hostile and abusive way, the reaction is hurt with the risk that we reject him. The key to "being available" is to communicate concern and availability to him so he knows and can respond when he needs to, as difficult as this is sometimes.'

Alexia agreed: 'It is sometimes difficult to sit back and watch the suffering, especially when you know there may be better ways. It makes me think of Rinpoche's words you said last session. I have become more sensitive to myself within the situation – this has developed quickly from sharing the previous experience. I catch myself saying to myself "this man is making me angry ... now, how am I responding for the best? What is prompting his anger?" I'll use the ideas of being proud and in control in de-briefing with the staff. That's really helpful.'

Chris picked up the use of empathy: 'The significance of empathy – how do we know the experience of the other and what meaning does the event have for the other? This experience illustrates the barriers that come between knowing the answers to these questions. Let me suggest something; a useful tactic at hand-over is to pose such questions as: What meaning does this event have for Mr Ali? and How do you know that? How is his wife feeling? Is it important to know this? If so – how can you find access? and How are you feeling? The idea is to turn hand-over into an opportunity for group reflection and learning.'

Alexia: 'We work with many Asian families and I do feel we are sensitive to cultural issues, so it would be good to surface these types of questions.'

Chris noted: 'Racial issues are often the most difficult to discuss and hence to resolve. It seems easy to stereotype Asian men as being hostile to women, as an explanation for their behaviour, and that white women cannot easily shrug aside their own perspectives to accept the arrogant Asian patriarch, even when we understand. We need to understand these issues and our own prejudices. We need to clear a space to see him and manage our own feelings without diminishing our caring concern. A fine balance to find and juggle. However, we need to give ourselves a break. Just because we come to understand things and understand them differently, does not mean we can easily change our embodied responses. Learning through reflection is essentially a holistic process of knowing and transforming self, not a cognitive activity. We are who we are for reasons that cannot rationally be shrugged aside.'

Reflection

By reflecting on her experience with the Asian man, Alexia built on the insights she had gained from session one. In particular, Alexia gained considerable insight into knowing who this man was within a cultural perspective. Whilst she couldn't condone his attitude she could better understand and accommodate it within her caring lens as necessary to be available to him and to likewise help her colleagues.

Learning the caring dance

In session three Alexia reflected again on the Asian man.

> *Alexia:* 'He's back in . . . my approach is very different. It is very positive. I felt a much greater connection with him which opened up possibilities to work together. The nurses all said "Oh no . . . why can't he go to another ward" when they heard he was coming back in. I confronted them with their negative attitude and helped them see him in terms of his needs and what we can offer him rather in terms of their own concerns They accepted that. A lot of our patients are back in with bad news – we have three in particular. I sensed that staff feel precarious at this time as a consequence. As one staff nurse said: "I don't want to be here this week".'

Chris' commentary   I noted the significance of Alexia enabling the staff to express their feelings in positive ways rather than as a whinge. I noted Lydia Hall's work (1964), whereby nurses needed to know and manage their own concerns so that they do not interfere with enabling the patient to see his own concerns. Negative labelling is a good example of this. Alexia shared how good she felt about her care although she did challenge herself whether she should feel good when working with people who were clearly suffering.

> *Chris confronted this perception:* 'Is it helping people with their suffering that brings your own satisfaction and suffering?'
> *Alexia reflected:* 'It's true, caring for these people brings me much satisfaction. It's what I became a nurse for. This satisfaction is increasing now I've found ways of being with these people in the ways I feel are caring. And I'm not absorbing the suffering as my own so much.'
> *Chris:* 'You highlight Benner and Wrubel's (1989) assertion that realised caring is the antidote to stress. They suggest that nurses are stressed because they have lost caring, and hence need to reconnect themselves to caring.'
> *Alexia:* 'I sense the wisdom in that . . . I have two positive experiences to share about connecting with families . . .'

Bob and Molly

> *Alexia:* 'Bob was trying to protect his wife by not talking about his feelings of his forthcoming death. I felt very close to this man: He talks about me as his friend. When he came in

he looked awful, dehydrated. I went home and worried about him over the week-end, resisting a strong urge to phone the ward to see how he was. On the Monday he was like a changed person – the colour back in his cheeks. I took his wife aside and asked her how she was feeling. She was fearful but anxious to talk with Bob about the future but felt she couldn't approach him with these needs. I had asked Bob – did he contemplate his death – what did he feel about that ... and brought them together – almost as if they had fallen in love all over again.'

Chris: 'You tuned in to them and there came a moment when the time was right to bring them together by gently confronting their restrictive attitudes rather than force the issue. The situation reminds me of Paul and his wife from our first session.'

Alexia: 'Yes. The second situation concerned a young man who had been severely beaten up, and my response to his older brother. I had taken the older brother aside so his parents didn't know. He was tearful, feeling guilty and angry about not protecting his younger brother. I was communicating on his level, calling the attackers "bastards", helping him to talk through and validate his feelings. When he left he gave me a hug to my surprise and that of his parents! Yet it felt right – a reflection of the connection between us.'

Chris: 'What has been significant in sharing these two experiences?'

Alexia was uncertain: 'Giving myself positive feedback ... building on the other experiences I have reflected on.'

Challenges to creating the caring team

In session four, Alexia shared her experience of responding to a D grade staff nurse whose 'wrong' attitude was threatening the well-being of the nursing team.

> *Alexia:* 'I've tried to understand where she's coming from so I can respond appropriately to her but it's not easy to challenge her.'
>
> *Chris clarified:* 'You want to confront her, to be tough on the issues but soft on the person?'
>
> *Alexia:* 'Yes. I have in my mind the ideal of the therapeutic team – a team that can effectively support our caring work with patients and families. I realise I have to confront her with her responsibility to this team.'
>
> *Chris:* 'I can see it's tough for you to be tough on the issues. I know from the many experiences that practitioners share with me, that interpersonal issues with colleagues are the most difficult type of conflict to take action on. It's if we have become entangled with our colleagues in ways that make it difficult to surface negative feelings and resolve conflict in positive ways. I have named this the harmonious team (Johns 1992, 2000). Consequently we avoid conflict and expressing negative feelings and they simply fester. You feel angry at her because she spoils things?'
>
> *Alexia:* 'She does spoil things and yes it does make me angry! And yes, I do not like conflict ... I have a bad taste with this from my previous work.'
>
> *Chris:* 'It's important to acknowledge this ... yet you cannot let it go. Your team look to you to role model leadership?'
>
> *Alexia:* 'I know ... I know!'

Chris' commentary   We didn't pick up the issue of Alexia's previous work and left the issue spinning in mid air for Alexia to take away with her and reflect on.

Becoming close

In session five Alexia said she had not taken any action with the staff nurse as 'things had quietened down'. I noted the conflict was contained but was simmering and would rear its ugly head again. Alexia felt this was true and did feel better prepared to tackle it more positively when that happened. She said she wanted to share her experience concerning Tom, a 47 year old man who had been readmitted to the ward with an abscess:

> *Alexia:* 'His wife had breast cancer – she was 45. They have two daughters. His major concern was her rather than himself ... he had wanted to go home to be with her when she died. She had visited the ward on one occasion – she had clearly been beautiful and now she looked so ill. He was a night club owner, had drunk and smoked a lot. I had kept him as long as possible for rehabilitation. He went home and she died at home the next day peacefully. I've become very close to Tom ...'

Chris' commentary   Alexia paused and reflected on this sense of connection and spoke about the way she talked with him about his feelings over what was happening to his wife. Alexia was animated and tearful in sharing this with me.

> *Alexia:* 'And now, this admission, he asked me yesterday whether the abscess was a reoccurrence of his cancer? I knew from the consultant that it was 98% certain, yet I have avoided telling him. I've felt uncomfortable and unprepared to talk with him about it even though I suspected he knew. I'm devastated by this ... gone home and felt guilt and angry at myself – why hadn't I handled it well? I felt he knew because he intimated that he would be spending some time in hospital now ... envisaging Christmas.'

Chris' commentary   I simply acknowledged Alexia's story and feelings and asked her what was significant to explore.

> *Alexia continued:* 'Talking it through now, I feel prepared to tell him ... that I can leave this session and deal with it. I'm conscious of the staff's reaction – a sense of "Oh no" – that Tom should have to go through this now. I see I have to spend time enabling Tom to talk through his feelings about his wife's death. That's where his head is ... he's been talking about the funeral and making connections between now and the past.'
>
> *Chris:* 'This is so important to understand; making the connection between what is happening now and the past is crucial in moving forwards. Marris' (1986) theory of change and loss helps us to frame this temporal connection – the need to make connection between what is happening now and the past before people can move on. Indeed – what did/could Tom look forward to right now?'

Chris' commentary   Alexia knew the significance of this temporal connection. Drawing on Marris' theory helped her frame it to see it more clearly and to bring it more into consciousness.

> *Chris gently prodded Alexia:* 'So why do you feel so entangled with him? What makes him different? Is it simply the immensity of this human tragedy – his wife dying, his cancer and the depth of your connection with him?'

Alexia: 'I don't pity him ... it's genuine compassion – so why do I feel guilty? Why do I blame myself? You've challenged me on this before to create a space to put these things. I feel I've always had an open relationship with him but I saw it wasn't the right time to respond to Tom's question and it needed to be the right time because I had to make sense of Tom's illness for myself.'

Chris: 'I may have challenged you before but the ways we see and respond to these things are not easy to change ... ways of responding and reasons for responding as we do are deeply embodied. We bring these things up to the surface and contemplate them. Tom would know how difficult that question was to respond to. You can now release your guilt and pick it up with him – Tom, that question you asked me yesterday ... I wonder whether the abscess was a reaction of Tom's effort to work out his grief and that being in hospital was an opportunity for him to be cared for/to give up a sense of responsibility?'

Alexia: 'Maybe that's true ... I'll take my feelings into the staff room and share/explore these.'

Chris interjected: 'And overcome your feelings of needing to protect him as a mother might for her hurt child ... Remember it is his life. You said you didn't pity him, but consider the difference between compassion and pity.'

Alexia could see that she had absorbed Tom's feelings and felt protective towards him and suffered because of this. Yet this was not to deny her genuine sense of compassion. She struggled to distinguish pity from compassion (Levine 1986). Alexia felt her vulnerability in the face of this man's suffering and suffered herself. Her concern for him was powerful, illuminating the way her concern made her available to him. Perhaps she struggled to manage herself within this intimate bond they had forged, reminding us of her earlier experiences. She wondered if she should feel so attached – and I left her to consider the nature of her relationships with patients.

Reflection

The session was very intimate, reflecting the intimacy between Alexia and Tom and highlighting guided reflection as a healing space. Whilst I had a great compassion for Alexia, I did not absorb her suffering. It lay in the space between us, just as she needed to learn not to absorb her patient's suffering. Alexia is a very experienced nurse and yet she struggled with this aspect of her work. Simply because it was new work for her. She had never allowed herself to get this close to patients before. Stepping over her own personal boundaries she had no markers to know the land and that gave her no ready ways for managing the strong emotions she felt. Yet she was exhilarated by this new found intimacy. She had unwrapped and connected to her caring self. Using transactional analysis (Stewart & Joines 1987) I helped her to redraw and explore her boundaries with patients.

Unloading emotional baggage

In session six Alexia talked about her miscarriage, relating it to a staff nurse she worked with on her last ward. Alexia reflected that she had not been caring enough when this nurse had had a miscarriage.

Alexia said: 'She annoyed me because she didn't want the child as she had two children.'

Chris' commentary   Alexia said she now felt guilty about her response. The staff nurse had needed six months off work for counselling. Alexia felt she had eked it out, gaining sympathy from every quarter.

Alexia said: 'But I should have been caring and I wasn't. People have been so caring towards her – fantastic midwives and I wasn't that fantastic to that staff nurse. I have spent a couple of days dwelling on it. I won't do anything about it now but at least I have worked through some of it.'

Chris' commentary   I again noted Marris's theory of loss (1986) that Alexia was connecting her present with the past, and trying to heal a broken thread so she could move on. We linked this experience to the way she was now endeavouring to establish the therapeutic team on the ward, a team that was mutually available to each other in ways that mirrored the caring approach to patients and families. In doing so Alexia had to come to terms with this dark shadow that haunted her. It was teaching her an important lesson; that in order to be available to the other we need to know and manage our own concerns. Alexia immediately felt 'softer' towards the staff nurse she had talked about in session 4, and reflected again on whether she knew this nurse well enough and whether her irritation blocked the view.

I noted my ideas about tuning into the other's wave-length and then managing the resistance between you and the other as necessary to be available to the other person. The other will acknowledge 'this nurse is on my wave-length', and feel understood and cared for. The wave-length may be faulty but can then be worked on so it vibrates at a healthier frequency.

Alexia noted: 'Too often we set the wave-length and expect others to tune into us. I can see that with patients and families. Sometimes we get close but at other times we are miles apart. They must sense that and feel uncared for as we impose our expectations without even acknowledging their own.'

Reflection

Alexia had been carrying her guilt about the staff nurse for some time. The session was like a confessional, enabling Alexia to unload this emotional baggage yet in ways that enabled her to understand why she had responded in the way she did, relating the experience to staff she currently worked with who resisted her in some way. I could see that Alexia's concern made her vulnerable to intolerance in others. Alexia could now see this in herself.

Working the system

In session seven Alexia had come prepared.

Alexia: 'I have two experiences to share – one frustrating and one "good". I'll start with the frustrating experience as it's been going on for some time about my role. I have been in post for one year this week in my dual role as ward manager and head and neck practitioner for the hospital and community. When the post was set up I was supposed to spend two days on ward and three days in the practitioner role. However I can't get away from the ward. I have fedback to my managers that I need an F grade nurse to support me. I have three E grades and one of them is taking a lead role. She should be paid for the role if she does it. She feels that way too. She said "I could get an F grade somewhere else", but she loves the ward, the work. I'm frustrated for her and she's feeling frustrated. When I broached the issue with my managers, they said they would look into it. My immediate manager agreed with me but the nurse executive doesn't believe I need an F Grade.'

Chris' commentary   I suggested that Alexia explored the nature of the role split.

> *Alexia responded:* 'The reason why I'm a few minutes late was because of a visit to a tracheostomy patient on another ward. I am getting a lot of consultant referrals to see patients but I'm finding I'm doing these in my own time, often in the afternoon when I'm tired.'
> *Chris clarified:* 'There seem to be two issues: managing your time and making a case for an F grade. Consider managing time – can you do an analysis of the use of your time within a vision for the practitioner role. Do you have a vision?'
> *Alexia:* 'No, but it's time I did, especially as the head and neck unit is becoming a regional centre.'
> *Chris:* 'Okay, first task. Second task, if I may give advice, is to plan the off-duty to accommodate your practitioner role and make the case for an F grade. Do you have budgetary control to allow for an F grade?'
> *Alexia threw her arms in the air, clearly exasperated:* 'They say you have the budget and then when you want to spend money differently they say you can't!'
> *Chris:* 'So real issues about who controls the budget.'

Chris' commentary   I suggested we explore her ability to effectively assert her position by working through the framework for assertive action (Johns 2000). In this framework, the practitioner's ability to be assertive hinges on a number of dimensions:

- A sense of the powerful self
- Having a focused vision of practice (claiming the moral high ground)
- Understanding the boundaries of authority and role responsibility
- Being able to make a good argument (the knowledgeable self)
- Being adept at interaction skills, most notably confrontation, catharsis and being catalytic
- Being adept at counter-coercive tactics against more powerful others
- Being able to monitor and manage emerging conflict ('pricking the bubble')
- Being able to resist becoming defensive ('staying in adult mode')
- Being able to 'tread the fine line' of confronting more powerful others without becoming marginalised
- Being able to create the conditions to maximise the effectiveness of being assertive.

I asked Alexia to stand and indicate how powerful she felt by the height from the floor she placed her hand on her body. She put her hand on her chest. I suggested that assertive people would place their hands at the level of the top of their head. Alexia agreed 'some room to grow'. I then asked her to visualise filling the room with her presence and suggested she did that at her next meeting with her manager.

Alexia clarified her 'good argument'. We then used French and Raven's sources of leadership power (French & Raven 1968, cited in Johns 2000, p. 172) to reveal the way management generally relied on authoritative sources of power, notable positional power and fear of sanction, reinforced on a daily basis through normal ways of relating. Such use of power was essentially parental to ensure subordinates were both docile and competent. (I noted the influence of Foucault (1979) in constructing this perspective.) From this perspective subordinates were viewed as essentially irresponsible and taught to know their place; 'seen but not heard'. In other words they didn't have a voice.

Alexia: 'Linking back to my feelings of anger at the staff nurse, I can see that I wanted to smack her for not being a good girl. That's really scary! I can see the significance of relational power in enabling staff to become responsible.'
Chris: 'Can you understand the need to be counter-coercive against such power gradients and how to best do this?'
Alexia: 'Easier said than done when normal ways of relating were based on authoritative sources, as if we are socialised to regulate ourselves and be "good" boys and girls.'
Chris: 'So – your task is to make the good argument, to play "the rational game", or, in other words, to speak "their" language in ways they cannot resist or easily shrug aside.'
Alexia noted: 'My manager is leaving which makes it difficult to press the issue with her. However, the doctors do value me highly and we could bring the doctors on board with their political "clout" even though it reflects how "small" the nursing voice is within the corridors of power. I could threaten to resign?'
Chris: 'Yes, a power-coercive tactic to call their bluff. We need to learn counter-coercive tactics as we have to assert against a power gradient. Another tactic is to take the moral high ground and outline the detrimental impact of their decisions on patient care and staff morale.'
Alexia: 'I feel like a conspirator against the empire. I feel much better about it. I no longer have a problem! I can see what I need to do. I'm back on the rails.'
Chris: 'That reminds me of a Bob Dylan album – *Blood on the Tracks* – the way conflict often ends in blood on the floor, especially when the peasants rise up in revolt. These sorts of issues wear us down, sap our energy, deplete our ability to care, erode our motivation. Yet we have to become political and fight for the resources we need. This type of experience is significant in reflecting on your leadership role, and contemplating how you can shift the conditions of practice to support caring practice.'

Chris' commentary   We then rehearsed the argument and how Alexia could assert it successfully, paying attention to the other criteria for assertive action.

Realising self as caring

Alexia continued: 'The good experience concerns Tim, a 39 year old man who has a tumour of his tongue. A 40 a day smoker, social drinker, barrister. He had a lump on his tongue for two months and he didn't do anything about it. He hadn't been to the dentist for ten years. A friend took him there and the dentist referred him to a consultant. He missed two appointments so eventually the dentist brought him here himself! In surgery they removed most of his tongue ... just a sliver left, reconstructed from muscle. After the surgery he was transferred to another hospital because of shortage of ITU beds. I was very disappointed because he did not get specialised head and neck care. I eventually got him transferred back when a bed became available. He was an absolute quivering wreck ... such a proud and intelligent man. For one reason and another I didn't meet him for one week after he got back. The girls said they had found him hard work. Then last weekend – I "took him" on a Saturday late shift – looked after him all day and started the "rap" ...

He was used to commanding but now felt out of control. He had never been in hospital before. I felt for him, the control issue – tuning into him. He couldn't speak ... he had to write everything down including his feelings. We spent four hours chatting and broke down the barriers, he bared his soul. He didn't want to die ... his children. His family came in – his wife was "stand-offish". She went at the end of the day and we could pick up our conversation. His biggest fear was not being able to talk again in court and as an after-dinner speaker. I was truthful – I never lied to him – I said to him that he would talk again although not with the voice he had before.'

Chris: 'What has he been told by the surgeons?'

Alexia: 'They told him he had up to five years. The cancer had invaded neck lymph glands. He will have radiotherapy after the surgical recovery. Next day, Sunday, I blocked off the tracheostomy and asked him to say hello – he said "hello" and burst into tears. He asked me to do it again when his wife came in. I did – he said to her "I love you". I was on cloud nine, "making a difference". It's a wonderful relationship.'

Chris basked in this intimacy and asked: 'And the moral?'

Alexia smiled: 'Enabling him to take control and reading the pattern and mutuality of relationship – he asked about me/cared about me.'

Chris: 'You said the staff found him hard work?'

Alexia: 'Yes, I will debrief with them and use my work with him to teach staff. The time is right to move to the Burford model (Fig. 7.1). I find myself using all the cues with him. They made sense!'

Chris: 'Tell me about his sons.'

Alexia: 'Tim's two youngest sons visit at the weekends, although they live a considerable distance away. His wife visits every day but always leaves after lunch to be home in time to collect the boys from school. The two youngest boys are very loving towards Tim and obviously both miss him and accept their father's new body image. They run down the ward with excitement and in anticipation of seeing their dad. The youngest boy sits on Tim's lap while the other sits on the bed beside him and they recount their tales of school and play time. Tim looks forward to their visits. The eldest son has only visited once. He seemed reluctant and afraid of seeing his father. His body language was close and his facial expressions

---

The 'Burford NDU model; caring in practice' was developed at Burford Community Hospital in 1989 grounded in reflective and holistic beliefs. Within the model a set of nine reflective cues were constructed to tune the practitioner into caring beliefs within each unfolding moment; Who is this person? What meaning does this illness/health event have for the person? How is this person feeling? How has this event affected their usual life patterns and roles? How do I feel about this person? How can I help this person? What is important for this person to make their stay in hospital comfortable? What support does this person have in life? How does this person view the future for themselves and others? (Johns 1994, 2000)

Fig. 7.1 The Burford model.

suggested that he felt very uncomfortable on the ward. Instead of greeting Tim and sitting close together as the rest of the family did, he hovered around the bed area refusing to sit down, hands in pockets, taking more interest in the television than his dad.

After the family left I asked Tim about his eldest son. He told me his behaviour was nothing unusual. He had kicked against school and family, and did not seem to grasp why his father was ill. Apparently he had expressed that he was embarrassed by Tim and had to be cajoled by his mother to visit. I suggested that maybe he couldn't cope with his father being ill and this was his way of dealing with it? Tim agreed that this might be a possibility. He hadn't thought of the situation that way. Tim's wife and two youngest sons remained in constant contact throughout his stay. The sons spoke daily with Tim on the phone but the eldest son was either out or refused to come to the phone.'

Chris: 'Your work with this man is profound. We can look back over the experiences you have shared and see this thread of holistic practice. Now you are beginning to shift the conditions of practice to accommodate and facilitate holistic practice through the ward.'

Still working the system

In session eight Alexia reflected back on the experience she shared in session five about Tom.

Alexia: 'Tom may be coming back in. He had an infection. I'm going to see him in out-patients this afternoon.'
Chris: 'Is it hard to think about him coming back in?'
Alexia: 'I have a fight with myself. I'm pleased to see him again and I don't like them to come back in. He sees us as his family now … like we are his daughters. His daughter Clare phoned us this morning. She said: "Dad isn't very good, another infection … he's really down just like when Mum died. What shall I do?" I felt awful because I lied to the bed manager in order to save him a bed even though he might not come in. If I had been truthful they would not understand.'
Chris: 'Is this an indictment of the system?'
Alexia: 'It is … on his last admission we didn't have a bed and he went to another ward for three days before we could get him transferred back to us. He was distraught.'
Chris: 'And what did that do to his health! But can you morally justify your action to manipulate the system to ensure the bed?'

Chris' commentary   We explored the bed manager's perspective – the bed is an object/the patient is an object. They do not see the person. Alexia's viewing lens is to see the person of the patient in all their humanness and suffering. The conflict of values was stark to the extent that Alexia had to adjust the system to cater for the human, or as I put it: 'Your moral justification to ensure your patient needs are met'. I reiterated this in challenging Alexia's prevailing sense of feeling awful: 'Where did this sense of awful come from? Was it fear of sanction for not playing the game?'

Alexia didn't feel it was this. Perhaps it was just because she felt she had lied and was feeling guilty as if a naughty child afraid of being caught. She feared sanction and so, could only respond to the patient's needs by being covert.

Chris' challenge: 'Why be covert? Why not simply be upfront and say no?'
Alexia: 'Why indeed! I don't think I'm ready to have my head shot off.'

Chris: 'You highlight the counter-coercive tactics necessary to act ethically and meet patient need without being viewed as unco-operative and the risk of being sanctioned and marginalised. The down-side is that the organisation can't learn through this situation because it is covert.'

Chris' commentary   Alexia continued by talking about the change in Tom's illness trajectory from night club owner and that lifestyle – the way the images had been stripped from himself – flash lifestyle to a person searching for meaning and finding meaning in a new set of values about the beauty of life and people met along the journey ... and for his daughters and personal assistant – from shiny clothes and immaculate hair to track-suits and roots showing through. I inquired whether Tom feared death?

Alexia: 'I don't think so ... he wants to live for his daughters and yet he looked forward to joining his wife.'

Chris' commentary   I felt as if Tom had 'brought himself home' to face and learn through his crisis in order to emerge at an expanded level of consciousness. (The expression 'brought himself home' is taken from the Objiway idea of 'Ain-dah-ing' – 'the home within your heart is where your primary essence waits' (Blackwolf and Gina Jones 1995).)

Reflection

Sharing Alexia's experience with Tom was another intimate moment between us, as we sat in awe of the realisation and power of caring in making such a difference to people's lives in the face of impending death. Yet to set up caring possibility Alexia had needed to confront and battle the system that would diminish the caring possibility. Alexia's experience exemplified that to be available to her patients and families she required to be heard along the corridors of power where decisions are made. It is pointless Alexia despairing that 'they' are uncaring. The reality behind the caring rhetoric of organisations is stark yet it can be successfully challenged.

Alexia became reflective and considered her journey since last May when she had commenced these sessions and the profound impact it had made on her personal as well as professional life; the way her husband said that she was a nicer person, less stressed and more fulfilled. Alexia said it was true but that she would never have imagined the impact of guided reflection in coming to know and transform self. She was more available and could live out her holistic beliefs with certainty.

Dealing positively with conflict

In session nine Alexia reflected on how she had confronted the staff nurse she had talked about in session four.

Alexia: 'The nurse, I had a chat with her. I told her how I felt and that I wasn't going to put up with it anymore. She dissolved into tears but I didn't feel bad about it. It's a step in the right direction. Before, I would have felt bad about it.'

Chris: 'Guilty?'
Alexia: 'Yes … now I don't! I'm proud of myself.'
Chris: 'And the consequences?'
Alexia: 'She knows how the rest of the staff and I feel about her and the ward is not going to put up with her behaviour any more. She knows what she needs to do. I've put it in a positive light and if she can't do that then she knows that I don't want her as a member of my team. *and* I don't feel guilty about that either! I couldn't have done that a few months ago. I feel I have the strength to do that now. I'm on top of the world again now.'
Chris: 'You remind me of a saying on a Renee Locks' brush dance card (Locks undated) – it says "and then the day came when the risk to remain tight in bud was more painful than the risk it took to blossom".'
Alexia smiled knowingly: 'I had been off for six days and when I returned to work I was met by a barrage of complaints about her. I asked myself: "What's going on with this nurse?" I didn't sleep last night because of it … and then I acted today. I feel free!'
Chris: 'The crisis had burst … now it becomes easier to deal with it again.'

Chris' commentary   Alexia felt this was true. She had commenced collecting evidence in a diary of events anticipating further struggle along the road. Alexia felt this staff nurse was an 'Ivy', one of Dickson's (1982) four stereotypes of women. These four stereotypes of women are: Ivy, the indirectly aggressive woman; Agnes, the directly aggressive woman; Dulcie, the door-mat; and Selma, the assertive woman. Ivy is characterised by the way the staff nurse acted indirectly aggressively to set staff against each other and saying things about Alexia which had got back to Alexia – that Alexia was insensitive and lacked compassion.

> *Chris:* 'Reflect on the way you have responded to her – can you be more compassionate to her. Do you know where she's coming from to act in these ways? Are we responding to her behaviour rather than trying to understand it? Draw links with the theory on "difficult" patients?'

Chris' commentary   Alexia confirmed she didn't like her although felt she was a good nurse, which inevitably raised my challenge of what was meant by a 'good nurse'? I challenged Alexia to consider whether she should be available to this nurse, to reach out and touch her in her humanness. Did she have a responsibility to explore the reasons for her behaviour?

> *Alexia:* 'She did say last time that she did have a lot of personal problems.'
> *Chris:* 'She has given you a cue to respond to. Do you need to show her the team does care for each other; even if she rejects your approach at least you can say you tried?'

Chris' commentary   Alexia felt uncertain as if she now faced a new dilemma, having thought she had solved the problem.

> *Alexia:* 'I feel I had an open door for my staff to approach me.'
> *Chris:* 'Saying my door is open is one thing but staff walking through it is another. Perhaps you need to extend a hand?'
> *Alexia:* 'I still feel good about this situation but you have challenged me. I think I will see her again.'

Chris: 'How is the F grade situation?' [from session seven]

Alexia: 'I went back to the consultants. They value me highly as the senior nurse on the unit. Their support is not yet active but will be. I'm gathering information from other head and neck units to support my argument. I'm seeing the acting senior nurse about levels of role responsibility.'

Chris: 'Which is a move towards dialogue and negotiation. So, the idea is not ruled out anymore. You are mobilising support.'

Alexia: 'Yes, to play the power game . . . they will not want to lose me.'

Chris: 'You are learning to play the political game with increasing astuteness!'

Honouring and closing relationships

Alexia then shifted the context of reflection.

Alexia: 'Paul [from session one] has died on the ward. Seven staff have gone to his funeral, reflecting the caring between staff. He was admitted as a medical problem and was going to be admitted to a medical ward. I heard he was in A&E but anticipating his need to be admitted here, I prepared a room for him. We wanted him to be admitted here as well. I knew he was dying but they said they had to sort out his problems. His wife and daughters were very distressed. They contacted me . . . told me he was going to a medical ward – can't he come here? I sorted it out – spoke to the medical SHO. He said Paul had arrythmias and other medical problems that required treatment, pneumothorax that needed chest drainage. He wanted him on the medical ward for 24 hours . . . wanted to do everything. I accepted this and explained to his wife and daughter that he would be transferred to us after 24 hours. The SHO promised that if Paul deteriorated he would not hesitate to get him back to us. I went to see him in A&E – he was clutching my hand saying, "take me to William Hart . . . take me to William Hart". You can imagine how I felt. I handed him over to the ward staff. I returned at the end of shift . . . he had taken a turn for the worse . . . he had none of the planned treatment . . . NFR [not for resuscitation] order . . . just for TLC. Therefore I asserted that they transfer him to us! This led to a full blown argument. I was getting nowhere so I contacted the senior nurse and she supported his move back to William Hart – he was with us within half an hour. He sighed: "I'm home". It was all I needed, a marvellous feeling. The staff were elated and the family were joyous. It was worth fighting for, to the bitter end.'

Chris: 'The way the power of caring smashed the petty politics. You took the moral high ground and caring triumphed. Brilliant!'

Alexia: 'I was not going home until I had won it and the staff knew that.'

Chris: 'Role modelling empowerment and assertiveness. Would they have been able to fight like this if you had not been on-duty?'

Alexia: 'Umm . . . I doubt it.'

Chris: 'Perhaps debriefing with the staff may help to empower them – "If I had not been on-duty?". This situation reminds me of the way you manipulated the bed system in creating the conditions where being available to Paul and Tom becomes possible. That's such a significant caring issue.'

Alexia: 'I did a double shift to support family, him and staff, to ensure he got the care he deserved. I did that for me as much as for him and the family, so I knew I had done my utmost. The staff were distressed that he was dying.'

Chris: 'Did you feel you were getting entangled, absorbing the family's distress?'

Alexia: 'I was conscious of that [giving me a knowing look]. The issue was knowing it and managing it. I did not feel distressed on his behalf. We did get him home for two hours so he could sit in his garden and listen to the birds in the sky. On the morning he died he said to me: "I'm going home today and take a very long walk". I knew what he meant, that he was going to die but I felt contented. He had spoken to each family member and each member of staff and thanked us. He waited for his family to be out of the room before "letting go". I was deeply honoured to be "in the room" and that he could talk openly to me. He really touched me. I'm not grieving for him, I'm happy for him. He said something similar to his wife. She came and said to me – "what's he talking about going home? He can't go home" – as if he was confused and rambling.'

Chris: 'It's easy to misinterpret what dying people are saying. For example, see the work of Callanan and Kelley (1993) – they highlight the way dying people wrap up important messages in an allegorical language. It is an important lesson to listen to what people are really saying, not simply what is said on the surface.'

Alexia: 'At the funeral his family were pleased to have us. I wondered if our presence would remind them of the past few days but the wife seemed to find it easier to be with us than with her family. She sought us out. She said to me: "You loved Paul didn't you? You cared for him every minute as if he was your father". She said: "I always thought of you as part of the family". It made me realise why I am a nurse and what I want to do in the future . . . to be a head and neck Macmillan nurse.'

Chris: 'And Tim . . . what's happened to him?'

Alexia: 'After his discharge Tim came back to visit us on a number of occasions. Unfortunately I was either not on the ward or on days off but the nurses told me how he looked and what he had said. Then, just recently, I was lucky enough to be working when he attended clinic and on hearing I was on the ward he came up. We greeted each other as old friends. I could not believe how great he looked. He had lost around two stones and it suited him. He had also cut off his moustache. I told him he looked years younger which he revelled in! I asked him about his family. He said his eldest son was still being very difficult which he and his wife found emotionally hard. He had given up his job to enjoy family life. As he put it, "we are financially secure and I just decided that my family were my life, not my job". I have to say this came as a shock as all he ever wanted when he was an in-patient was to get back to work. He asked me the latest on the nursing staff and how I was – our reciprocal relationship speaking up again! As he walked down the ward I watched him and felt proud, I felt he had made it and we had helped him. I felt positive that in the future he would set things right with his eldest son. I look forward to the next instalment with him.'

Chris: 'Your story illustrates how people come to seek and find meaning in their lives triggered by the crisis of illness and the spectre of death and the significance of the nursing role. It also gives meaning to the Burford model cue – "what meaning does this health event have for Tim and his family". Your caring dialogue with him was grounded in responding to this cue.'

Alexia: 'I can see that's so significant. We need to set another date.'

Footnote

We didn't set another date as Alexia shortly went on extended sick leave related to her pregnancy. The space between sessions eight and nine had been three months, because of circumstances. Yet it provided a space to look back and draw together the threads of the various experiences extending through the narrative and to celebrate Alexia's sense of achievement in becoming more available to her patients and creating a supportive ward environment.

References

Benner, P. & Wrubel, J. (1989) *The Primacy of Caring*. Addison-Wesley, Menlo Park.

Bolen, J.S. (1996) *Close to the Bone: Life threatening illness and the search for meaning*. Touchstone, New York.

Callanan, M. & Kelley, P. (1993) *Final Gifts*. Bantam Books, New York.

Dickson, A. (1982) *A Woman in Your Own Right*. Quartet Books, London.

Eakes, G., Burke, M. & Hainsworth, M. (1998) Middle-range theory of chronic sorrow. *Image: Journal of Nursing Scholarship*, 30, 179–84.

Foucault, M. (1979) *Discipline and Punish: the birth of the prison* (trans. A. Sheridan). Vintage/Random House, New York.

French, J. & Raven, B. (1968) The bases of social power. In *Group Dynamics Research and Theory*, 3rd edn (eds D. Cartwright & A. Zander). Harper and Row, New York.

Hall, L. (1964) Nursing – what is it? *Canadian Nurse*, 60(2) 150–54.

Johns, C. (1992) Ownership and the harmonious team: barriers to developing the therapeutic nursing team in primary nursing. *Journal of Clinical Nursing*, 1, 89–94.

Johns, C. (ed.) (1994) *The Burford NDU Model: caring in practice*. Blackwell Science, Oxford.

Johns, C. (2000) *Becoming a Reflective Practitioner*. Blackwell Science, Oxford.

Jones, Blackwolf & G. (1995) *Listen to the Drum*. Commune-a-key Publishing, Salt Lake City.

Levine, S. (1986) *Who dies? An investigation of conscious living and conscious dying*. Gateway Books, Bath.

Locks, R. (undated) Brush Dance card #2089. Brush Dance, 100 Ebbtide Avenue, Bldg. #1, Sausalito, CA 94965.

Marris, P. (1986) *Loss and Change*. Routledge & Kegan Paul, London.

Rinpoche, S. (1992) *The Tibetan Book of Living and Dying*. Rider, London.

Stewart, I. & Joines, V. (1987) *TA Today; A new introduction to Transactional Analysis*. Lifespace Publishing, Nottingham and Chapel Hill.

Chapter 8

Finding a New Way in Health Visiting

Yvonne Latchford

'An alternative perspective, posed by Prawat (1993), is to view impasses or dissonance in experience not as obstacles to be eradicated, but as possibilities for creation.'

(Fenwick & Parsons, 1999, p. 60)

My journey began on ENB A29 with the experiences I reflected on about my work with two families with child protection concerns. I became increasingly aware of contradiction and conflict within my role, which became the driving force behind my determination to find a better way for health visiting in child protection work at a time of turbulence within health visiting.

The Government consultation document *Supporting Families* (DoH 1998a) launched in November 1998, urges health visitors to rise to the challenges of developing a modern approach and a 'high quality early investment', shifting the focus of health visiting from dealing with failure towards prevention. This involves questioning traditional roles and working styles in order to find new ways of working that involve 'new partnerships and inter-agency and multi-disciplinary working to deliver high quality and effective services to address the challenges of inequalities, parenting and family policy'. This renewed Government commitment to expansion of family support services is an extension of the underpinning philosophy of the Children Act 1989 that placed a new emphasis on family support and formalised the notion of working in partnership with parents. These Government initiatives have placed early family support interventions firmly at the heart of the challenge for health visitors to find a new way.

Historically this has not been the first major Government challenge to change health visiting practice. Welshman (1997) suggested that health visiting remains 'a prisoner of its history' due to its inability to extend its scope of practice. Welshman charted the course of resistance by health visitors to expand their role, that eventually resulted in expansion of social services provision to the detriment of health visiting during the 1950s and 1960s. Despite increased opportunity due to 'wider economic, social and medical changes' and, despite Government encouragement to expand the 'traditional field of work with mothers and infants', health visitors on the whole did not expand their work into the newer arenas of preventative work. If resistance to change has become woven into the fabric of health visiting history, then it is essential that positive, enlightened responses to new challenges are developed to ensure the future survival of the profession. Health visitors must choose to proactively meet these challenges or passively accept that nothing can be done.

Reactions to the new Government proposals provide some early indication of the current professional mood. Initial response to the *Supporting Families* consultation document supports the need for an expanded role of health visitors whilst recommending that there needs to be a substantial increase in the number of health visitors in order to achieve this goal. Welshman (1977) also outlines Government recognition that in order to expand its role, health visiting needs a fundamental change. The article entitled '*Family policy doomed without increase in health visitors*' (Anon 1999a) chooses however to de-emphasise change, and focuses instead on the need to increase health visitor numbers. Although such increase may be relevant, it could nurture a passive response in health visitors. Accepting that nothing can be done without more health visitors will deter an alternative positive debate on change and action.

Although disguised, the more disturbing suggestion is that health visitors who do not change will fail to become involved in new policies. As these policies are going to determine the nature of future provision of family support in the community, a passive stance may affect the way the Government considers the future role of the health visitor. In the light of the wider acceptance that work with young families remains a priority and still dominates the workload, how can health visitors afford to sit back and ignore these new initiatives in primary care? We know through past experience that if health visitors do not rise to the challenge of change then others will. These are important issues for the future of our profession.

There are strong influences within health visiting that traditionally nurture a sense of passivity, so it becomes even more crucial to find a way to create the conditions of empowerment within the ranks. There is a need to find a way to challenge resistance that will potentially 'act as a counterweight to the desire for change and will induce people to accommodate themselves to the discontent they are suffering' (Fay 1987, p. 29). Within this research I have taken up the challenge to find a new way. I will illuminate the way I have become empowered to change my everyday practice and question and actively participate in changing an entire working culture through the medium of guided reflection, through my ongoing relationship with Helen and her family.

Helen

Helen is separated from her profoundly handicapped husband and lives with her two children, Natasha aged four years, and Robert aged six years. Helen suffers from manic depression that is presently controlled by lithium. Helen is a devoted and loving mother and when she is not ill she copes with the children very well. Acute bouts of illness have occurred twice in the two years I have known her. The first time was just before I met her. At this time the children had been placed on the child protection register and Helen had been taken into hospital. Soon after her recovery the children were taken off the register and were returned home to their mother.

My early experiences of guided reflection were set against a background of Helen's mistrust and anger stemming from her sense of not being heard, a metaphor for her powerlessness. Belenky *et al.* (1986) suggest that women's sense of voice can be used as a metaphor for their experience and that the 'development of voice, mind and self are intricately intertwined' (p. 18). At this stage, Helen's sense of self and inner voice was struggling to emerge and was being denied. I found it necessary to find a way to peel back these layers of anger in order to connect with her and to build a relationship with her. Her anger at this time was preventing any significant access to the family by social services or health visitors. Helen viewed any access as an intrusion and was immediately resented. At this time she was taking steps to sue her previous health visitor and social worker. Her anger was due to her feelings that she had been misrepresented, misquoted and misunderstood during the child protection process. My early aims with her were to find a way of regaining trust and building a caring relationship that could empower her to move forward in her life.

Guided reflection provided me with a safe clearing so I could see around me. I realised that I had been frightened of Helen and I wondered why this should be so. I began to question the way she had been labelled, noting in my journal that 'it would have been difficult for anyone to see the real Helen under such a dense fog of negative labels'. This inner questioning represented my first determined steps towards coming to know my true self in context of my work with clients. I pondered over her words – 'I don't mind you, it's health visitors I don't care for'. I asked myself why this should be, and in doing so began to scrutinise the role of the health visitor in child protection work. I gradually became aware of feelings of tension and contradiction between my sense of self and my sense of role.

One example of an issue I explored at this time was the increasing emphasis on risk assessment and assessment of vulnerability, including the use of clinical guidelines and check lists in health visiting child protection work. Although this was accepted practice, I saw that according to research, this was at odds with more tacit, intuitive ways of knowing, to which health visitors would rather pay attention. I also looked at the ways that child protection work encourages health visitors to act in covert ways (Dingwall 1982; Taylor & Tilley 1989), and how this was at odds with the need for health visitors to develop 'open and honest ' relationships (DoH 1995). Through guided reflection I had begun to expose contradictory ways of working within my practice. It was a time of sudden clarity, a time of enlightenment 'marked by the emergence of a disposition which is intent on subjecting social arrangements to rational inspection, and which is bent on breaking with the done thing when examination shows it to be unwarranted' (Fay 1987). It became clearer that I needed to break with the old order to find a better way for health visiting in child protection work, a way that enabled me to realise personal and professional beliefs and values in actual practice.

Research process

'It has been said that it is possible only on the page, in stories, that we can be so tender to one another, so free, so humane, so brave and so pure' (Okri 1997, p. 43). For all these reasons, in my early days as a reflective practitioner it was a profound experience to be able to give expression to my personal feelings and perceptions within the pages of my journal. With the benefit of guided reflection however, the true significance of Okri's words in terms of my health visiting practice soon became much clearer to me. I became aware of the limitations of self guided reflection as I gradually realised that becoming 'true' and 'free' were not as straightforward as I had first perceived.

I did not journey alone. I had a guide. Sharing my stories with Chris I found that my practice began to change in ways more congruent with my ideals of desirable practice. In choosing to record and share certain experiences I opened myself to the possibility of gaining new insights and understanding, opening the possibility to show 'the lived quality and significance of the experience in a fuller and deeper manner' (Van Manen 1990, p. 10). Engaging in a free and open dialogue with Chris enabled me to peel back the layers of interpretation even further as he introduced his own perspectives and understandings. Through discussion and drawing on literature I came to understand why things were as they were and what they might become. Together we are able to co-construct new meanings and new possibilities, the 'dialectical play which Gadamer calls the fusion of horizons' (cited in Weinsheimer 1985, p. 210).

My motivation became focused and I became increasingly empowered and knowing to act on new insights. I became liberated. Within education the conditions of liberation can only be achieved when the educator's efforts 'coincide with those of the student to engage in critical thinking and the quest for mutual humanisation' (Freire 1972, p. 49). Freire believed that the relationship must be primarily one of partnership based upon a profound sense of trust in the student's ability to act as a conscious and creative being. As such my journey became our journey. We contracted to meet for one hour every month. In total we met seven times between August 1998 and April 1999. Between these sessions I used a journal to reflect on my visits to Helen which became the basis for our dialogue within guided reflection. I took notes of our dialogue which I wrote up immediately after each session to capture the essence of what took place, and these are used to unfold my journey.

Introducing Helen

In our first session I talked about Helen:

> *Yvonne:* 'I visited Helen at home. She was warm and friendly and readily talked about how she was coping. I asked whether she had heard anything from social services regarding obtaining access to her conference notes. She said she hadn't and became angry. She talked about going to see her solicitor again. I remember thinking how sad it was that we were still having the same conversation after all this time.'
> *Chris:* 'It reminds me of Butterfield's paper (1990), 'Thinking upstream', as if Helen keeps falling into a stream and you keep pulling her out. The problems that cause her to fall in are upstream and not being adequately dealt with.'
> *Yvonne:* 'Yes, although Helen knew I shared her frustration it was not enough. I tried to talk to her but she became even angrier. I wasn't afraid although I felt concerned for Natasha who was playing nearby. She said "Mummy is angry with you" and I said "Yes, mummy is very angry, but I don't think she's angry at me". She then went to play upstairs. She had said "You always make me feel so angry" and asked me not to visit any more. Then she lifted a large plastic box over her head and slammed it down on the floor next to me. I didn't feel frightened but was unsure what to do next. The force had split the box in half. I remember wondering if this was taking catharsis too far. Then it happened. She began to talk to me

between copious fears. She talked to me about feelings of despair and hopelessness. I asked her how she now felt. She said that she had only ever broken out like that once before in her life and then apologised, asking me how I felt. I said I was glad she had been able to release some of her anger but that perhaps it was a bit too threatening for me. I said it was also a shame about the box. She smiled at this comment and seemed much calmer.'

Chris: 'I'm sure we could find literature on the therapeutic value of humour.'

Yvonne's commentary   We discussed the value of catharsis as a therapeutic intervention. Chris pointed out that an intervention could only truly be cathartic if it was followed through to the end, as had happened during my visit. He then challenged me to consider whether or not I had been in danger or had placed myself at risk. Although I had not felt frightened, I felt there had been an element of risk due to the intensity of Helen's anger. Chris encouraged me to reflect on this anger.

> *Yvonne:* 'All it would take is a letter from social services or some demonstration of concern to neutralise this anger. Instead they choose to ignore her and this compounds her feelings of helplessness. It's not access to the notes she really needs, its recognition. She said she would write another letter to them and I said I would write to support her if she felt that would help.'
>
> *Chris:* 'It may be that Helen can't have access to her notes, in which case all you can do is clarify that. It would be better to have this in writing so Helen can see that action has been taken. This raises another issue though – why can't she have access to the notes? What is there to hide?'
>
> *Yvonne:* 'It seems that social services are just paying lip service to their espoused philosophy of empowerment. If they wish to be empowering, why not allow her to see the notes . . . what harm would it do? She would be able to have her say, and respond to their comments and move on. They have not even replied to my letter. It seems nobody is listening to either of us.'
>
> *Chris:* 'The challenge to be listened to or in Belenky *et al.*'s terms (1986) to develop a more powerful voice?'
>
> *Yvonne:* 'I felt the pattern of our mutual powerlessness. I felt the powerful and controlling influences of social services on us. I wondered why I have never before considered my relationship with social services in terms of power?'
>
> *Chris:* 'Summarise what's been significant in this session.'
>
> *Yvonne:* 'I understand Helen's anger and feel we are more connected. It would be useful to reflect on the lack of response by social services and the nature of relationships between health visitors and social services.'

Interpretation

I had reached a turning point with Helen. Within the safe space of guided reflection her smashed box had emerged as a metaphor for my inner cathartic feelings of release. It jolted something deep within me as I became aware of a deep frustration and anger that after all this time the causes of Helen's anger had not been resolved. As I look back over my relationship with Chris, I can see the way we have endeavoured to peel back the layer of Helen's and my own anger so I could better know and connect with Helen, to become more available to her. It was only when I had begun to look at myself and to question my beliefs and values that Helen had started to trust me. Although she still had nothing good to say about health visitors or social workers, her trust gave me access to the family. Now this trust was threatened by her renewed anger.

Becoming aware of my silence was revealing. Belenky *et al.* (1986) link women's silence with oppression, ways in which silent women 'see blind obedience to authorities as being of utmost importance for keeping out of trouble and ensuring their on survival' (p. 28). Keeping out of trouble and surviving may have become a way of being for myself, and health visitors in general. I need to unmask this spectre of oppression. It's not just Helen who is struggling to emerge and find an authentic voice. In becoming empowered I can better enable Helen to become empowered.

There is a prevailing lack of understanding about the health visitor role and much seems to depend on individual perspective. One study that set out to consider consumer perspective uncovered a lack of knowledge about their health visitor's role (Collinson & Cowley 1998). In this study, health visitors had failed to explain their role and this had created a mismatch of client and health visitor perceptions resulting in a failure to fulfil client expectations. This in turn had generated negativity towards the health visitors. It seems that health visitors themselves are uncertain of their role and therefore experience difficulty in explaining it to others. This uncertainty may be exacerbated due to the increasing pressure for health visitors to make their role explicit within service contracts for purchasers. Health visitors for example are resorting to the use of clinical guidelines despite evidence to suggest that these tend to be unsupported by research, lead to an increased use of scoring indices based on invalidated material and potentially constrain and erode professional judgement (Appleton & Cowley 1997). In this way, health visitors are denying and disguising the true nature of their work and are therefore contributing to the prevailing lack of understanding of the health visitor role.

This is bound to affect the way that health visiting is valued in the community. In terms of understanding power relationships, it is feasible that within this prevailing climate of vulnerability and uncertainty, health visitors may feel less able to assert themselves. These conditions are far more likely to reinforce the feelings of passivity, reactivity and dependency that bear all the hallmarks of oppression (Belenky *et al.* 1986). Freire (1972) suggested that self-perception is impaired by 'submersion in the reality of oppression' (p. 22). Freire maintains that at this level, the oppressed are more likely to attempt to identify with the oppressor than to recognise or to struggle against contradiction. Perhaps within this climate of vulnerability, health visitors have internalised a feeling of subordination in their relationship with social workers whose powerful, statutory role in child protection work has steadily grown as health visitor numbers have steadily fallen. Perhaps we have found it necessary to align ourselves more with social services in order to survive.

Shifting attitudes towards Helen

In our next session:

> *Yvonne:* 'I spoke with Jo, a social worker. She was interested in the way I was working with Helen. She agreed that Helen should either be given access to her notes or at least a response. It was such a relief to speak with someone on my wavelength. I said I couldn't understand

why social services were blocking Helen's attempts to see her reports if they were genuinely concerned with empowering clients. Jo agreed and said she wanted to pursue this issue with her manager in her own supervision. At last someone is listening! Some colleagues asked me about my research with you. I said it was concerned with finding a new way for health visitors in child protection work. This provoked curiosity. They asked me what I thought was wrong with the way things are now? I explained that over the past 18 months guided reflection had helped me to see and examine things I had never questioned before. I gave examples of the ways I had changed my perspectives and in turn my practice, notably shifting from covert ways with which I felt health visitors worked when dealing with families in child protection. Initially they all disputed this. I stood my ground noting that this had become clear to me after I had been guided to expose contradictions between my beliefs and the way I had practised.'

Chris: 'What was significant about these two interactions?'

Yvonne: 'I was amazed at the strength I drew from giving examples of my personal experiences from guided reflection. When I said I had questioned my beliefs, something in the atmosphere changed. Both Jo and my health visitor colleagues warmed towards me. I think my words were effective because they were honest. They paid attention to me because the purity of striving to realise beliefs was irresistible to them as caring practitioners.'

Chris: 'You took the moral high ground?'

Yvonne: 'Yes, I realised that my experience of guided reflection had somehow set me apart from various colleagues. I felt so powerful. I was powerful!'

Interpretation

Sharing my feelings about these two conversations enabled me to set my increasing awareness of power and powerlessness into the context of the awareness of others. It soon became clear that my awareness was at odds with that of my health visitor and social work colleagues as I had found a way of turning my beliefs and values about practice into a reality which did not seem to be their experience. I realised that this had given me a feeling of control over my practice that had altered my self-perception. I had been able to assert myself in convincing ways and had felt powerful within these interactions. Kieffer (1984), in his study of the emergence of citizen leader empowerment, described four distinct and progressive phases of skills and insights leading to attainment of a 'real and self-perceived sense of participatory competence' (p. 12) (Fig. 8.1). At the first phase or 'era of entry', Kieffer believes that empowerment is provoked through a sense of 'outrage' or 'violation of the sense of integrity' and is a time when 'individuals are first discovering their political muscles and potential for external impact' (p. 19). This was my era of entry. It was my emergence from my sense of anger, frustration and helplessness. This session marked my transition from a sense of moral outrage (Pike 1991) intensified by the constraints that were blocking my attempts to empower Helen into a sense of freedom to act in congruent ways. Guided reflection had not only enabled me to become aware of my inner struggle but was now fuelling it in order to sustain my emergence.

Flowing with Helen's resistance

In session three I shared the following:

Phase	Development
Era of entry (Birth of struggle against conflict)	Birth of emergence of participatory competence. Integrity violated, provoking and mobilising sense of frustration and powerlessness towards an empowering response.
Era of advancement (Continuing struggle)	Maturation of empowerment through extension of involvement and deepening understanding through intensive self-reflection with the help of an external enabler.
Era of incorporation (Continuing struggle)	Reconstructs sense of self as author and actor in environment. Learning to confront and contend with barriers to self-determination leads to a sense of mastery and competence in the individual's sense of being.
Era of commitment (Continuing struggle)	Adulthood of participatory competence – integrates new abilities and insight into reality in meaningful ways.

Fig. 8.1 Attainment of participatory competence through four phases of involvement (Kieffer 1984).

Yvonne: 'Helen cancelled our appointment to meet at the nursery. She angrily said to my colleague that she didn't see the point of meeting. I felt so despondent. I called it 'the black hole', in my journal. I can't see how I can move forward. She blames health visitors and social workers for her anger. She tars us all with the same brush. On reflection, I know I am being negative but can rationalise her reaction. Her anger has always been bubbling away and this is just another eruption. It's a catch 22 situation though. I can't easily arrange to see her when she's so angry, but I need to see her to help her move through her anger. Her anger is preventing me from gaining access to the children. How can we protect children if we don't have access?'

Chris: 'At the centre of this is her inability to have access to her notes. Perhaps we could use ethical mapping (Johns 1999) to clarify your situation about what would be the "right thing" to do and reconsider your position within this dilemma?' (see Fig. 8.2).

Yvonne's commentary   Considering how I had reacted in the past, I realised that it would have been so easy for me to withdraw and to feel powerless to act in this situation. Instead I decided to telephone Helen and suggest that we go to social services together.

Interpretation

Applying the ethical grid enabled me to clarify and understand my position but also realise that understanding in itself was not enough. I could feel the contradictions and imagine ways that I could confront these people whom I perceived to be more

Patient's/family's perspective	Authority to act?	Doctor's perspective
Helen believed she has a right to be heard and wants to be given the opportunity to respond to the accusations on the document	I can't show Helen the notes but I can support her attempts to gain access to them	I think the GPs would support me in this; perhaps I should ask them
Is there conflict of values?	**The situation/dilemma**	**Ethical principles**
Both Jo and I seem to share the same beliefs and values about empowerment of clients	Helen's inability to gain access to the reports and to seek redress	Social workers said Helen would be more upset if she read the report. I feel it is her right to decide whether or not she will be upset
Nurses' perspective	**Power relationships?**	**Organisation's perspective**
My colleagues agree I should support Helen. They feel I should not visit her on my own while she is so angry	I wonder to what extent social service management influences my actions as a health visitor in child protection work	My line manager has already let Helen see some paragraphs of the report but she was not allowed to take a copy home so she still could not respond. Access has to be permitted by social services

Fig. 8.2 Ethical mapping.

powerful than me. Using the grid helped me to sustain and build on my sense of inner struggle against conflict, so essential to sustain my emergence at Kieffer's level of advancement and incorporation (see Fig. 8.1). This now embodied sense of awareness was enough to propel me out of a 'black hole of passivity towards determined action'. As Fay (1987) said, 'it is only when acting on the basis of considered reflection, when one's actions express one's rational judgements as to what is best, that one can be said to be truly free' (p. 76).

Without guided reflection I wondered if I would even have attempted to find a way to maintain any form of intensive, preventative intervention. Still, it would have been professionally acceptable at this point to revert to the recommended core surveillance programme that currently frames health visitor intervention (Hall 1996) and tends to represent the minimum level of health visitor intervention with pre-school children. Yet Helen's children were not on the child protection register and there were currently no concerns about the children's well-being. As Hall pointed out, child surveillance is only part of the recommended child health promotion programme and is secondary prevention. Hall envisaged 'more emphasis on primary prevention' (p. 223).

If I had withdrawn, my ability to continue working with this family in a primary preventative way would have been compromised. In some ways the core programme has made it easier for health visitors to withdraw from primary prevention. I could, for example, have left a calling card suggesting that she come to my clinic. I may have chosen to view this as empowering in that it enabled Helen to make up her own mind about whether she needs to see the health visitor. In terms of primary prevention however, how can I expect Helen to anticipate her health needs without any help? Isn't anticipatory guidance my role as a health visitor? The first principle of health visiting is the search for health needs and this 'is based on the outreach nature of health visiting when unacknowledged needs may be identified' (Orr 1990).

The new public health white paper, *Supporting Families*, together with the Acheson Report, *Inequalities in Health* (DoH 1998b), have placed primary prevention at the heart of Government policy. The clear expectation is that health visitors will move away from a problem-solving approach and move towards intensive, effective primary care support (Turner 1998/9). Health visitor support has now not only been recognised as an effective primary care intervention, it is now being actively encouraged within health policy. There is however, mounting evidence to suggest that health visiting may not rise to these new challenges. In terms of being able to move forward in my work with Helen, this requires further investigation.

In her spirited keynote speech to the Health Visitors Association (HVA) annual professional conference in 1988, the HVA General Secretary, Shirley Goodwin made an impassioned plea for a 'virtual revolution in some of the basic tenets of health visiting' and for health visitors to create the climate for radical change necessary for health visiting to become relevant to the needs of the people (Goodwin 1988). This plea was in anticipation of the recommendations of the pending report of the third joint working party, commonly known as the Hall Report (Hall 1996) that set out to systematically review and to improve child health surveillance. In her speech, Goodwin described health visiting as a 'gloomy picture of a beleaguered even demoralised profession, frustrated about what it would wish to do but cannot'. Recognising the need to move away from directive, secondary prevention child health screening and surveillance approaches, she urged health visitors to become involved in identification of individual parental needs in order to create participatory opportunities for primary care and 'support of parental confidence and competence' in line with the Hall Report recommendations.

Although it has been 11 years since that landmark speech, there is evidence to suggest that health visitors remain trapped in the narrow and restrictive strait-jacket of health visiting practice that she first described. There still remain tensions between participatory and directive styles of practice even though there is now renewed emphasis on primary care and the need for a shift in the relationship between parents, children and health professionals to one of partnership, rather than supervision, in which parents are empowered to make use of services and expertise according to their needs (Hall 1996).

A study for exploring ways of determining effectiveness of health visiting interventions unmasked conflicting tensions between participatory and directive styles of practice and suggested that some professionals were still setting their own agendas as opposed to empowering people to set their own agendas (Dolan & Kitson 1997). This study drew attention to recent evidence that suggested that health visitors were still viewing their 'workload' as being a constraining element to developing their role. 'Workload' has traditionally been given as a reason for inability to expand and develop the health visitor role even though there is evidence to suggest that modifications of workload have positive and empowering outcomes.

Health visitors in Nottingham's Strelley Nursing Development Unit became the first community based project to win a substantial Kings Fund grant for targeting resources to areas of greatest need and for finding ways to work in partnership with clients (Jackson 1994). An alternative health visiting framework was proposed and developed focusing on family health promotion and child health, high intervention work and public health. These were all primary care health strategies. In order to make any impact within these areas with no extra funding, the health visitors initially decided to reduce and to prioritise and redistribute caseloads. Other health visitors during a Sure Start funding bid, found that they too were able to develop and innovative, targeted practice after consciously deciding to reduce routine case work (Bidmead 1999).

These projects provide good examples of what can be achieved when health visitors decide to actively tackle the problem of workload. These endeavours may become essential as the very 'bread and butter' of health visiting practice is being threatened. Sure Start core services, outreach and home visiting, support to families and parents, primary and community health care and advice about child health and development and family health, and support for people with special needs including help getting access to specialised services – all these are remarkably similar to the core services that many health visitors would consider to be their everyday practice.

However, the Government has recognised that the nature of intervention varies greatly between health visitors. In recognising that 'some health visitors are already able to provide support for the family' (Dolan & Kitson 1997), the Government also recognises that some health visitors are not. Despite this, the Government now expects that all health visitors will 'extend and improve what they already do' (Sure Start document, p. 12) and will develop innovative proposals to ensure a lasting support to families that is 'long enough to make a real difference' (p. 6). The Government also expects that health visitors will develop this support within existing resources and that is why radical and innovative changes are being sought. Health visitors recognising that Sure Start is 'exactly what health visitors have been trying to do for many years with too few resources' (CPHVA News 1999) are also failing to recognise that without innovation there will be no extra funding. If health visitors do not change and refocus their work, new models of support will evolve to usurp the health visitor role.

Indeed there is already evidence of this happening. Recently in Hackney, the views of 202 family members were sought as part of some research funded by the Department of Health. It is unsettling, as Cook (1999) noted, that although these families had access to an individual health visitor, many still 'expressed a wish to have open access to a family adviser in general practice who could listen to and discuss concerns and possible responses' (p. 69). In response to the survey, it was felt necessary to develop a new 'Well family service' for the 6800 people within those caseloads.

The key elements to this new approach were described as being home visiting, a consistent relationship on the user's terms, parenting education, emotional support and advocacy. Most health visitors would probably list all of these as being key elements to the 'old' approach of health visiting. The developers of this new approach however, have no such expectations, declaring that 'with larger caseloads, higher levels of statutory child protection work, increased routine tasks and extended development testing, health visitors are not in a position to offer a targeted service to vulnerable families' (Cook 1999, p. 171). Even more worrying, the key target group of 'families with children in need to fall below the current threshold for social service support' (Cook 1999, p. 169) are currently just those families that represent the 'holding work' or 'grey area' that increasingly takes up much health visitor time. More families are being supported in a holding relationship by health visitors who find that social services departments are 'often only accessible if a referral is described as a child protection issue' and who find that social workers are putting less effort 'into intervening and working preventatively at an early stage with families (Appleton & Clemerson 1999, p. 134).

In reality, the important emotional work that health visitors are involved in with families at best is undervalued and at worst remains invisible, thus contributing to the perceived need to develop 'new' services that mimic and supplement the health visitor role. If such a significant proportion of health visiting work remains invisible, then it becomes essential to develop a sense of clarity about what we are actually doing with health visiting practice. Without such clarity, negative assumptions are flourishing and successfully disguising the true therapeutic, primary care nature of health visiting intervention. Without such clarity I would have been unable to move forward out of this self-induced silence of hopelessness towards a sense of inner certainty and confidence. As Freire (1972) said, 'as critical perception is embodied in action, a climate of hope and confidence develops which leads men to attempt to overcome the limit situations' (p. 72). To again cite Freire (1972), in challenging the 'concrete historical reality' (p. 72) of my health visiting practice and within the wider profession, the only real 'black hole' or 'strait-jacket' to practice is likely to be a self perceived one. Through guided reflection I have moved my perceptual goal posts, have readjusted my sense of reality and am now ready to move forward in my work with Helen with a sense of inner certainty and confidence that I have never experienced before.

Moving beyond Helen's resistance

In session four:

Yvonne: 'I phoned Helen today but early in the conversation she made it clear she didn't want to talk to me. She said she had given up on health visitors. I used the model of structured reflection cue – "how is she feeling" – to remind myself that she had never accepted me as a health visitor but had always done so as a person. I drew strength from this and staying with her, empathised saying, "I know how you feel. It's like we're banging our head against a brick wall." I encouraged her to think about the ways we were slowly making progress. Gradually she opened up and talked to me and eventually decided that she would like me to accompany her to social services. I said I would be away for the next two weeks and we could go when I returned. I'm dismayed at the lack of response by social services. I ask myself, "why is it so difficult? Helen doesn't ask for much at all".'

Chris: 'She doesn't ask for much at all? Perhaps you should reflect on this some more.'

Yvonne: 'Just what is everyone afraid of? It's such a struggle for me, let alone for Helen. We're both battling against the odds ... but why?! However, in so far as social services are concerned, I now feel resolute and decisive. I know my continuing support will help to strengthen Helen just as your guidance gives me strength to do it. I do wonder why it feels as if I am entering into battle!'

Interpretation

By repeating the words 'she doesn't ask for very much at all', Chris gave me the opportunity to reconsider them not just in terms of my frustration, but also in terms of their true significance. The more I thought about it, the more incomprehensible the situation became. If health visitors and social workers really wish to work in partnership with families, then this level of openness and honesty should surely be less difficult. In wishing to challenge the contents of a report written about her, all Helen was really asking for was a chance to take back some control, and yet this goal had for the last year been unachievable. I could now see that this was unacceptable and that it was time to question why this should be.

However, health visitors being open and honest with clients has proved to be problematic. Following a pilot study within six primary care teams, a child protection working group decided to conduct a study to develop a tool that would encourage an open and honest relationship with clients (Glew & Heron 1998). As part of the study, health visitors were asked to broach the subject of child abuse with families at the six week development check. Not only was there a low response rate to the study at 35%, some of the remaining sample admitted that they found raising the subject of child abuse difficult. Although the authors put this down to the stressful and distressing nature of child protection work, it is feasible to make a further assumption that this level of openness and honesty was too difficult to contemplate. Bell (1995) identified the therapeutic benefits of encouraging parents to become involved at the initial child protection conference, but also highlighted how health visitors 'had greater difficulty than social workers in presenting negative information about parents and children in front of them' (p. 256). It is strange that even within the prevailing climate of partnership building with families, health visitors are experiencing such incongruence between their espoused beliefs and values and their actual practice in child protection work. This in itself is revealing and so worthy of further critical scrutiny.

Focusing on the ability of health visitors to act in self-determined ways, it is clear that a high degree of structural autonomy (Batey & Lewis 1982) exists within health visiting as health visitors are 'expected in the context of their work to use their judgement in the provision of client services' (p. 15). Although health visitors cannot expect complete autonomy, as they function as part of an organisation, freedom to make independent decisions exists in almost all settings where nursing is practised. The more complex the patient's problems and the more persons involved in the patient's care, the greater the need for independent decisions by nurses related to the practice of nursing (Singleton & Nail 1984). Despite this, it is clear that under certain circumstances health visitors feel constrained and unable to realise their caring beliefs in actual practice. Within the child protection arena it seems that health visitor ability to maintain levels of self-determination is significantly reduced. It may be that attitudinal autonomy is being compromised because health visitors do not perceive themselves to be free to use their judgement in decision making (Batey & Lewis 1982). I recognise that I may have been labouring under this type of constraint in my work with Helen. Reflecting on my experiences I can now see the impact of social service interventions on both Helen's life and my practice. My attempts to help her gain access to her notes have been to no avail. In this disempowered state of silence I can now see how I have unwittingly colluded with social services and how, in doing so, I have compromised my professional integrity. Holden (1990) highlighted that nurses have a tendency to collude with doctors who are practising in unacceptable ways although this in turn 'strikes at the very core of their personal and professional integrity' (p. 402). This becomes intolerable to nurses and causes conflict between the medical and nursing professions. Collusion with social services has encouraged me to give up my sense of autonomy and power and to act in ways that are against my beliefs and values. It seems therefore that increasing child protection work merely serves to contradict the very nature of health visiting practice and that this may be the reason why these interventions have so often seemed intolerable to me and to other health visitors.

In my silence I have also unwittingly reinforced a perception that social services are relatively more powerful than health visiting and this may be contributing to my feelings of disempowerment. Holden (1990) suggests that to take back the reins of responsibility nurses need to prioritise their desires in order to decrease frustration, to employ a critical awareness in order to act on their own convictions and to develop a strength of will in order to maintain a sense of personal integrity. I am now able to prioritise my desire to become more therapeutic and am developing the critical awareness necessary to help me realise these desires in actual practice. Developing an inner strength is my next challenge if I wish to restore a sense of self-integrity. Indeed this is the next major challenge for health visiting if health visitors genuinely wish to embrace the notion of true partnership with clients. However, within child protection work, there seems to be a weakness of professional identity and attitude that has resulted in collusion with the perceived values of social services and this needs to be further explored.

Collusion with social services may have been facilitated due to the increased bureaucratisation and rigidity of framework for health visitor involvement in child protection work since the publication of the Children Act 1989. This act outlines the duties and responsibilities of health authorities and NHS trusts in relation to child protection work. Significantly, the act recommended the 'identification of the senior nurse with a health visiting qualification as a designated senior professional to become a member of the Area Child Protection Committee' and also the 'identification of a named nurse/midwife for child protection matters' (DoH 1998c, p. 3). These new posts, together with the act's emphasis on duty to comply with requests for help from a local authority, have laid a foundation for increasing links between health visiting and social services in child protection work. This has been to the extent that health visiting is increasingly and mistakenly described as being a statutory agency (Browne 1994). Although it is recognised that the Children Act 1989 imposed no statutory duties on health authorities, there has been a strengthening of bureaucratic links with statutory agencies especially those with social service departments and this may account for the misconception of the health visitor role. Increased bureau-cratisation may also have contributed to the weakening of professional autonomy in health visiting.

Hall (1968) has suggested that there is a tendency for autonomous professions to be less not more bureaucratic and that a 'rigid hierarchy of authority seems more incompatible with a high level of professionalism' (p. 103). The increasing rigidity of framework to health visitor intervention in child protection work may have con-tributed to the perception of less autonomy and control. It may be that health visitors who have not been given the space or time to consider these issues have become blinded by the reality of this oppression, and so believe that becoming more like social services is the most effective way to gain power and control (Roberts 1983).

Freire's (1972) work suggests however, that identification with the oppressor results in a loss of sense of individual awareness, self-esteem and confidence. This ensures that a cycle of oppression is set in motion, which in turn perpetuates the perception of subordination. It is possible to see that within this cycle a weak sense of professional identity could emerge. Hall (1968) suggested that some 'established professions have rather weakly developed professional attitudes', the strength of which 'appears to be based on the kind of socialisation that has taken place both in the profession's training programme and in the work itself' (p. 103). It therefore seems that both in training and practice, health visitors must find a way to unveil, examine, and challenge dominant values in order to break the cycle of oppression and to strengthen professional attitude (Watson 1990). Restoring a sense of professional integrity will enable a caring morality to emerge and to shape future practice con-gruent with our beliefs and values about the nature of desirable practice.

Guided reflection strikes at the very core of an oppressive cycle by providing the safe place necessary to facilitate awareness and fuel conflict (Johns 1998). I can see the source of oppression at face value so that although my own position is intolerable it is within my power to change the situation. Within my continuing struggle for self-determination, it is a time of creativity, strength of purpose and strength of will. This developing sense of inner being relates well to the attainment of a sense of self-mastery and self-competence within the 'era of incorporation' (see Fig. 8.1). I have rejected the misplaced, negative images of health visiting in favour of a truer, clearer under-standing of my position in terms of relative power. That in itself is strengthening and in becoming strengthened I know that I am now far more likely to be able to sustain an empowering, therapeutic relationship with Helen.

Facilitating Helen's empowerment

By session five I had talked to Jo [social worker] again about Helen and had also seen Helen during a visit to the nursery and I chose to discuss the outcomes of these contacts within guided reflection.

> *Yvonne:* 'Jo telephoned to let me know the outcome of her supervision session. She said she felt disgusted at the response of her manager. She felt there had been no co-operation. Her

manager had said that Helen was definitely not allowed to have access to the records, which made Jo angry. She was also anxious and said "I could get the sack for talking like this". She had tried to express her view, that is very similar to mine, but this had been to no avail. She said there was nothing more that she could do and said that unlike me, she would not be able to surface her feelings of disgust about it in supervision. We compared supervision experiences. Jo was supervised by her line-manager, who was far more likely to scrutinise her practice than to help her clarify her beliefs and values. I explained that my supervision experience had been empowering and had encouraged me to focus on finding ways to empower my clients. Jo wanted to support me. She said that she had not realised health visitors became involved in advocacy work with clients. We talked about this and other types of therapeutic interventions in health visiting.

I told her that Helen said she had made an official complaint to social services over 18 months ago, and that although the complaint had been acknowledged, there had been no further response. Jo said that she would ask her manager to write to Helen and that she would telephone Helen to talk about this. She gave me names of the people she thought Helen could contact to make a complaint and said she would send me a copy of the "complaints" procedure. She wished me good luck.

A few days later I met Helen and the children at the nursery. Jo had explained to her that she couldn't have access to the notes because they were officially the children's notes. She seemed pleased she had at last received a letter but said she was still angry and concerned about the possibility of her son gaining access to the notes in the future. She wanted to be given the opportunity to clear her name. She seemed a lot calmer today and more receptive to my help. We talked about the possibilities of recommencing counselling sessions in the New Year. She said she found it difficult to focus on counselling when she was feeling so angry but was willing to try when Natasha had settled into the nursery. I suggested that she put her thoughts and complaints down in writing and gave her the list of names Jo had given me. Helen seemed keen to pursue this and so we arranged to meet after Christmas in order to allow time for a response.'

Chris: 'So what feels significant about this session?'

Yvonne: 'Comparing our styles of supervision was eye opening! Her frustration and suppressed anger at being constrained in practice were powerful.'

Chris: 'Yet you seem to be helping her to work through these feelings in positive ways to resolve her emergent understanding of the contradictions in her practice?'

Yvonne: 'We shall see.'

Chris: 'Try using the framing perspectives [Fig. 1.6] to untangle the significance of your conversation with Jo.'

Yvonne's commentary   Following Chris' advice, I used the framing perspectives to generate a number of questions to focus my understanding and action:

Philosophical framing	How do the constraints and oppression experienced by Jo impact on Helen and my desire to be an empowering practitioner?
Role framing	Why was Jo so unclear about the health visitor role? Does this lack of understanding affect my relationship with her?
Theoretical framing	What theory, research or information do I need access to, to help me clarify these issues?

Reality perspective framing	Why was it so difficult for Jo to actualise her beliefs and values in practice and how can this influence the work of the health visitor?
Problem framing	How can I make people listen and respond to Helen?
Temporal framing	Have I internalised similar feelings of constraint and until now have not been aware or questioned them?
Parallel process framing	What are the differences in health visiting and social work styles of supervision and how do these affect the way each practises? In what ways do Jo's feelings of constraint impact on health visiting and hence our clients?

Interpretation

The session had generated many more questions than answers, but I could begin to see the common thread of oppression and empowerment that linked the sessions. It became clear that I was so much further along than Jo in my journey or struggle towards self-determination as reflected in our contrasting supervision styles. Jo had indicated that the underlying emphasis of her supervision was concerned with ensuring she responded in normative ways, reflected in her sense of being monitored and controlled. It had been a revelation for her to realise that the emphasis of supervision could be empowering. My conversation with Jo had fuelled her sense of conflict to the extent that she began to articulate her own sense of powerlessness and this had been a revelation to me. Up until this point it seemed to me that Jo had passively accepted these constraints and they were so powerful that even with an increased awareness, she had still felt unable to support me in an overt way. Her supervision silenced her to the extent that she could only speak with her supervisor's words rather than her own. Freire (1972) believes that in doing this the 'oppressor' who has stolen the words of others will begin to develop doubts in the abilities and competence of others and in turn will become 'more accustomed to power and acquire a taste for guiding, ordering and commanding' (p. 104).

In contrasting our supervision, Jo felt her position to be intolerable and that she had nowhere to go to explore this dissatisfaction in a critical way. She felt trapped within a cycle of oppression where there was no opportunity to find a way towards emancipation from the conditions of domination. I can now more easily comprehend why Helen and I have often felt it has been an uphill struggle to gain support from social workers. It must be difficult for social workers to become empowering as practitioners under such a regime. In the light of my understanding of the increasing influence of social services on health visiting, it was now important to further consider the impact of Jo's experience on my desire to become an empowering practitioner.

While comparing my supervision with Jo's had been illuminating, I knew my experience was by no means universal. Supervision within health visiting child protection work has historically developed in a way that mimics social work supervision (Bond & Holland 1998). Scott (1999), a health visitor child protection advisor, declared that 'the value of supervision in child protection work is constructively to challenge, guide, and direct the contribution of all practitioners in the multi-disciplinary prevention of abuse' (p. 762). Scott highlighted the way supervision can be linked to the annual individual performance review to help identify weak practice. She clearly demonstrates her support of the notion that supervision in child protection work can be used to monitor and control.

There is evidence that this style of supervision in child protection work is being imposed on health visitors in the same way that it is currently imposed on social workers. Health visitors in Bedfordshire received a proposal for a mandatory protocol for supervision of child protection work and management of poor practice. The protocol stated that supervision sessions would become mandatory for all professionals who have completed a CP1 (initial child protection referral form) and for those with children on their caseloads who are on the child protection register. It also stated that 'in the event that poor practice is identified during a supervisory session the matter will, in the first instance, be discussed with the individual and then referred on to the child protection advisor for further consideration'. The aim of this style of supervision is obviously to 'police' and to control the workforce, and as such, is disempowering by nature.

Braye and Preston-Shoot (1995) note 'for empowerment in social care to have meaning, the organisational culture must move away from that of power (control of expert) and role (emphasis on given tasks and procedures) to that of community (learning with users). Such a culture would seek to use and enhance the power and authority held by users, while recognising that professional power and authority remain legally mandated, and may have to be exercised' (p. 115). My work with Helen has helped me to understand the ways in which, as a health visitor, I can unwittingly collude with oppressive forces and so compromise my professional practice. Especially in child protection work where organisational aspects become more complex due to a blending of ideologies, it is essential that we are able to maintain a sense of control over our working culture if we are to succeed in becoming empowering practitioners. In order to achieve this goal an empowering type of supervision would seem essential.

Breaking through

Before I met Chris again in session six I sent him an e-mail:

> *Yvonne:* 'Dear Chris, yesterday something wonderful happened. I'm still reeling. When I went into work there were messages from various people who were all very concerned about Helen and her children. From the moment I picked up the messages I tuned into you and I thought of all the things you have taught me in guided reflection. I thought of Helen and began to draw together all the fragmented strands of knowing. I looked into myself becoming more and more in harmony with her. It felt like nothing I've experienced before. I just knew that whatever I did next would be good for Helen and would protect the children. *And it worked!* It is a long story that I cannot wait to tell you. After a very long and tiring day with Helen, the children, child care social workers, mental health care social workers, psychiatrists and managers, the children were protected and happy in a foster home and Helen was in hospital receiving the care she desperately needed. None of this would have happened if Helen and I had not been so connected.'

Yvonne's commentary   This had been an emotional and passionate communication. It had felt like stars were colliding. All our work within supervision had come together in a way that enabled me to intervene in time to prevent harm to the children. This work had become living evidence of a new and effective way to protect children through health visiting and guided reflection.

I described the intervention by reading my last journal entry to Chris:

Yvonne: 'The messages I received had been from the school nurse and the headmistress (Mrs Johnson) of Robert's school. Luckily the school nurse was in her office and I was able to talk to her. She said that Mrs Johnson had become increasingly concerned about Helen's mental health over the last two weeks. She said Robert was coming into school late, sometimes not arriving until lunchtime. Helen had been striking up strange, inappropriate conversation full of sexual innuendo with members of staff, and writing long, confused letters to Mrs Johnson.

I telephoned Mrs Johnson who confirmed her anxieties. She said she had contacted the duty child care team at social services. I contacted the duty officer (Lynne) who had taken Mrs Johnson's referral. Lynne said she had received two referrals expressing concerns about the family. The other referral was from a worried neighbour. Despite this, she had decided to pass these referrals on to the mental health care team. I registered my concern by saying that I wished to refer the family back to the child care duty team. I explained that the children had both previously been on the child protection register and that although no longer registered, there were still child protection concerns in relation to mum's mental health. The social worker explained that a visit had been organised for Monday afternoon by a member of the mental health care team.

I telephoned Helen. I asked her how she was feeling and she said 'awful'. I asked her if she needed help and she replied "yes". I asked her if she would like to go into hospital and again she simply replied "yes". She began to cry. I said that I would like to come straight over to see her and bring a social worker with me. She agreed saying, "I'm not coping with the children". I could hear them laughing and screaming in the background.

I immediately telephoned social services and they agreed to visit that (Friday) morning. I took the mental health care social worker (Kay) in my car and we arranged to meet Lynne at the house. When we arrived, Kay said she would rather wait for Lynne to arrive. I said I felt uncomfortable sitting outside Helen's house and I went to knock on the door. I was shocked when I saw her. She looked so tired and drawn. Her hair was greasy and lank and her clothes were dirty and had been put on inside out. As soon as she saw me she started to cry and I still remember the sadness I felt as she led me through the house.

Although Robert is six years old, he was running around wearing nothing except a nappy, a T-shirt and a crucifix tied around his neck by a boot lace. Both he and his sister were wild, running and screaming among chaotic piles of toys, wet laundry, remains of food and other debris. One minute Helen was crying and the next she was laughing. Robert was eating a biscuit and I asked him if he was hungry. He took my hand to show me "what Mummy cooked for dinner". It was a saucepan full of the charcoal remains of a wooden spoon and a newspaper. He said "we all watched the fire until it went out". By this time the social workers had come in and Kay had started to assess the state of Helen's mental health. She concluded that it was not necessary to admit her to hospital. In disbelief I showed her the saucepan and said that although I was not trained in mental health nursing, it was obvious to me that she needed help and could not be left alone to cope with the children. Eventually it was agreed that Helen should be admitted on a voluntary basis and that the children should be taken into foster care. However Helen refused to sign the document. To my amazement, Lynne responded by saying that there was nothing more she could do if that was the case and stood up as if she was ready to leave! I offered to read the document to Helen and after some moments she said that she would only sign it if I read it to her. There was so much trust between us.

Soon after this there was a flurry of telephone calls and the children left quite happily with Lynne. Robert seemed relieved. He said "You are taking mummy away to make her better aren't you?". Kay and I took Helen straight to hospital and the consultant later decided that she was suffering from an acute episode of manic depression. I attended a decision making meeting at social services the other day and was shocked to find out that it had been organised even though Helen was still in hospital and so was unable to attend. I immediately expressed my concern that this meeting should go ahead without her and they agreed to cancel and reschedule the meeting. It was so easy. The whole feeling of the meeting was somehow different.'

Chris: 'What do you think was different?'

Yvonne: 'The social worker that chaired the session seemed to know everything about the history of Helen's case. She may well have read my letters to social services and comments I had made at meetings over the last year. They may at last have had an impact. Anyway something had changed and it was more empowering for Helen so I was pleased.'

Interpretation

Within those moments my responses had been natural, confident and in harmony with the needs of the family. Helen and I had worked together in true partnership. Yet without the trust and connection that had been nurtured in guided reflection, I could not have intervened in such an effective and preventative way in this acute time of need. The session demonstrates how I have developed a critical awareness within the supervision process that has brought about a sense of maturity and competence as described by Kieffer's fourth phase of involvement (see Fig. 8.3). At this level, Kieffer considers that it becomes more possible to integrate and apply personal knowing in a meaningful and proactive way. He points out that this awareness can be difficult to achieve without the support of an external enabler.

In moving as I move, in tune with my needs, my supervisor has been a dynamic and strengthening influence and has mirrored my desire to become empowered in practice. Such is the parallel nature of work within supervision and clinical practice when the underlying commitment is to become more available to work with others in therapeutic ways. Whilst I am aware that the struggle towards emergence will always continue, I also have an overwhelming feeling that I have moved on, have chosen a good path and that things will never be quite the same again.

Asserting my new voice

In session seven I reflected:

Yvonne: 'Since our last session Helen has been discharged from hospital. She and the children were well. I have attended two case review meetings at social services. One was a positive experience, the other one was very negative. The first review meeting went very well for Helen. She had been allowed to bring her friend into the meeting to act as an advocate because she had said that sometimes she was unable to explain herself clearly and was consequently often misinterpreted. The chairperson encouraged her to talk throughout the meeting and listened attentively to the advocate. In the end, the decisions made were based primarily on Helen's wishes. It was decided that she would continue to have increasing access to the children and they would return home when she had fully recovered. She seemed relaxed and happy. It had been the first time that she had ever truly participated at a meeting in my experience.'

Chris: 'Something has changed?'

Yvonne: 'There has been a noticeable shift in perception and attitudes. It has been a gradual shift that has recently gathered momentum. When I think back to my first piece of reflective work with Helen, I recall the ripple effect of my own change of perception. Looking at labelling theory helped me to understand the ways Helen had been affected. Labelling had negatively influenced our early relationship. This and other early reflections helped me to critically question my perceptions and to see the true Helen. Gradually, others began to change their perceptions and became more sensitive and co-operative towards her. I attribute the more recent changes to our joint determination to continue to be seen and heard. We are both emerging with a sense of inner confidence. At the case review meeting, everyone took great care to ensure she had her say. It was wonderful.'

Chris: 'How did it differ during the next meeting?'

Yvonne: 'The next meeting was awful. I was told that the chairperson, Mrs Granite, was a social services child protection team leader. Things started to go wrong from the outset. When Helen explained that she had brought an advocate, Mrs Granite said the advocate could support but not talk.'

Chris: 'Did you question this?'

Yvonne: 'Not at that point. I was quite shocked. We were asked to read through the care assessment carried out by Helen's two social workers. As Helen began to read it she became quite agitated. Due to her past experiences she feels very threatened by this kind of document. She didn't agree with some points but was firmly denied the right to comment. Mrs Granite reminded Helen that she had already been given time to read through it. I suggested to Helen that it might help her to write her feelings down on paper. She agreed and so I asked Mrs Granite if it would be possible to include her comments in the report. Mrs Granite's reaction was startling. Reminding me that she was the chairperson and had not asked me to speak, she entirely disregarded the idea.

I resolved to have my say in the meeting when it was my turn to speak. During the discussion about Helen however, I was not asked to contribute at all. Instead I was asked to comment about the children. As it was apparent to me that the discussion regarding Helen had ended, I said I would like to discuss the outcomes of a conversation between Helen and I regarding future support. She had told me of her fears and concerns about the future and we wanted to make sure there was a safety net of support in operation in case she suddenly became ill again.

At this point Mrs Granite asked me to clarify my involvement with the family. I explained about the nature of my supportive work with Helen. I must have used the word "therapeutic" because suddenly she exclaimed "you are a health visitor and you do not have a therapeutic role! Your job is to assess children's development. I've been a social worker for 20 years and I should know the role of the health visitor by now!" Although shocked at the inappropriateness of this outburst, I felt confident and talked to Mrs Granite about the nature of health visiting interventions with parents and children. I offered to send her a recent paper that uncovers the therapeutic role of the health visitor (Cody 1999). Suddenly Helen said "I have no problem, I understand her role".'

Chris: 'A profound moment?'

Yvonne: 'I felt very calm. I found myself using the Burford cues [see Fig. 7.1] that I now use so naturally within interactions. I thought of Mrs Granite and asked myself "how does this person make me feel?". I visualised the space between us. I was able within those moments to remind myself of our separate roles, especially in terms of power. She suddenly seemed far less threatening. I asked myself "who is this person?" and thought of her role in child protection. The previous chairperson had not been a child protection social worker and their styles were so different. I wondered whether her oppressive style arose from her beliefs and values about her practice or from the culture she worked within. Perhaps it was a bit of both, but whatever the cause she could have been overwhelmingly powerful.'

Chris: 'But she wasn't?'

Yvonne: 'No. Both Helen and I were able to respond in a convincing and assertive way. My comments about the safety net were acknowledged and discussed and everyone listened to Helen talking about her fears for the future. I then went on to discuss the children's general development. We had our say despite the odds and actually we were the powerful ones!'

Chris: 'So what's been significant?'

Yvonne: 'The second meeting was not as awful as I thought. I managed to shift the balance of power which enabled a positive outcome for Helen, chipping away at the same old block and it finally paid off. Helen has become increasingly confident, able to assert her own ideas about the future safety of her children, and people are listening! I feel very optimistic that we will be able to protect the children from harm in the future.'

Chris: 'Your mutual sense of empowerment shines through your words.'

Yvonne: 'It's true. I do feel empowered and it has rubbed off on Helen.'

Interpretation

The 'awful' second meeting had been revealed in a truer light. Despite the odds, Helen and I had articulated our wishes and contributed our ideas with a heightened inner clarity and confidence. It was a time of transition into a newer way of knowing. Through the empowering and parallel nature of guided reflection we had both found a way to reclaim our sense of self. Belenky *et al.* (1986) refer to this as speaking with a 'constructed voice', where women have learnt to speak with a unique, authentic, informed and passionate voice. This voice transcends the 'subjective voice' whereby women have an increased sense of private authority but lack the 'tools for expressing themselves or persuading others to listen' (p. 134). As my story reveals, there is a 'transition from sense of self as helpless victim to acceptance of self as an assertive and efficacious citizen' (Kieffer 1984, p. 33). Fay (1987) describes this combination of power and will as emancipation, or a 'state of reflective clarity in which people know which of their wants are genuine because they finally know who they really are, and a state of collective autonomy in which they have the power to determine rationally and freely the nature and direction of their collective existence' (p. 205). Helen and I were both developing this sense of self-determination. Our work was now taking the form of cultural action (Freire 1972) witnessed in the transformative change in others' attitudes and in the shift in the balance of power in our favour.

Conclusion

I have repeatedly referred to my experiences of guided reflection as having been an unfolding journey. It felt as though I was at the foot of a hill that obscured my view but only needed to be climbed to reveal new and exciting pastures. It turned out to be a long and steep climb. My interpretative analysis of the guided reflection sessions became increasingly involved and complex as new insights emerged into my consciousness, peeling back the layers of self-distortion in order to reveal myself to myself, and clear the path to reach my goal. The turning point came just before Christmas between sessions five and six when I felt as if I had reached the top of the hill revealing a whole new vista. I have been able to construct a better way for health visitors. My work demonstrates that child protection work often contradicts the espoused philosophy of health visiting and so becomes a source of tension for health visitors. Perhaps health visitors feel uncertain about their role, which leads to a lack of confidence and a passive acceptance of the status quo. This has resulted in an increasing alignment with the secondary preventative 'detection work' that has traditionally been the focus of social work. This alignment is apparent in the way supervision within child protection work is currently being developed, that mimics the style of social work supervision which is fundamentally disempowering.

Significantly, examination of current Government initiatives reveals that there is an opportunity for health visitors to become proactive and creative and to develop a new way of working based on intensive and effective primary care interventions. It is therefore time to take stock of our position within child protection work. My work indicates that in forging blindly ahead and increasing our surveillance role and crisis intervention work, we are increasingly departing from our espoused beliefs about desirable practice.

The experiences I continue to share in guided reflection affirm my new way of health visiting as if I am free-falling down the hill. I have become more positive, confident and assertive. In many ways I realise this story is just the beginning. As Belenky *et al.* (1986) note 'even amongst women who feel they have found their voice, problems with voice abound' (p. 146). The ongoing struggle for constructivist woman is not to find voice but to make others listen. This must mean developing a collective voice that can effectively challenge not only perceived internal constraints but oppressive and disempowering work cultures. It is my assertion that this can be achieved through the empowering and transformative process of guided reflection.

References

Anon (1999a) Family policy doomed without increase in health visitors. *Community Practitioner*, **72**(7) 190.

Anon (1999b) News. *Community Practitioner*, **72**(7) 190.

Appleton, J. & Clemerson, J. (1999) Family-based interventions with children in need. *Community Practitioner*, 72, 134–6.

Appleton, J. & Cowley, S. (1997) Analysing clinical practice guidelines. A method of documentary analysis. *Journal of Advanced Nursing*, 25, 1008–17.

Batey, M. & Lewis, F. (1982) Clarifying autonomy and accountability in nursing services: Part 1. *The Journal of Nursing Administration*, **12**(9) 13–18.

Belenky, M., Clinch, B., Goldberger, N. & Tarule, J. (1986) *Women's Ways of Knowing: the development of self, voice and mind.* Basic Books, New York.

Bell, M. (1995) A study of the attitudes of nurses to parental involvement in the initial child-protection conference, and their preparation for it. *Journal of Advanced Nursing*, 22, 250–57.

Bidmead, C. (1999) Bidding for success: making a Sure Start application. *Community Practitioner*, 72, 166–7.

Bond, M. & Holland, S. (1998) *Skills of Clinical Supervision for Nurses*. Open University Press, Buckingham.

Braye, S. & Preston-Shoot, M. (1995) *Empowering Practice in Social Care*. Open University Press, Buckingham.

Browne, K. (1994) Preventing child maltreatment through community nursing. *Journal of Advanced Nursing*, 21, 57–63.

Butterfield, P. (1990) Thinking upstream: nurturing a conceptual understanding of the societal context of health behaviour. *Advances in Nursing Science*, **12**(2) 1–8.

Cody, A. (1999) Health visiting as a therapy: a phenomenological perspective. *Journal of Advanced Nursing*, **29**(1) 119–27.

Collinson, S. & Cowley, S. (1998) An exploratory study of demand for the health visiting service within a marketing framework. *Journal of Advanced Nursing*, 28, 499–507.

Cook, A. (1999) The Well Family Service: a new model of support. *Community Practitioner*, 72, 168–71.

Dingwall, R. (1982) Community nursing and civil liberty. *Journal of Advanced Nursing*, 7, 337–46.

DoH (1995) *Health Visiting: Working in the Community*. The Stationery Office, London.

DoH (1998a) *Supporting Families*. The Stationery Office, London.

DoH (1998b) *Independent Inquiry into Inequalities in Health* (The Acheson Report). The Stationery Office, London.

DoH (1998c) *Child protection for senior nurses, midwives, and their managers*. The Stationery Office, London.

Dolan, B. & Kitson, A. (1997) Future imperatives: developing health visiting in response to changing demands. *Journal of Clinical Nursing*, 6, 11–16.

Fay, B. (1987) *Critical Social Science*. Polity Press, Cambridge.

Fenwick, T. & Parsons, J. (1999) Boldly solving the world: a critical analysis of problem-based learning as a method of professional education. *Studies in the Education of Adults*, **30**(1) 60.

Freire, P. (1972) *Pedagogy of the Oppressed*. Penguin Books, London.

Glew, A. & Heron, H. (1998) Child protection: developing a personal child health record. *Community Practitioner*, 71, 328–9.

Goodwin, S. (1998) Whither health visiting? *Health Visitor*, 61, 328–32.

Hall, R. (1968) Professionalization and bureaucratization. *American Sociological Review*, 33, 92–104.

Hall, M. (1996) *Health for all Children*. Oxford University Press, Oxford.

Holden, R. (1990) Responsibility and autonomous nursing practice. *Journal of Advanced Nursing*, 16, 398–403.

Jackson, C. (1994) Strelley: teamworking for health visiting. *Health Visitor*, 67, 28–9.

Johns, C. (1998) Opening the doors of perception. In *Transforming nursing through reflective practice* (eds C. Johns & D. Freshwater). Blackwell Science, Oxford.

Johns, C. (1999) Unravelling the dilemmas within everyday nursing practice. *Nursing Ethics*, 6(4) 287–98.

Kieffer, C. (1984) Citizen empowerment: a developmental perspective. *Prevention in Human Services*, **84**(3) 9–36.

Okri, B. (1997) *A Way of Being Free*. Butler & Tanner, London.

Orr, J. (1990) First principles. *Health Visitor*, 63, 368.

Pike, A. (1991) Moral outrage and moral discourse in nurse-physician collaboration. *Journal of Professional Nursing*, 7, 351–63.

Prawat, R.S. (1993) The value of ideas: problems versus possibilities in learning. *Educational Researcher*, 22(6) 5–16.

Roberts, S. (1983) Oppressed group behaviour: implications for nursing. *Advances in Nursing Science*, 5(4) 21–30.

Scott, L. (1999) The nature and structure of supervision in health visiting with victims of child sexual abuse. *Journal of Advanced Nursing*, 29, 754–63.

Singleton, E. & Nail, F. (1984) Autonomy in nursing. *Nursing Forum*, 3, 123–30.

Sure Start document (1999) *A Guide for Trailblazers*. DfEE Publications, Suffolk.

Taylor, S. & Tilley, N. (1989) Health visitors and child protection: conflict contradictions and ethical dilemmas. *Health Visitor*, 62, 273–5.

Turner, T. (1998/9) The family way. *Community Practitioner*, 71, 398–400.

Van Manen M. (1990) *Researching Lived Experience*. State University of New York Press, New York.

Watson, J. (1990) The moral failure of the patriarchy. *Nursing Outlook*, 38(2) 62–6.

Weinsheimer, J. (1985) *Gadamer's Hermeneutics: a reading of truth and method*. Yale University Press, New York.

Welshman, J. (1997) Family visitors or social workers? Health visiting and public health in England and Wales 1890–1974. *International History of Nursing Journal*, 2(4) 5–22.

Chapter 9

Working with Deliberate Self Harm Patients in A&E

Background

Jane approached me (Chris) to guide her undergraduate dissertation using guided reflection. She had previously studied with me on the ENB A29 course (as did Aileen and Yvonne). Jane writes as follows.

The subject of this narrative was 'stumbled' upon during my first guided reflection session with Chris. We were discussing the changes that reflection had made to my clinical practice, which prompted me to surface and explore my negative attitude towards deliberate self harm (DSH) patients when working within a busy A&E environment. I shared an experience (see below) which illuminated what I meant about my attitude and which prompted me to decide to focus my research on this topic. I chose to work with Chris in a guided reflection relationship because reflection had become such a meaningful learning milieu for me. Reflection enables me to access and analyse my practice, leading to insights that influence my future practice within a reflexive spiral of development. The narrative is structured through a series of seven guided reflection sessions that spanned six months.

Narrative

Focusing deliberate self harm

In our first session, issues surrounding DSH patients were not on my mind, or so I thought. On reflection I realise that I had concerns about this area of my practice. These thoughts or anxieties had lain dormant, waiting for the right time to be expressed. Chris began by simply asking how I was. I had not anticipated what might result – to my surprise my anxieties about DSH patients tumbled out.

Jane: 'Something happened a few weeks ago. I haven't really thought long and hard about it yet. I have some "nagging" doubts about what happened, I think it's been easier to ignore it and put it to the back of my mind. On a recent shift I dealt with a man who had deliberately cut his arm. I still feel uncomfortable about the way in which I responded to him. It was a night shift at around three in the morning. I went into a cubicle to carry out a treatment. Until this point I had not met this man, all I knew about him was that he had deliberately cut his arm. He required sutures and I went into the cubicle to carry out his treatment. On reflection

I am aware that I pre-judged him, stereotyped him. His deliberate act of self-harm irritated me before I met him. I went into the cubicle and communicated necessary information with him; I was professional, and I tried to hide my feelings but felt "empty". He was excluded from any feelings of compassion that I am able to feel for other patients. Prior to treatment commencing he asked if it would hurt. I felt this was a ridiculous question, why should he care if it hurt? I found my irritation bubbling to the surface and in answer to his question I replied, "The local should numb the pain of the stitches, but it must have hurt when you did it!" I wasn't asking a question that required an answer, I now realise it was a way of communicating my feelings, a reprimand for his behaviour. Although my response makes me uncomfortable I wonder if compassion would encourage him to continue with such futile acts again and again; mutilating your own body is such an alien concept. It seems such a waste of time to stitch someone who is going to repeat the injury.'

Chris: 'Do you have any idea why you feel this way?'

Jane: 'I've never really thought about it. It's frustrating when you see the same patients returning over and over again; they never seem to recover.'

Chris: 'Perhaps you don't see the ones who recover because they don't come back for treatment. Perhaps your frustration lies with your inability to put things right? Perhaps these patients are manipulative. You may want to examine whether the boundaries of your role require you to "patch up the damage", whether DSH patients require a more therapeutic approach?'

Jane: 'I don't feel that I have enough knowledge to distinguish between manipulative and non-manipulative patients. They obviously have reasons for their behaviour, but I find it difficult to respond.'

Chris: 'What sort of reasons?'

Jane: 'I don't know. There could be a million different reasons. The environment doesn't help. The A&E environment is very challenging, for example a nurse may find herself comforting grieving relatives one minute and the next trying to come to terms with the fact that the person in front of them has tried to take their own life, or has inflicted harm upon themselves.'

Chris: 'Are some people more worthy of care than others?'

Jane: 'I think I should treat everyone with the same care and compassion, but in reality I do treat these people differently. The very fact that I do this is upsetting; it doesn't meet my own philosophy of care and they are not feelings I expected to have when I embarked on my nursing career. I care, that's why I entered the profession; it distresses me that I cannot be more therapeutic with this patient group.'

Chris: 'Does anything else influence your reaction to such patients?'

Jane: 'I've spoken about my mother in the past. She suffers with a progressive debilitating condition and I constantly witness her failing health; she doesn't deserve it. Why do fit and healthy people injure themselves?'

Chris: 'Do you think this subject will be too emotive to tackle?'

Jane: 'I think it will be very emotive but I really think I should attempt to understand why I feel this way and change the way in which I deliver care to this patient group and hopefully deliver care in a therapeutic way.'

Interpretive analysis

Sharing my experience resulted in asking various questions of myself such as, why do I have difficulty with offering the same level of care to this patient group? The realisation surfaced that my detachment in caregiving with this group may well affect these patients' overall well-being. Watson (1999) highlights this:

'We see glimpses indicating that the nurse's presence and consciousness, attitude and behaviour can affect the patient, for better or for worse.' (p. 225)

Reflection has enabled me to realise that there is a fundamental contradiction between my practice and what I want it to be. From this session I take with me the 'need' to know more about DSH. I will use my experience in a positive way and remember what I have learnt when caring for the next patient. Chris utilised the being available template (Fig. 3.1) (Johns 2000), in particular 'concern' for another person. This enabled me to confront and begin to clarify my beliefs and values. I realised during this guided session that I do care about DSH patients; if I did not care this research would not have evolved. Benner and Wrubel (1989) state:

'Caring (Having things matter) puts the person in a place of risk and vulnerability. Relationships, things, events, and projects do not show up as stressful unless they matter.' (p. 1)

Realising that I didn't care for these patients in the way I felt I should was distressing, and even though I may find this research difficult and lay myself open to vulnerability, I care enough about my practice as a whole to eliminate this contradiction in my practice.

Deliberate self-harm (DSH) is a term used interchangeably with parasuicide. Arguments surround the various terminology used. Fairburn (1995) criticises terms such as parasuicide believing they are used to suggest a person's intent to die, when arguably the range of injury a person can carry out upon themselves is wide ranging and not always life threatening. For the purpose of this research the preferred term will be DSH. Anderson (1999) also utilised this terminology in a review of self-harm and suicide, stating:

'The term deliberate self-harm encompasses behaviours where the patient can be considered suicidal, such as taking an overdose, self suffocation, self strangulation, wrist cutting, drowning, etc. However the term is also used to refer to acts a young person may engage in, but where suicide may not be the intention.' (p. 92)

I began a literature review to enhance my knowledge of deliberate self-harm. It is one of the top five causes of acute medical admissions for both males and females and is a known risk factor for suicide (Hawton & Fagg 1992); 150,000 attendances occur per annum (Hawton & Catlin 1997), the majority presenting at general hospitals. McLaughlin (1994) notes that:

'The casualty department is usually the first port of call for these patients. Such high incidence rates can cause stress on both nursing and medical staff and could influence the attitudes they hold in relation to attempted suicide.'

It is estimated that in the UK one person every day contemplates suicide (McLaughlin 1991). The Government green paper *Our Healthier Nation* outlines targets for the reduction of suicide rates (DoH 1998). Research and literature surrounding the attitudes of nurses and other health professionals in both A&E and, surprisingly, psychiatric units suggests that an improvement in attitudes is needed to improve patient care and reduce suicides. How then is this to be achieved if the literature suggests that attitudes are incongruent with desirable practice? Alston and Robinson (1992) state that when responding to a suicidal patient: 'The nurse may hold attitudes which lead to fear, anxiety, absence of empathy and anger' (p. 206). Whilst exploring literature I found an article written by Fiona Lynn (1998) a woman with a history of self-harm, in which she states:

> 'Needing stitches was a nightmare. I felt embarrassed and shamed about being stitched up by a nurse whose comments, or lack of comment, made me want the ground to open up to swallow me.' (p. 56)

The nurse's 'lack of comment' she knew; she heard the nurse's attitude without a word being spoken. Her words really encourage readers to view things from a different perspective.

Avoidance

When we next met in session two Chris asked me: 'What has happened since we last met?'

Jane: 'Nothing, I've had no contact with any DSH patients at all.'
Chris: 'Why?'
Jane: 'I don't know really, interactions just haven't happened.'
Chris: 'No patients have been through the department when you were on duty?'
Jane: 'Well yes, plenty of patients, there always are. I was busy with other patients. That's not really true. I suppose if I'm honest I've been avoiding them.'
Chris: 'Why?'
Jane: 'I haven't really thought about it; on reflection I suppose it's easier isn't it?'
Chris: 'Perhaps you have deliberately used avoidance as a mechanism that allows you more time to unravel your belief system before you attempt another interaction. Do you think this might be the case?'
Jane: 'I have been avoiding them but haven't analysed why. I do feel that I need to grasp more understanding of the subject. I don't want to hurt anyone by saying the wrong thing.'
Chris: 'I think this period of avoidance is a positive step towards understanding yourself; we will discuss it again next time we meet.'

Interpretative analysis

The session began with negative feelings about avoiding contact with DSH patients. During and post supervision this was turned into a positive feeling that I was making progress. During supervision came the realisation that I had been avoiding DSH patients for a specific reason; it was also a relief to admit that I feared the next interaction. Chris suggested that I had used avoidance as a mechanism because I needed more time, that it was a step towards unravelling my belief system. Chris realised this period of avoidance was a necessity and that it was significant to my journey of reflection. Carveth (1995) believes avoidance is used by nurses when the prospect of dealing with a difficult patient arises. Whilst avoidance provides a protective mechanism for the nurse from life and death issues, avoidance can be painful for the patient who may already feel isolated (Eldrid 1988).

I realise that 'I am not alone'. Many nurses have difficulty with this patient group. The work of Corley and Goren (1998) identified the way in which nurses stigmatise certain patients, including those who are suicidal. This results in nurses distancing themselves from patients and minimising the contact they have with them. Jameton (1992) described this as the 'dark side of nursing'. Reflective practice and work such as Corley's enabled me to see that on a personal level I needed to understand why I responded in the way I did, and that without understanding DSH I could not change. I conclude from her work that amongst other reasons the overriding factor for my thoughts/feelings/actions is my upbringing, my nurse training, and my life as a whole; all have moulded my beliefs/moral opinion. I now understand that I need to view patients and respond beyond the 'label', to see these attempted suicides/self-harmers as people/individuals needing help. Chris has challenged me to examine my boundaries as an A&E nurse, whether my role only required that the damage was 'patched up'? I answered that I knew my feelings, however well hidden, were picked up by patients and this ultimately affected their care. Corley cites Younger (1995) as suggesting that nurses protect themselves from being overwhelmed by suffering by distancing themselves from the sufferer. I feel that I distance myself for more than one emotional reason; fear, anger, resentment and lack of empathy come quickly to mind. Distancing myself from patients has certainly been a tactic I have used in the past. I am beginning to understand that I have used this in the past as a way of protecting myself.

In the session Chris had challenged me to consider ways of framing my growth of effective practice. I felt that one significant issue was a growing sense of empowerment to act according to new beliefs and changed attitudes. He introduced me to some 'empowerment models' that I could review. Of these I chose to use Kieffer's (1984) 'stages of availability' model. I am currently in what Kieffer describes as the 'era of entry'. He explains that an individual who moves through this stage is motivated because they have experienced an emotionally significant or symbolic episode. Particularly significant was my comment that the wound must hurt when he cut himself, so why was he worried about the pain of stitches? Kieffer states that this symbolic event triggers or initiates a period of reactive engagement.

Moving from avoidance towards connection

In session three Chris picked up on the issue of avoidance from the last session.

> *Chris:* 'When we last met you realised that you had been using "avoidance" as a coping mechanism, has anything new developed?'
> *Jane:* 'Becoming conscious that I was using avoidance was a step forward in itself; I had been using that time of "avoidance" to "get my thoughts together". I wanted to work out how I would overcome that first hurdle and try and care for DSH patients in a "better" way.'
> *Chris:* 'Have you had any patient interaction since we met?'
> *Jane:* 'Yes I have. In fact I went out of my way to nurse a DSH patient. I spoke to my colleagues on shift and asked them if I could "take" DSH patients ... it wasn't what I expected at all. I took handover of a DSH patient and went into the cubicle explaining what clinical

procedures were needed. I acted in a way that I wouldn't usually. I gave what I hoped was a warm smile. I pushed negative feelings to the side.'

Chris: 'Just remind me of those feelings you usually experience when dealing with a DSH patient.'

Jane: 'That it's a cry for attention, not as "deserving" of my attention/care as other patients. They are often time wasters; I could be helping someone who really needs it!'

Chris: 'We have already discussed why you feel this way?'

Jane: 'Yes, I understand my past experiences that make me feel this way. I do want to do something about it; it is hard though… I asked Andrew very directly why he had taken an overdose. He said his life was a mess, his mother didn't care. He was thin, a little emaciated, I did feel sorry for him.'

Chris: 'How did it feel to ask him why he had taken an overdose?'

Jane: 'I felt very, very clumsy. I stumbled over my words, I felt hot and uncomfortable.'

Chris: 'Why do you think you felt this way?'

Jane: 'I know that if he had answered my question, I wouldn't have known how to respond. I didn't do any psychiatric training; I wouldn't be able to fulfil his needs. He might ask for something I can't give.'

Chris: 'What do you usually do when you don't have an answer? Usually if something happens at work that you don't understand, what would you do?'

Jane: 'Well I suppose I ask someone for help.'

Chris: 'So if a DSH patient asks for something that you don't understand you could refer to a colleague who could help, couldn't you? I think your statement that "he might ask for something I can't give" is more significant. Is this more to do with your beliefs?'

Jane: 'I suppose what I really mean is that he/she may ask me to understand them, have knowledge of whatever disorder/mental illness they have. I don't think I have it inside me to understand. I want to change, I want to give more than clinical care, but I find these patients mentally draining. It's scary to think that someone can be so desperate.'

Chris: 'This time you have given more than clinical care. You asked Andrew why he had taken the overdose, didn't you? Ok, so you felt clumsy but that must have been important to Andrew. Has he a past history of this type of thing?'

Jane: 'Yes, he's done it several times before.'

Chris: 'What does that tell you? Do you view him less seriously? Or more seriously? You said you felt sorry for him, why?'

Jane: 'Previously, before looking at the facts and figures in literature, I would have viewed him as an attention seeker, taken him less seriously than another patient. I have discovered since we last spoke that individuals may inflict harm many times, sometimes over long periods of time. Eventually a significant number will actually commit suicide, so maybe this helps me to understand a little. I felt sorry for him because, apart from his appearance, he was very apologetic; he was compliant with his clinical care.'

Chris: 'He was a good patient?'

Jane: 'Yes, he was, I suppose.'

Chris: 'There is literature that explores the concept of "good and bad" patients. Patients who comply, "do as they are told" by the nurse or doctor. Perhaps you might be interested in exploring this for yourself. It is rather interesting that you liked him and stated that he was compliant. Perhaps if he had been non-compliant in some way or abusive you may not have felt so warm towards him. Is there anything else you want to discuss?'

Jane: 'No, I'm happy with what we've covered. I think any more would be too much for me to take in.'

Chris: 'So, to recap. Although you felt clumsy, you feel positive about your interaction and feel that you can learn from this experience, and move on? Perhaps you could think of a way

to ask patients why they have self-harmed in a different way, perhaps you could try a cathartic approach, perhaps ask what has upset them so much today that they felt the need to hurt themselves? Or perhaps a very direct approach is appropriate for a particular patient?'
Jane: 'I think I would be happier to frame the question in a different way, but my nerves got the better of me.'
Chris: 'Andrew didn't mind from what you've told me. I think the most important thing is that you wanted to ask, and you asked.'

Interpretative analysis

This was my first contact with a patient since the interaction described in session one. The dialogue reveals that this interaction, although not perfect, was a positive experience. The main clinical issue is my lack of knowledge surrounding psychiatric nursing; however I now feel empowered to change. Chris suggested that I explore the concept of 'good and bad patients'. I have begun the process of exploring literature and have previously discussed the work of Corley. I have also read the work of Kelly and May (1982) who critiqued the theory of 'good and bad patients' and explain that it is typically assumed that negative attitudes, held by nurses due to educational or technical reasons, can be corrected at the training stage. However, it would appear that for many nurses this issue is not adequately addressed. If negative attitudes had been successfully corrected surely there would not be an abundance of literature highlighting negative attitudes amongst nurses? Sociologists such as Conrad (1979) claim patients are treated according to class/attitude or illness. Kelly and May state:

'It is unlikely that problems in nurse-patient relationships will prove amenable to simplistic prescriptions since the cause of those problems is endemic of social interaction itself.' (p. 154)

The literature led me to the same answers: 'the answer is not simple', 'a wider view must be taken', 'medical models are too rigid'. I am constantly led to reflexivity; it would seem that to reflect, to know self, to be open to all the possibilities will ultimately resolve my original questions and unravel my belief system. Chris suggested that I consider why I liked Andrew and asked if it was because he was compliant with his treatment. Trexlar (1996) described 'difficult' patients as those who are perceived to act in a deviant manner, and goes on to suggest that such patients respond by adopting expected role behaviour which results in:

'stigma and social isolation that reinforces the original behaviour and may lead to secondary deviance and validation of the nurse's judgement of the patient.' (p. 132)

If Trexlar is correct in his assumption, perhaps nurses and society play some part in patients who repeatedly self-harm. Perhaps as nurses we perceive such behaviour as unacceptable, and this is picked up by the patients who continue with 'deviant' behaviour, or at the very least they do not know how to respond in any other way.

Perhaps Andrew 'tuned' into me. Here was a young man with a past history of harming himself and who was familiar with the attitude and responses of medical staff. Perhaps he manipulated the situation by turning himself from what Trexlar describes as a deviant patient to a compliant patient that provoked a caring response from his nurse. Keisler (1983) validates the concept that Andrew acted in a certain way. Nievaard (1987) cites Kiesler's classification of interpersonal behaviour, describing how attitudes of hospital patients are divided into four main groups:

- Dependent
- Self-reducing
- Co-operative
- Rebellious

Whilst understanding that Andrew's 'compliance' did affect my response to him I also believe that I felt some empathy towards him, and this comes with the dawning of understanding. I have learnt that not all individuals who attempt self-harm do so with the intent of dying. The reasons for self-harm vary and it is carried out under differing circumstances across a broad spectrum of individuals (Roberts 1996). Hawton and Catlin (1997) state that:

> 'Someone who has attempted suicide is a hundred times more likely to commit suicide than the general population within the following year.' (p. 1409)

This interaction is part of an ongoing process, I may not ever understand DSH but perhaps I will be able to change how I interact with this patient 'group'. Previously I would have dealt with this 'type' of patient differently. I would have carried out their clinical care; never before have I asked a patient 'why?'. I feel empowered to bridge the practice/theory gap, as well as being confident to examine myself. I would have said that my beliefs did not affect patient care. I now know my beliefs *do* affect not only my ability to care, but the way in which that care is delivered. Furthermore I now believe that previous patients have been aware of my feelings, something I would previously have denied.

Confronting my resistance

In session four:

> *Chris asked:* 'When we last met, you said that you wanted to continue your interaction with DSH patients and you would be cathartic in your approach?'
>
> *Jane:* 'I have had an interaction with a patient that made me feel really angry. Karl had taken an overdose. His notes revealed that he had taken a near fatal overdose twelve months previously. This really brought home the seriousness of Karl's feelings to me. I am attempting to view all DSH patients as "serious", but it was easier to view Karl seriously because of his history. I went into his cubicle, feeling open, wanting to help, wanting to be cathartic. I asked: "What upset you so much today? Something must have really upset you to do this to yourself." Karl didn't want to talk to me. He ignored me, he didn't even look at me, and his face was averted to the wall. I looked at the situation and asked myself: "How is Karl feeling, what is his main concern?" It was then I realised that his mother and brother were in the cubicle; perhaps he didn't want to talk in front of them. I asked if they would mind leaving the cubicle. I asked Karl again, he ignored me. I asked could he at least look at me, I felt my anger rising, but felt that I was managing it well.'

Chris: 'Why did you feel so angry? . . . was it because Karl wouldn't tell you why he did it?'
Jane: 'Yes and he wouldn't even look at me. There I was making all the effort, a big effort. I felt like I was falling flat on my face. Why was I even bothering? The fact that I wanted to help had no effect on Karl, he wasn't interested.'
Chris: 'You say you managed your anger, that's great. You were able to understand your anger and manage your frustration. What happened next?'
Jane: 'I told Karl that I could see he was upset, but if he wanted to talk later, I was there. I told him I would come back in a while and would be available to talk if he wanted to.'
Chris: 'So you sent a very positive message to Karl, didn't you? You let him know that you cared, you let him know you were available to him. You told him you cared enough to go back and see him later. Are you placing great emphasis on the fact that he wouldn't talk?'
Jane: 'A couple of days later I revisited the experience when I wrote in my journal. I had calmed down by then and realised that one of the reasons I wanted him to talk was because I had a need to understand. I know that Karl's reason for DSH is not the same as everyone's, but I thought he could give me some insight. The other reason for feeling angry was simply that it had taken courage on my part to offer myself, to make myself available to Karl.'
Chris: 'But you managed yourself within the unfolding moment that is a change in you, you have managed yourself with a DSH patient within the unfolding moment. You negotiated both your own resistance and Karl's resistance. It might be useful to chart this with a diagram. It will demonstrate the progress you are making.'

Interpretative analysis

I now feel happier, more comfortable and appreciate my interaction with Karl through new eyes. I understand that I rushed in with a cathartic approach with high expectations. I realise it's all right that Karl didn't want to talk. It wasn't the right time for him, maybe it was too soon, and I can reassure myself that he will have the opportunity to talk when he is ready because, in this particular case, admission to hospital was required. Again the empathy that I am beginning to feel is in itself motivating me towards achieving more. The most important issue is that Karl knew that I cared. I felt I managed my rising anger well and did not let it affect Karl's care. I reinforced the fact that I cared by telling him I was there if he needed me. My anger came from the fact that he didn't need me in the way I had anticipated; I understand he just needed a caring response and nothing more. Now my residual negative feelings have evaporated. I can now explore my self at a deeper level and go beyond my anxiety, as if facing a great white shark in a steel cage. I utilised the being available template (Johns 2000) as a way to view myself moving along each of the six markers that determine how available I was with Karl:

(1) *Knowing what is desirable*
    I knew that 'desirable' practice was to treat Karl in the caring way in which I would treat any other patient. I was able to manage my own concerns in order to care for Karl in the most therapeutic way I possibly could. I knew this because I had thought deeply about my personal philosophy of care and realised that to adhere to that meant changes in my practice.

(2) *Knowing the person*
    I had made a huge effort to try and make some sort of connection with Karl – an 'unpolished' effort but the intent to know him as a person was there.

(3) *Concern for the person*
     I feel that I genuinely had concern for Karl.
(4) *The aesthetic response to the patient*
     I was responding to the contradiction in my practice.
(5) *Knowing and managing self's involvement with the person*
     I feel that I used new knowledge of my own feelings/thoughts and attitudes to become more aware of my response to Karl as a person.
(6) *Creating and sustaining an environment where being available is possible*
     In managing my own concerns I was able to negotiate my own resistance as well as Karl's. I tried to provide the best environment in the given circumstances. He was in a private cubicle, I asked his relatives to leave allowing him more privacy and I let him know that I wanted to care for him.

I am experiencing a great sense of motivation. Using the reciprocation-resistance scale I could see the way that both Karl and I resisted each other because I had not tuned into his wave-length adequately (Johns 1999). As Chris suggested, I need to imagine a space between us so I can see these things unfolding, yet remain available to Karl even as he resisted me.

Nurturing my concern

I had been looking forward to sharing and examining my thoughts and feelings with Chris in session five, possibly because I felt that I'd made real progress. He started session five by asking what I had to share since our last meeting and I was able to tell him about the literature I had discovered and read.

Jane: 'I have been reading literature surrounding the attitude of nurses with regard to DSH. I've also experienced another patient interaction. He's a man in his 40s, who had taken a large overdose. He had visited his estranged wife and when she refused to let him into the house, he sat down in her garden and took a massive overdose. She wasn't aware that he was still in her garden and some hours later a passer-by called an ambulance. To say that I interacted with him is debatable. I carried out his clinical care, but he was unconscious, quite ill in fact so I didn't actually speak to him.'
Chris: 'How did you feel about this man?'
Jane: 'I felt really sad. Sad that he had felt so desperate. Sad that he could die. Sad that maybe he didn't mean to kill himself, perhaps he just wanted his partner to come outside and talk. I felt sad that his estranged wife would probably feel guilty and blame herself. I just felt incredibly sad. I think I saw the seriousness of DSH, the desperation, and the waste.'
Chris: 'This is new for you isn't it, this sympathy?'
Jane: 'Obviously I felt sad when DSH patients have died in the past, but perhaps not as sad as, for example, a victim of a road traffic accident, or a child.'
Chris: 'You feel differently now?'
Jane: 'Reflection has made me think differently about all sorts of things, not just in the workplace; it's "bigger" than that! A combination of these sessions, keeping a journal and learning about DSH are beginning to affect my thought processes and the way in which I interact with this patient group.'

Interpretative analysis

I felt this experience was very significant. I found myself caring for this man at a time when everything I've been thinking about is falling into place. As a result of more understanding my whole attitude is changing. The belief system and moral opinion is being replaced by new values, brought about new insights.

I have now entered Kieffer's (1984) second stage of his 'stages of availability', known as 'maturation of empowerment'. Kieffer identifies three key elements needed to successfully move into 'maturation of empowerment'. The first of the three quite distinct and necessary elements is the focus and stability of a mentoring relationship. The relationship I have with my supervisor has been extremely stable and has focused on relevant and significant issues. The second distinct element is supportive peer relationships within a collective organisational structure. My practice area is the organisational structure and most of my peers/colleagues have been curious and supportive of my research. I hope that my research on an individual level will induce a collective action towards change. The third documented element is a more critical understanding of social and political relations. Literature has provided a deeper understanding that I have and am constantly critically analysing.

Realising right attitude

Chris started session six by reviewing our last meeting and asking about new interactions. I felt very comfortable, relaxed and exhilarated; I had been waiting to tell Chris about an interaction that had gone very well.

> *Jane:* 'I've had another interaction with a DSH patient. A young man in his twenties, he arrived in the early hours of the morning. He had taken some paracetemol tablets, not many; he was very distressed. He kept saying "sorry" and apologising for wasting the nurse's time. I found that instead of offering no reply to this statement or giving a half-hearted "you're not wasting anyone's time" I actually wanted to talk to him. I sensed that he wanted to talk; he had financial worries and girlfriend problems. It all tumbled out very quickly. I was only supposed to be carrying out triage (a two to three minute assessment in order to categorise his problem, which dictates how quickly someone should be seen by a doctor), but found myself talking to him for at least 15 minutes. The department was not busy, so instead of handing his care over to someone else, I took him into a cubicle and continued to talk. At all times during my interaction, I was aware of my concern for him. I felt tender towards him; I had a strong desire to help by simply listening. I know that he appreciated my concern for him and I know that he felt I was genuine in my concern. He had to stay in the department for several hours awaiting results of blood tests; he was assessed by a doctor who discharged him (his friend was going to stay with him overnight, and ensure he attended an out-patient appointment in the morning).'
>
> *Chris:* 'This sounds like a very positive experience for you. Why do you think you "wanted" to talk to him, what surfaced your concern, why did you feel tender?'
>
> *Jane:* 'Well I was very conscious of "reflecting" within the moment, of reading his pattern. The more concern I felt, the better I felt. I wasn't hiding anything from myself. I viewed him as a person, not a condition. I used the model of structured reflection, asking myself who is this person? What does he need from me at this moment, how can I help him? Using those cues really helped me to focus on an individual human. By focusing on him

and him alone, I was able to ignore any misconceptions about patients who deliberately self harm.'

Interpretative analysis

My belief system is very different now. I feel happier within myself now I am more available to patients. Focusing on the third element of the being available template, 'concern for the person', highlights that I now feel motivated to care, to express my empathy and am discovering that such expression opens up new possibilities for the relationships I develop with patients. While I believe my care giving remains balanced, I am discovering the more I 'give' the more I 'get' from shared relationships. My beliefs and values have been exposed and examined for their meaning and relevance. My response to DSH patients has changed; there is a positive shift towards more congruent practice.

Knock back

In session seven I was feeling quite 'down' about my recent experiences but felt comfortable enough about my relationship with Chris to discuss what I considered to be fairly negative interactions.

Jane: 'I feel as if I've taken two steps forward and three back! I don't quite know where to start. I've had what I consider a very "negative" experience and a positive one, and I don't understand why. I know that I shouldn't blame myself, but I do feel guilty about the negative interaction I had.'

Chris: 'Describe the negative experience first.'

Jane: 'Well the shift was really busy; it was over the New Year period that a young girl presented in the department after taking an overdose. Her friend had recently committed suicide. She was hysterical, and I could not calm her down. At the start of our interaction, I reminded myself that here was a young girl who had lost a friend in traumatic circumstances. As I've already said the shift was busy, and there were other patients close by who were very ill. In order to be fair to this patient and other patients in the department I needed to calm her down. I had conflicting priorities: my other patients needed a quiet calm atmosphere, but I needed to take control with this patient and I was failing. The more hysterical she became the more irritation I felt; my anger was rising up inside me. I thought she was silly, a "drama queen". Obviously I understood she was grieving for her friend, but I was under pressure, it was two o'clock in the morning and I think alcohol played a part in her behaviour.'

Chris: 'So she wasn't a "good" patient?'

Jane: 'No! Her father wasn't any help either; he had also been drinking and their relationship did not come across as particularly close. I hoped that her father would calm her down, but he seemed to cause yet more hysteria. I felt she needed to be told her behaviour was unacceptable. I told her that I wanted to help but couldn't if she wouldn't let me. Nothing I tried worked.'

Chris: 'What happened next?'

Jane: 'I thought it was in the patient's best interest to hand over her care to someone else. I felt that I had made no connection with her and that I could not manage my feelings. It was best for the patient and myself to be removed from the situation. She was moved away from the poorly patients, the second nurse was firmer than I was, she eventually calmed down, and I don't know what happened after that.'

Chris: 'Do you think you adopted a parental role with her because her mother was absent and her father "useless"? That you took on the role of a critical mother? You perhaps wanted to tell her off?'

Jane: 'I wasn't conscious of taking on a parental role but being a mother myself it's an easy role to fall into. Anyway if I unconsciously took on a parental role it didn't work, did it? I didn't even get to the point of thinking about deliberate harm!'

Chris: 'What about the other patient you mentioned?'

Jane: 'This is where my confusion lies. A few days later another young girl, about the same age, came to the department. She was at school, brought in by the class teacher; she had taken a small overdose. I was completely different with this patient; I was able to talk to her and let her know my concern was genuine.'

Chris: 'What factors changed the outcome of this interaction? Was it late at night? Were you tired? Were you busy?'

Jane: 'It was a day shift 9 or 10 in the morning. It was quiet in the department.'

Chris: 'Do you think the business of the department makes a difference in the way self-harmers are treated?'

Jane: 'I'd like to say no, but every ward, every department works under pressure. When it's busy it's impossible to give that little bit more. As awful as it sounds, time can be an influencing factor. We all try to make time, to make the most of our time, but sometimes it isn't enough.'

Chris: 'Have you come across any supporting literature?'

Jane: 'Yes an abundance of literature suggests that time influences attitudes of nurses towards DSH patients.'

Chris: 'We know that "time" affected you; with the second girl you had more time, you've also said it was a day shift. Perhaps you were more receptive to her needs because you weren't tired yourself?'

Jane: 'I was able to ask her why she had self-harmed and we discussed other things that she could have done instead of taking the tablets. She had taken them because her mum wouldn't let her visit her boyfriend the night before. I don't think she did it to manipulate her mother. I think she did it because she felt so desperate about not seeing him. She agreed that a preferable course of action would be to talk to someone, a nurse, a teacher, her mum, or a friend. I think she actually learnt from the experience, she took something positive away with her.'

Chris: 'Do you think that again you took on a parental role?'

Jane: 'In this case I think I did.'

Chris: 'Apart from time constraints, could anything else account for the difference in your interaction with these two young girls?'

Jane: 'Yes, I was definitely conscious of my previous interaction. I didn't want to get it wrong again.'

Chris: 'So you learnt from your previous experience, you reflected on it and from what you describe as a negative experience comes a positive one?'

Jane: 'That's perhaps a better way to look at it.'

Interpretative analysis

I felt that my response to the second patient in this instance was more congruent with my newly developed values. With the first patient, within the unfolding moment I felt that I could not manage my own concerns and care for the patient. It was in the patient's best interests to receive care from another nurse. Guidance encouraged me to examine the variables. The variables are as follows:

- Time constraints
- Concern for other patients in my care
- Workload
- Time patients present to the department.

Greenwood and Bradley (1997) state that the majority of DSH patients present to A&E departments 'out of hours' and confirm this with an audit of DSH time presentation. They suggest this may contribute towards negative attitudes due to difficulty in accessing psychiatric services 'out of hours'. Speaking from a personal perspective I agree that most DSH patients present during the early hours of the morning or late at night. This means on a night shift it is typical to care for at least one patient who has self-harmed. During a night shift 'enthusiasm' may not be at the same level as during the day, thus making it easier to respond in a negative, incongruent way. Time constraints come hand in hand with workload, more patients to care for, resulting in less time for each patient. The human response is to critique each other on meeting for the first time. McLaughlin (1994) states: 'Nursing can readily lend itself to the rapid formation of attitudes towards those who come into contact with it' (p. 1111).

McLaughlin further suggests that initial contact, in addition to confidential information about the patient, can lead to negative attitudes, resulting in influencing the quality of care and jeopardising the nurse-patient relationship. In a busy department, variables such as time constraints and workload can easily produce dysfunctional attitudes that can lead on from initial patient interactions. This is something I have come to understand, and armed with this knowledge, aim to change. Concern for the other patients in my care was also an influencing factor. On reflection, all patients, including the young girl, benefited from being moved from one room to another. Initially she was in 'resus' (a large room equipped with several beds used for patients requiring life saving interventions) and on reflection, the room may have been very frightening for her; she was moved into a separate cubicle, which provided privacy for not only her and her family but for the other patients. She also benefited from receiving care from a nurse who was able to manage her own concerns and was tuned into the patient. I gained from the interaction because I reflected on the interaction, and learnt from the experience.

Only a few days later I met another girl, also around 15 years of age, who had overdosed and this time I was really happy with the way in which I responded and cared for her. I was able to do this because guided reflection had produced a new insight into the previous interaction, in addition to all of the other interactions. Mezirow (1981) states:

> 'Our meaning structures are transformed through reflection, defined here as attending to the grounds (justification) for one's beliefs. We reflect on the unexamined assumptions of our beliefs when the beliefs are not working well for us, or where old ways of thinking are no longer functional. We are confronted with a disorientating dilemma, which serves as a trigger for reflection. Reflection involves a critique of assumptions to determine whether the belief, often acquired through cultural assimilation in childhood, remains functional for us as adults. We do this by critically examining its origins, nature, and consequences.' (p. 223)

My belief system was not working for me; this triggered reflection, which has changed the meaning in the way I deal with patients. The meaning is revised and is still changing with each experience and new knowledge. This is made valid by the very fact that the next interaction provoked a caring response. Obviously variables were different. It was during the day, quite early in the shift, the workload was light and I could concentrate on her care. Throughout our interaction I remembered the other teenager. Again I dealt with a teenager verging on hysteria, quite difficult to deal with; our interaction could easily have spiralled into a negative experience for both of us. However, whilst managing my own concerns I successfully met her needs. I no longer fear involvement with such patients. As Benner and Wrubel (1989) believe, connecting with my caring is one of the most effective coping resources.

Reflection

At the outset I was concerned that any changes I made to my practice (in relation to DSH patients) would leave me in a vulnerable position. Benner and Wrubel (1989) believe that emotions can no longer be viewed as interruptions. By this they believe emotions have significance and content in their own right and that respect for knowledge and wisdom is gained if the individual allows their emotions to direct their thoughts and attention. They state:

> 'Attending to emotion offers the possibility of bringing a past interpretation of the situation into the present, where past history can be reinterpreted and reconstituted.' (p. 96)

How true. As a result of my understanding about my beliefs, a host of factors including cultural and religious beliefs emerged that influenced the way I was responding to DSH patients. Being brought up in a predominately Christian society with strong cultural beliefs about self-harm and suicide has obviously affected my belief system. As recently as 1961, suicide and attempted suicide fell into the same category as murder and there were a number of prosecutions.

Decriminalisation in 1966 did not lead to any great change to the belief systems that existed. McLaughlin (1994) states: 'In the Judeo-Christian cultures there has always been a belief that suicide is reprehensible and ethically wrong' (p. 1112). Other factors contributing to my previous belief system included lived experiences with patients. Accepting my mother's failing health and the seriousness of her condition dissolved some of my anger. I recognised that because I worked in an acute area, I had fallen into a trap of measuring, quantifying or prioritising patients and their conditions. Fear that lack of knowledge would make 'a bad situation worse' played a part in my incongruent practice.

A debate was held with colleagues when they expressed an interest in my research. They were divided on their own feelings about DSH patients. Whilst some felt they firmly understood and treated the patient group in exactly the same way they would any other, not all felt this way. Some found themselves, perhaps like myself somewhere in the middle, lacking real knowledge of self-harm and experiencing difficulty with caring for such patients. Some felt that DSH patients were time wasters who manipulated both nurses and the medical system. One co-worker stated that she was 'resigned' to nursing DSH patients. I asked her to explain and she said that the only DSH patients we ever met were those in crisis. She further explained that we never saw patients that 'got better', 'recovered'. The comments made are similar to those documented by Anderson *et al.* (1999) on the attitude of medical staff towards the suicidal. Data was collected by age, gender, profession and length of service. Anderson *et al.* state that 'nurses and doctors do not support the notion that suicidal behaviour reflects mental illness' (p. 8). One staff nurse who took part in the research stated:

> 'Sometimes I think they are time wasters – occasionally, and quite selfish – if you have a good reason to self harm then that's that … but if not then I think it's quite selfish.' (p. 6)

These were some of my own thoughts prior to researching the subject. The debate allowed thoughts and feelings to rise to the surface and whilst I was not able to change my colleagues' opinion, perhaps a seed was sown, a seed that may surface later, at a time that is right for the individual to address their own contradictions. When others choose to address their own contradictions perhaps a paradigm shift from the normal approach to a different approach will occur. Anderson *et al.* (1999) cites Oppenhem's (1992) definition of attitude as 'Reacting in a certain manner when confronted with a specific stimuli' (p. 2). Anderson *et al.* suggest that attitudes towards DSH are complex, multidimensional, and the interaction between nurse and patient will depend on their belief system of each other. Repper (1999) discusses the importance of the role of A&E staff, given that they work at the interface of all other components. Repper highlights the fact that:

> 'Poor information and communication systems, lack of knowledge about suicide, negative attitudes towards people who self-harm do not help the rising number of patients presenting with DSH.' (p. 11)

Repper advises that A&E staff become more involved with education/training and that negative attitudes are challenged.

I have gained new knowledge about self-harm and this has helped to create a shift in attitude; I hope that my research will present a challenge to others, create a new paradigm enabling others to find a more therapeutic way of responding.

These factors accumulated and merged together and this led me towards superficially questioning the value of my intervention, and the little or no return I anticipated from such a patient group. Without reflection I could go no further than to superficially question my contradiction; without reflection I was left to ignore the contradiction in my practice that bubbled beneath the surface. Moss (1988) states:

> 'If nursing is to attain the status of an independent profession it must identify and rectify the factors that influence nursing attitudes.' (p. 616)

I feel that I have addressed the factors that have influenced my attitudes, and quite possibly the attitudes of other nurses, and in doing so have redefined my belief system. In recognising the biases I had previously anchored in my belief system I have discovered myself as a person and have found that this in itself naturally leads to 'tuning' into others and their needs. My learning and understanding have travelled full cycle, described by Gadamer (1979) as an oscillating cycle that continuously evolves. My empowerment to act came from within because I had experienced enlightenment. Empowerment brought with it the knowledge and courage to act in ways that brought about changes to my practice. Emancipation, or the realisation that I had achieved it, came quite recently. My arms around a woman in great distress, crying a steady stream of tears, I found myself reflecting-within-the-moment (Johns 2000), suddenly realising I genuinely cared. I had not needed to prompt myself for the best verbal response. We were talking as I carried out clinical observations, but I was so in 'tune' with this woman I instinctively knew what she wanted from me. I sat next to her and her tears began. She physically moved towards me; I believe she sensed my empathy and the genuineness of my caring response. As I encircled her in my arms I felt emotional, I felt sadness for her, but realised the truth of Ramos' (1992) words when she stated:

> 'Nurses described an emotional identification which was real, not devastating to the nurse, but a motivator' (p. 504).

I felt very positive, I felt that a burden had been lifted from my shoulders. Ramos describes such a relationship as a reciprocal relationship and the very cornerstone of nursing care. I wanted to hold this woman because she needed me to hold her and I felt very comfortable about doing so. With this interaction came the realisation that I had entered Kieffer's (1984) final stage – the 'era of commitment'. Kieffer believes individuals may struggle at this stage as they try to integrate personal knowledge and skill into everyday situations. The reader will already be aware of my struggle to integrate newly acquired knowledge through shared dialogue and patient interaction. I see beyond any previous understanding and I have evolved into a practitioner that has found a therapeutic way of responding.

References

Alston, M. & Robinson, B. (1992) Nurses' attitudes towards suicide. *Omega*, 25(3) 205–15.

Anderson, M. (1999) Waiting for harm: deliberate self-harm and suicide in young people – a review of the literature. *Journal of Psychiatric and Mental Health Nursing*, 6, 91–100.

Anderson, M., Standen, P., Nazir, S. & Noon, J. (1999). Nurses' and doctors' attitudes towards suicidal behaviour in young people. *International Journal of Nursing Studies*, 37, 1–10.

Benner, P. & Wrubel, J. (1989) *The Primacy of Caring*. Addison-Wesley, Menlo Park.

Carveth, J. (1995) Perceived patient deviance and avoidance by nurses. *Nursing Research*, 44, 173–8.

Conrad, P. (1979) Types of medical social control. *Sociology of Health and Illness*, 1, 1–10.

Corley, M. & Goren, S. (1998) The dark side of nursing: impact of stigmatising responses on patients. *Scholarly Inquiry for Nursing Practice: An International Journal*, 12(2) 99–121.

DoH (1998) *Our Healthier Nation: a contract for health*. Department of Health, London.

Eldrid, J. (1988) *Caring For The Suicidal*. Constable, London.

Fairburn, G. (1995) *Contemplating Suicide: The language and ethics of self-harm*. Routledge, London.

Gadamer, H-G. (1979) *Truth and Method*, 2nd edn. Sheed & Ward, London.

Greenwood, S. & Bradley, P. (1997) Managing deliberate self-harm. the A&E perspective. *Accident and Emergency Nursing*, 5, 134–6.

Hawton, K. & Catlin, J. (1997) *Attempted Suicide: a practical guide to its nature and management.* Oxford University Press, London.

Hawton, K. & Fagg, J. (1992) Trends in deliberate self poisoning and self injury in Oxford 1976–1990. *British Medical Journal*, 304, 1409–11.

Jameton, A. (1992) *Nursing Ethics and the Moral Situation of the Nurse.* American Hospital Publishing, Chicago.

Johns, C. (1999) Caring connections: knowing self within caring relationships through reflection. *International Journal for Human Caring*, 3(2) 31–8.

Johns, C. (2000) *Becoming a Reflective Practitioner.* Blackwell Science, Oxford.

Keisler, D.J. (1983) The 1982 interpersonal circle: a taxonomy for complementarity in human transactions. *Psychological Review*, 90, 185–214.

Kelly, P. & May, D. (1982) Good and bad patients: a review of the literature and a theoretical critique. *Journal of Advanced Nursing*, 7, 147–56.

Kieffer, C. (1984) Citizen empowerment: a developmental perspective. *Prevention in Human Sciences*, 84(3) 9–36.

Lynn, F. (1998) The pain of rejection. *Nursing Times*, 94, 27.

McLaughlin, C. (1991) Parasuicide counselling in casualty departments. *Nursing Standard*, 6(8) 15.

McLaughlin, C. (1994) Casualty nurses' attitudes to attempted suicide. *Journal of Advanced Nursing*, 20, 1111–18.

Mezirow, J. (1981) A critical theory of adult learning and education. *Adult Education*, 32(1) 3–24.

Moss, A. (1988) Determinants of nursing care: nursing process or nursing attitudes. *Journal of Advanced Nursing*, 13(5) 615–20.

Neivaard, A. (1987) Communication climate and patient care: causes and effects of nurses' attitudes to patients. *Social Science and Medicine*, 24(9) 777–84.

Oppenheim, A.N. (1992) *Questionnaire Design, Interviewing and Attitude Measurement.* Pinter, London.

Ramos, M. (1992) The nurse-patient relationship: theme and variations. *Journal of Advanced Nursing*, 17, 496–506.

Repper, J. (1999) A review of literature on the prevention of suicide through interventions in Accident and Emergency Departments. *Journal of Clinical Nursing*, 8, 3–12.

Roberts, D. (1996) Suicide prevention by general nurses. *Nursing Standard*, 17, 30–33.

Trexlar, T. (1996) Reformulation of deviance and labelling theory for nursing. *Image: Journal of Nursing Scholarship*, 28(2) 131–6.

Watson, J. (1999) *Post Modern Nursing and Beyond.* Churchill Livingstone, Edinburgh.

Younger, J. (1995) The alienation of the sufferer. *Advances in Nursing Science*, 17, 53–72.

Chapter 10

Working with Women Following Traumatic Childbirth

Bella Madden

This research is a reflective journey on my own practice, in order to more fully comprehend the nature of a specific series of events. Using journal entries I made over a six month period whilst in clinical practice, I have attempted to uncover the political nature of the care in question – listening visits to women requiring some form of 'debriefing' post childbirth. This is not research about the issues raised by these women at the time, but rather the effect they had on me as a practitioner as I examined my interaction with these women during 'listening visits'. This is a story about my own development as a practitioner, triggered by the stories these women were unfolding to me as they struggled with their own journeys. This is a story about how their voices led me to challenge my own practices and beliefs about midwifery, and about the realisation of the political nature of all practice interventions and innovations. This is a story about finding a different voice.

Background

Recently within midwifery, there have been moves to explore the value of debriefing or listening services for women following childbirth (Lavendar & Wilkinshaw 1998). This movement arises from a cluster of related developments asserting that listening to women is inherently good (Audit Commission 1997; Butler & Jackson 1998); that it gives women a chance to have a voice and also provides feedback on the quality of caregiving within organisations (Marchant & Garcia 2000). Linked to this is a growing body of research showing that the childbirth experience itself can have far-reaching, traumatising concequences for women (Ballard *et al.* 1995; Menage 1996) and that we should be offering services for women who require a safe place within which to offload their memories, fears and anxieties (DoH 1999; Axe 2000).

Visits typically lasted between one and two hours, and took place as soon after referral as possible (usually within two weeks). The offer of a visit at home was always readily accepted, the rationale being to minimise the influence of a medical environment on the dialogue. On reflection, many of these women would not have been willing to come to the hospital, as there were too many painful, negative memories associated with it. It also seemed to be a more sensitive response to their needs to move the interview away from the hospital, as being a guest in someone else's house diffuses the medical gaze. Following each visit I wrote notes of the discussion and my impressions of the meeting that are the data for this research.

If the core concern of this research is the quality of caregiving, then a range of professional and government agendas support the endeavour. *Changing Childbirth* (DoH 1993) calls upon the maternity services to ensure parity of power and choice between women. The push for the provision of 'women-centred care' finds its first authoritative expression through this report, and is echoed again in subsequent follow-up reports (Audit Commission 1997). Our duty as midwives to care for others is one of the fundamentals within the Midwives Rules and Code of Conduct (UKCC 1998), and *Practitioner Client Relationships and the Prevention of Abuse* (UKCC 1999) provides us with detailed insight into all the possible forms of abusive relationships within healthcare settings, and our duty to identify them in order to eradicate abuse.

From a moral standpoint, a democratic healthcare system would be one in which people all have a voice. This is where this research originated, with the attempt to create an official space for women's voices. Having created this space however, it is imperative that the released voices are not shouting into the wilderness – there must be listening and meaningful dialogue. The current emphasis within midwifery on the setting up of listening/debriefing services (DoH 1999) requires closer scrutiny. There is a dearth of evidence that such services are of any benefit, and some that they may even be harmful (Robinson 1998). But equally, there is confusion as to what exactly 'debriefing' is in the context of these particular services springing up within the maternity sector (Alexander 1998). While this research cannot hope to answer the first question (is it useful?) it should go some way towards an exploration of the second (what is it?).

What I hope comes out of this is a greater understanding of the possibility of the visit being therapeutic. For although the interest here is in my own part of the dialogue, it is also true that I am looking at my responses to the needs and distress of others – and these needs will be an important part of the research also. What I am looking at is the process of allowing those concerns to be voiced into an environment that acknowledges them, values them, and uses them to change practice. From a 'common sense' viewpoint, listening or debriefing services are seen as unproblematic. I have spoken to many colleagues whose idea of such a service revolves mainly around 'telling the woman what happened and why', or worse, 'finding out which midwives are upsetting women, and reprimanding them'.

I am still left with a crisis of confidence though, as I oscillate between believing passionately in the worth of such a venture, and worrying about the levels of introspection involved. Jack Whitehead helps me out (Johns & Whitehead 1999):

'My responses to the questions "Why bother?", "To what purpose?", engage with my fundamental values, purposes and understandings ... My reasons for holding this particular space ... include my values of social justice. I am thinking of social justice in terms of enabling the voices to be heard, of those whose embodied knowledge has been eliminated from academic discourse through the imposition of technical rationality.' (p. 109)

The fundamental values, purposes and understandings I hold are embodied not only in the research focus, but also in the methodological choices I have made.

Within the confines of this research, reflection was initially a guided process between myself and my tutor/supervisor as I undertook the initial listening visits. I have no data from these sessions upon which to draw in this analysis, but acknowledge their importance as setting a blueprint for the subsequent self-directed journey.

The data and data analysis

The journal is an interplay of texts: a woman's articulation of the memory of her baby's birth, and my interpretation of this articulation. Analysis of the journal could therefore be from a variety of perspectives and levels. In the first, there are the stories themselves, expressions for the most part of distress and discomfort. Self-selected samples of women needing to be heard have relayed their narratives to me. The notes arising from these narratives, however, whilst conveying something of their stories do not capture their experiences in sufficient depth for an analysis of common themes and categories (and I might question the underlying agenda of normalisation inherent in such an exercise).

Of direct relevance to this research process is Holbrook's (1995) assertion that:

> 'personal document research not only liberates the client's voice from the often oppressive assumptions of the scientific method, it can also liberate the practitioner's voice as well.' (p. 751)

But what exactly can be gained from reflection on the written word, in this context? To what do we look in order to decipher the meanings inherent in text? I propose that the following doors are available to us:

- Words reflect the values of the person uttering them; they are chosen (whether consciously or unconsciously) for their appropriateness to the moment, as judged by the author (Stewart & La Nae 1990). They are political devices in so far as they can express participants in passive or active terms, they can neutralise or activate the stories of others.
- Integrated into the language are expressions of group convention, in as much as data is filtered through pre-understandings, and the text produced by the researcher becomes the authoritative interpretation. Certain pre-understandings have social precedence over others, elevated by powerful ideologies to positions of dominance (Crowe 1998; May & Fleming 1997). In this context, I am referring to the assumed role of the midwife in the dialogue, which can be accessed by examining some the actions or behaviours that I display.
- Writing is therefore a way of creating, not merely representing, knowledge (Rolfe 1997). The issues that are addressed, as well as those left unresolved or ignored, are both significant as they signal my own priorities in the listening visit.
- There is also the question of the openness or otherwise of the journal entries. How

far do they attempt to define, restructure and control the voices of others? How collaborative are they? (Holmes 1997). I have called this factor 'permeability' in the frame in Fig. 10.1.

These questions may guide the analysis of the journal, with the intention of unearthing the ideologies competing for prominence within the text (Fig. 10.1).

Role expressions →	*What assumed roles are visible? How is this story being interpreted?*	**Words** ↓
What is not said? What is ignored? What is left unresolved?	**Personal document research: the clinical diary**	*What words are chosen and what intent do they reveal? How are people and action represented?*
↑ **The unsaid**	*How open or closed is this interpretation to the voices of others? Are all utterances filtered, or given direct expression?*	← **Permeability**

Fig. 10.1 Guide for unearthing the ideologies competing for prominence within the text.

Access to the circle can occur at any point, and the revelatory quality of each aspect will not necessarily be constant. The framework provides a hook upon which to hang the analysis; it is not presented here as a blueprint, or as exhaustive in its analytical facilitation. The desired outcome of analysis is to reach some conclusions as to the assumptions underpinning the text, the cultural templates from which they spring, and thus the interests they serve. In so doing, it is hoped that some conclusions can be drawn, in this case, as to the nature of the dialogue being represented, or the form of the intervention and the role the midwife and the woman play together.

The journal entries and analysis

Each story will be presented here as a vignette, with analysis and discussion following on two levels. The first is an analysis of my reaction to the stories, contained in the discourse created by my notes, and the second is an abstraction of themes and issues as they emerge from clusters of vignettes, according to the analytical template above.

The overall aim here is to unearth assumptions and beliefs guiding my own practice throughout the course of these visits, and for that reason the stories are presented in chronological fashion.

Ruth, Sarah and Jane

Ruth

'Ruth felt traumatised by her delivery, which was arduous. She felt that she had lost control of the events that beset her and that she could not 'move on' until she had more fully understood and come to terms with the events of her labour. I spent an hour and a half listening to her concerns and anxieties and taking her through the case notes in some detail, and she said she felt a lot happier at the end of the session. She came to a fuller understanding of the combinations of causes that led to her forceps delivery and could put her anxieties in context, and thus hopefully in perspective. I urged Ruth to contact me again should she need more help, but will make a follow-up call in approximately two weeks to see how she is.'

Immediately, a number of assumptions arise from a reading of these notes. I wanted Ruth to 'move on', to allow me to fix her perceptions through increasing her information and understanding. There is an underlying belief here then, that she was ignorant of the forces operating on her (that she had 'misunderstood' their origin) and that filling in the gaps with reference to the hospital notes had solved the problem. I sense a pedagogy at work here – that it was Ruth who needed to 'move on' and not us (health professionals). There is also a reliance on the official documentation (the hospital notes) for the answers – these notes are credited with a truth value that is not really questioned here. I have no reason to doubt that the information the notes contained helped Ruth understand her experience within the context of modern medicalised birth, but I wonder now if the issue alluded to at the start, lack of control, was addressed within this meeting. The following assumptions therefore, surface here:

- Women need more information
- Understanding and information emerge from the official story (hospital notes)
- Understanding, information and explanation will heal the hurt.

Sarah

'Sarah immediately launched into her worries about her second delivery (six years previously) – I assured her that the meconium stained liquor was not abnormal, and that her baby's Apgar [method of assessing baby's state] scores (6, 10) were satisfactory. I explained that from the notes it appeared that her blood loss at delivery was due to a relaxed uterus which was quickly rectified by IV syntocinon and Hartmanns to replace fluid loss. I explained that the loss did not constitute haemorrhage (300 ml) and that the loss had quickly subsided. Sarah wanted to discuss her first delivery also, as the epidural had not worked and she was left in pain (the epidural was eventually resited, and worked second time). She says she has had headaches ever since the epidural, which she never had before. I reassured her that others have expressed similar anxieties and traumas; Sarah said it made her feel much better to realise that she is not alone and that whilst not absolutely trouble-free, her labours were not life threatening. She now better understood the chain of events and wishes that this service had been available when she needed it six years ago!'

The discourse inherent in this entry is overwhelmingly normalising. I have concentrated on her baby's 'satisfactory' Apgar scores, and her blood loss that was 'quickly rectified' (and did not amount to haemorrhage anyway). I 'assured', 'explained' and 'reassured', all of which appeared to lead to Sarah feeling 'much better' and grateful for the service. The three assumptions listed above are present again, with the emphasis on information-giving and a reliance on the hospital notes. There seems also to be a fourth assumption:

- Women do not understand what traumatic really is; if only they knew how bad it could get, they would be more prepared.

This last assumption is evident in the penultimate sentence, when I refer to the anxieties and traumas of others, and the fact that her labour was not 'life threatening'; underlying that assertion is the idea that only life-threatening labours are the ones to get really worried about.

As far as I have recorded, I have ignored the problem of Sarah's headaches, which are noted but not addressed. Additionally, there is the repeated use of the term 'loss' instead of bleeding, or blood. I wonder if that was the term I actually used when talking to Sarah, as it seems to be a device that sanitises the physical and emotional reality of bleeding. It is probably even more significant that I used it to myself – significant of a 'professional' (and medical) stance that denotes a certain distance from the messy reality of vaginal bleeding during childbirth.

Jane

'Nothing really specific here – no complaints about care – praise for her second midwife who looked after her in labour particularly. Left shocked and "traumatised" by degree of pain. Was very tense in labour but felt this was due to personal politics between her labour companions. Explained effects of tension on pain levels. Took Jane through labour chronologically to sort out any misunderstandings or gaps in memory. Reassured her that a second stage of one hour 20 minutes not at all unusual for first vaginal birth, and explained reasons for midwives wanting IV access (previous c/section). Jane did not appear "let down" – I felt that she was relieved knowing that everything was "normal". Interview ended abruptly when her partner came in and Jane obviously felt uneasy and signalled for us to finish.'

Reading this entry, it seems clear to me that I may have been missing a huge clue as to the reason for the visit. I write 'no complaints about care' and this seems to leave me feeling a little out of place. Again, I am concerned to explain, 'sort out gaps in her memory' via the hospital notes, 'reassure' and help Jane to realise that everything was normal. I cannot help but feel that my opening phrase – 'Nothing really specific here' – belies my agenda. I was there actually to manage complaints (even though I did not see my role as such at the time), and when there was none, I was not sure what I was listening for. This woman was shocked and 'traumatised' (why did I put that word in speech marks?) by pain, was tense due to 'personal politics' around her (and I remember that her birth companions were her partner and her sister), and the interview ended 'abruptly' with a signal from Jane to stop because she felt 'uneasy'. If I had seen the message at the time, I did not act on it. Jane's behaviour could quite easily be interpreted as the desperate summoning of help from someone in an abusive relationship. Even now, I remember the odd feeling in that house, and the forced jollity and Jane's ever-present nervousness and constant watching of the door, even though she was very articulate and outgoing. It is only in retrospect that I can articulate this, but I feel a frustration that I cannot return and ask Jane the questions I believe she may have wanted to have been asked. I am normalising, informing, explaining, and am rather perplexed when Jane does not seem really to require it.

Summary: Ruth, Sarah and Jane

Taking these three visit entries together, what can be learnt about the way I saw my role, and the 'cultural templates' (Fig. 10.2) that informed my actions and behaviour at the time, as well as my recording of these events?

Role expressions →	Midwife as expert/leader Midwife as fixer/healer	Words and language ↓
Ruth's loss of control Sarah's headaches Jane's relationship	**Ruth** **Sarah** **Jane**	Assured, reassured, explained Loss rectified
↑ **The unsaid/ignored**	No direct expression of others' voices. Filtered emotions and feelings	← **Permeability**

Fig. 10.2   Ruth, Sarah and Jane's cultural template.

There is a feeling now, looking back on these visits, that it was important for me to leave with a sense of completion, of resolution. I wanted a beginning, middle and end; a referral, a visit and a woman healed of the scar of her experience. I believed that information and education would provide the balm, and that women did not realise just how traumatic birth was. It was as if my approach was, 'Yes, I hear you had a dreadful time, and I am sorry, but that is only to be expected'. I had not as yet seen this assumption within myself, and could not monitor the effect it had on the listening activities. I am not arguing that there is no merit in such an approach, but I would argue that it de-politicises both the woman and the midwife. In a sense my approach was pedagogical – the midwife as expert, the woman as lacking enough knowledge to put her experience in a wider context, and thus 'in perspective'.

Dawn, Flo and Wilma

The entries for Dawn, Flo and Wilma show, I believe, a slight shifting of my concerns.

Dawn

'General lack of direction within the delivery process – i.e. fetal distress to decision for c/section to preparation for c/section to consultant review and much 'heated discussion' in the delivery room, back to decision to go for vaginal delivery. Dawn and partner felt uninformed and traumatised by the event. Dawn had been on medication for PND (postnatal depression) and cannot think of hospitals and medical personnel without having flashbacks. We went through Dawn and partner's perception of events and tied them into the notes. I tried to answer any queries they had regarding reasons for certain decisions and the nature of midwifery/obstetric care, i.e. constant re-evaluation of care and management as labour progresses. Peter and Dawn were given the opportunity to relay their concerns in detail – it was clear that Peter felt quite traumatised by the events. Dawn had been suicidal two weeks ago, which was when the GP became involved, and she had started antidepressants. Dawn was unwilling to see her CPN [community psychiatric nurse] – I reassured her that there would be no stigma involved, and that she may find their help very useful.'

The noted departure here from the previous entries is my statement in the first sentence of delivery of poor care, that is, around the confusion. I have attempted to explain this, by saying that the nature of midwifery care is one of constant re-evaluation as events proceed. However, I allude to a 'lack of direction' and the effect this had on Dawn and her partner. Also, there is an attempt at negotiating the story in the tying of the two versions of events together, rather than a stating of how things were from the hospital records. Although therefore, there is an effort to defend practice here, it is less certain, more tentative, and credits Dawn and her partner's story with a greater truth value. The hospital records have not been used in the same way; faced with the depth of Dawn's distress, they take second place, and the information they contain has less power to heal.

I remember feeling out of my league here, very worried lest I should inadvertently add to the trauma this couple felt, hence the dialogue about getting help from the community mental health team. My power to 'fix it' was diminished, and I knew it. This left me feeling rather shaky about my role, and there is a suggestion that I did more listening than talking when I state that Peter and Dawn were 'given the opportunity to relay their concerns in detail'. I could not normalise this story, I had not previously encountered suicidal ideation generated by the experience of childbirth (as it would have clearly been bizarre to assert that most women felt this way). Whilst I offer information that is specific (what happened according to the notes), and a little that is general (the nature of midwifery/obstetric care), I am mediating rather than normalising their experience. Of the assumptions underlying the previous entries, I would say that only the first two (women need more information, and this can be found in the hospital records) are really present, and then in a weakened form. The fourth, (women do not understand what traumatic really is) is blown out of the water. Dawn understood only too well.

Flo

'Talked through previous induction of labour (IOL) – reasons, methods, time taken. Explained that second IOL more likely to respond quicker – that second stage should be easier – more likely to have SVD (spontaneous vaginal delivery) without episiotomy. Explained differences between primip and multip labours – was very reassured. Drew up birthplan regarding, if possible, greater mobility, use of bath in labour for pain, baby delivered straight onto tummy and put to breast asap.

Encouraged Flo to ask for staff she knew if possible. She said she was very reassured. Booked for IOL this week.

Follow-up: Seen post delivery. Flo felt that second experience not much better – at least for first stage. Had epidural – but did not work totally. One hour 17 minute second stage. Says she feels disappointed but less traumatised.'

This visit was initially more comfortable for me, as I revert to explanation and information giving. There is the beginning also of an idea that, although the past experience is beyond fixing, the future one is not. The drawing up of a birth plan, and the encouragement to Flo to ask for a midwife she knew, holds within it the beginnings of a resistance to depersonalisation and disempowerment of women within the maternity services. My concern is still to reassure, but there is little concentration on the past events. Flo's story is not addressed in any depth, as perhaps it is beyond fixing, and perhaps I am beginning to feel less of a requirement to fulfil that role. There is more collaboration happening here.

The crunch comes at the end, when our efforts do not have the desired effect. Flo's second birth was hardly any better and I can still remember feeling hugely disappointed when I spoke to her on the ward the day after her baby's birth. It was a flat, resigned, emotional response. We did not discuss the birth in detail (amazingly) as we both felt there was nothing now that could be done to improve the experience.

The pedagogical midwife sits alongside the midwife facilitator, hoping to empower an individual woman to get the birth experience she wanted. What is lacking is an attempt to understand the reasons why this failed in both instances.

Wilma

'Wilma had PPH (post partum haemorrhage) from a cervical tear last time, and after seeing Dr J. in antenatal clinic (now 20 weeks pregnant) was concerned about the possibility of having another transfusion. Was considering asking for c/section. Suggested earlier appointment to see consultant, but did not want it – reassured by talking it through. Biggest fear is having blood – it gave her nightmares last time – "felt possessed". Reassured her that tear appeared to happen because of baby's hand last time and we will discuss possible positions to aid full dilatation this time, i.e. mobility; left lateral position when lying down. Wilma happy to learn that the room has a bath and would like to use it in labour. Said that no guarantee could be made about the dilatation of the cervix, but that she would do well to assume that all will be OK and take events as they arose. Wilma happy with this – no longer wants c/section. Left my phone number – Wilma now really looking forward to labour. Discuss possibility of being "on call" for Wilma nearer the time and get back in touch.'

There is tentative information giving here, alongside a positive plan of action for the coming birth. I remember my concern here was to open up to Wilma the option of a vaginal delivery, as I felt the caesarian section option was somehow missing the point. In other words, it failed to really address Wilma's fears, and ran the risk of creating complications that would only serve to deepen her distress. Her fears of a second blood transfusion were, in my mind, the root of her concern about this next delivery, and I remember her vivid accounts of the terror she felt as 'ghosts floated above her bed while she was awake'. Whatever the reason for the apparitions, they had a profound effect on her, and had reduced her in this pregnancy to a state of perpetual anxiety. I was worried for her, and wanted very much to be available when she went into labour. I was beginning to want to be 'on call' for all the pregnant women I saw, but was concerned that this would not be acceptable from the unit manager's perspective. In fact my feelings of connection to the unit were weakening; I was aware of a growing sense of unease with the culture of care it represented as I witnessed these women's stories from the outside world. At the time, however, I could not articulate this. All I remember feeling was that I was in some way engaged in a surreptitious activity, and that if I started looking after referees I risked casting myself in an isolated, possibly threatening role. I was anxious not to be seen as such to those who had authority over me.

Summary: Dawn, Flo and Wilma (Fig. 10.3)

Less emphasis on the hospital records in these three visits leaves more space for the stories themselves to emerge; there is greater permeability within the journal entries. Whilst I stay with my role as expert, as educator and informer, there is more concern here to avoid a repetition of these experiences for the women involved. I am not actually engaged in changing practice, but more in the setting of strategies to prevent recurrence.

Role expressions →	Midwife as expert Midwife as mediator Midwife as facilitator	**Words and language** ↓
Reasons for Flo's bad experience Hospital records (Flo/Wilma)	**Dawn** **Flo** **Wilma**	Reassured/explained Talked through/tried to encourage
↑ **The unsaid/ignored**	No direct quotes, but less dilution of story (Dawn) and less reliance on hospital notes (absent in Flo and Wilma)	**← Permeability**

Fig. 10.3 Dawn, Flo and Wilma's cultural template.

Birth plans figure in two of these visits to some extent, as well as the possibility of putting myself 'on call' for Wilma. I would argue that there is the beginnings of resistance here, at least at the level of the individual woman. This resistance does not direct itself at the heart of the institution, but is proposed as an add on. Interestingly, it fails to make a difference for Flo, and I am left wondering why – no attempt is made to uncover the details of Flo's birth story. This may have been an unconscious reason for wanting to be on call for Wilma, in that I was losing trust in the hospital to care for these women I had met. This is not because I lacked trust in my colleagues, or felt that

I was somehow a better practitioner, but it was linked to the fact that in these cases I had spent a couple of intense hours in their company. I felt (rightly or wrongly) that I understood their concerns, and accepted them as valid. This was born of the opportunity to view the institution from the outside, as I slowly built up a picture that was initially unfamiliar to me. How was it possible to practise in ways that respected women's needs, and also fulfilled all the requirements of the employer? This, and related questions, are at the core of the next entries for Anne, Alice and Lynda.

Anne, Alice and Lynda

Anne

'Anne was angry when we talked on the phone – she felt that she and her husband had received no care on the ward because of the shortage of staff and that the midwife who was there "did not know enough" to inspire her with confidence. She told me that she had not trusted the midwife on the ward. When she *did* get to the labour ward she was "dumped" and left for 20 minutes before her new midwife arrived, in whom she had every trust and confidence. However, her labour was progressing too quickly for an epidural. She proceeded to a normal delivery. When asked what was the worst part of the experience, she said being left unsupported. I pointed out that she had obviously coped well with the pain, as this *had* been her greatest fear. Anne agreed that the lack of support was the central concern. She said she would *never* have another baby. We talked about her fear of being left unsupported again and I tentatively suggested that home delivery was a possible option if she were to get pregnant again. Both Anne and her husband responded very positively to this suggestion (even though it would rule out an epidural) and we talked about ways of ensuring good quality support second time around either at hospital or home. She was not sure that she felt any better for talking things through – she/they are still angry. Anne looked very tired – she is still being visited by her health visitor – I shall make a follow-up call in a week or two.'

The language here is more powerful, more emotive than in previous entries. Anne was 'angry', she had been 'dumped', she would 'never' have another baby. I am quite overwhelmed by her rage, making no attempt to defend or explain the care she had received. The emphasis of certain words signals my own irritation, as well as the depth of Anne's emotion. I actively sought out the worst aspect of the experience from her, probably a risky business given her anger, and am taken aback by her determination never to have another baby. I remember getting tired of hearing about lack of emotional support from midwives, that it made me feel powerless and implicated by occupation. The resistance offered here is to opt out of the institution altogether; although the personnel involved would be from the same service, the care would take place at home. I am concerned that Anne looks so tired, and wish to monitor her progress; I do not really want to let go (a development from being 'on call').

Anne starts angry, and ends angry. There is no resolution here, in fact there is the suggestion that the visit may have made things worse. I remember this as a very uncomfortable visit; I was not sure how to manage the anger that they both felt, and did not know where to put it. When I left the house I also remember feeling rather beaten, and lost as to what I should do next. I telephoned her health visitor to express my concerns for them, but remember a rather curt response of surprise as to why I should possibly be worried. Anne is tired, they are both angry, I am worried and the health visitor is distant.

Alice

'Using data available (Alice's description of labour/CTG [cardio tocograph]/notes) explained probable cause of long labour and persistent back pain – i.e. occipito posterior (OP) position. Alice described feeling lonely and unsupported – her waters broke on the ward and it was *one hour* before someone saw her (although this may have been due to midwives not being told specifically of SROM [spontaneous rupture of membranes]). She felt the severity of her pain was invalidated by lack of response and action by midwives. Labour care – poor communication and little trust in main midwife (although second midwife relaxed her). Lack of information – was not told about OP position until the end. Lack of help with breastfeeding (suffered very sore nipples). Did not like her community midwife – found her patronising. Broken down perineum added to her distress. Suffered PND for most of the first eight months – now feels much better. Supported by health visitor. Reassured Alice that second labour is usually more efficient. Stated that various positions/strategies could be used a second time to aid progress and efficiency of labour. Listened to and validated Alice's feelings of lack of support – her perceptions matter. Offered apologies. Alice has good HV (health visitor) support – encouraged her to use this in future. Gave hospital phone number for Alice to contact me again if need be. Informed her that community midwife is now changed, and that she can always ask for another in labour – although this is hard.'

The 'data available' begins with Alice's description; the hospital notes are subordinate to Alice's voice, although it is not represented in the first person. I apologised for the poor care and lack of support she had received, underscoring again the *one hour* time lag between her waters breaking and someone seeing her. All I could offer was a reassurance that second labours were usually easier, and various strategies to aid progress. I felt the need to write that 'her perceptions matter' and to tell Alice this, offering my future support. I give less information than in some of the previous entries, emphasising that I validated her story. How did I think this had been achieved?

There is a weariness in this entry, and no attempt to normalise her experience. All labours are not like this, and what transforms them is not necessarily the physical mechanisms at work, but the context of care in which they take place. However, I was beginning to hear similar stories repeatedly, in some sense it had become normal for me. I remember feeling immersed in the grief, anger and depression of others generated by an event that, I felt, could have been different.

This must have affected my attitude towards both the maternity unit, the current practice of midwifery and the nature of the intervention I was undertaking. I felt less powerful as a midwife, and more powerful as a woman speaking to another woman. Why was there a demarcation between the roles? Why did I feel unable to truly support another woman when I adopted the mantle of the 'expert midwife'? If 'midwife' means 'with women', then why were so many midwives clearly anything *but* 'with women'? Was I seeing reflected back to me, in the stories these women told me, aspects of my own practice?

Lynda

'Lynda had many complaints about her care: these are being dealt with through the complaints channels. What I attempted to do was to keep the session focused on the delivery. Lynda was very affected still by this, and was tearful whenever she talked about it (the delivery). She described the joy of holding her baby – and felt the actual moment of birth was handled according to her wishes – very positive for her. She did, however, feel a lack of communication between Dr S. and herself regarding the reason for the forceps delivery (lack of progress and fetal distress). I felt she needed reassuring, and needed a way of moving forward from the experience. So:

- Discussed strategies to employ next time (Lynda is trying for a baby now), i.e. mobility, positions to encourage labour, staying at home as long as possible.
- Reassured her that there was no disproportion, i.e. no moulding, and was "easy" delivery from mechanical point of view. Lynda agreed. Discussed using bath next time if possible.
- Discussed six hour discharge – early return to known carers.
- Discussed possibility of my being on call for delivery if possible next time.

Lynda felt better offloading to someone not involved with her recent complaints – we talked openly about the problems inherent in giving truly individualised care within an institution, i.e. meeting both individual and institutional needs. I expressed my concern that she was still tearful about the birth and that I felt she wanted to move forward but could not. Lynda divulged that she dealt with negative experiences by containing them tightly, and that her reactions were normal for her. I left my work number and urged her to contact me as she needed to, particularly when she became pregnant again. Lynda seemed more relaxed as I left.'

I remember this visit with clarity. Lynda's hospital notes were copious, she had put in a lengthy complaint to the midwifery managers about various aspects of her care. My manager was keen that I should visit her, as she had already done so and felt that Lynda would benefit from being listened to by someone without a management agenda. I wondered at the time whether my manager had felt too constrained by her position within the institution to connect with Lynda.

As soon as I entered Lynda's house, there was a wall of what I can only describe as 'need' to meet me. Lynda needed to tell, and tell again, her story. I set her notes down instantly, underneath the sofa. I felt they would be a distraction, particularly as they were so weighty. Lynda was friendly, outgoing, trusting and tearful as she tore through her pregnancy, delivery and early motherhood. While I 'attempted to keep the session focused on the delivery' I was not always successful, but it did seem to be the hub for much of her distress. I remember feeling that Lynda was very alone, that she needed someone as a guide, that she was floundering with so many experiences and emotions, she could not sort a way through the maze. I could not sort out for myself why she was so upset when she thought of the delivery and yet was so pleased with the actual care she received at that precise moment. I wanted to move her forward from the experience, probably because I felt unable to deal with her emotional response.

All I could offer was some midwifery knowledge, as a way of reassuring her prior to a second pregnancy, and a few strategies to resist another experience of poor care. But I never got near to the root cause of Lynda's distress, I knew it then and I know it now.

Lynda needed much more than I could offer, and this at least was apparent to me from very early on in the visit. I was unable to fix and heal this experience, as it went beyond both my role as I saw it, and my knowledge and expertise. I was constrained to offer only one visit, or risk setting myself up as a counsellor, and this was unacceptable in terms of both resources and accountability. The one thing we had done was talk about the difficulty of receiving individualised care in institutional settings; this was becoming a favourite theme of mine as I searched for the reasons behind the distressing narratives I was witnessing.

I simply could not offer any fixing measures here, and felt disempowered while I remained in 'expert midwife' role. My expertise as a midwife seemed less relevant to Lynda's distress, and somehow prevented me listening to her. If she was not unhappy with the management of the delivery by her midwife (and she said this had not been problematic), then what was the basis for her complaint? I was keen to find a discourse within which I could offer something positive, within which I could feel powerful. This was, I believe, behind my reasons for focusing on the delivery itself, rather than the wider processes of pregnancy, birth and motherhood. Looking back now, the sentence 'Lynda divulged that she dealt with negative experiences by containing them tightly, and that her reactions were normal for her', is revealing. I remember her saying this to me, and I remember that it felt like standing on a precipice as we both peered down, wondering if we had the courage to jump in. But 'I left my work number' and stayed on safe ground. Perhaps that was the best course of action at the time, perhaps neither of us could take that jump on a first meeting.

Developments within the listening role

It was after seeing Lynda that I began to feel frustrated with the service. I felt reined in, and constrained by the 'one visit only' guideline that had been agreed at the outset. I knew that there was much more happening within these visits six months into the service than had been allowed to emerge at the beginning, and that I was becoming both concerned by the boundaries of this role (where were they?) and the effect these stories were having on my own beliefs about practice. I was aware that those involved with the service had different agendas, and that they were not always congruent with each other. I believed that I was developing something of my own expertise within this field, and was anxious that this should be used and disseminated to others coming into the service as 'listeners'.

However, I was also feeling that my exposure to these women's voices, and the trust they placed in me to tell their stories, was a weighty responsibility. I was concerned that in order to maintain good relationships at work, and my growing passion for the continuance of the listening work, I needed to steer a careful course between a variety of agendas, or discourses. These agendas pivoted around the purpose or aims of the service and the personnel within whom these agendas dominated. As I saw it, the following could be identified:

(1)   The service as a method of complaints management
(2)   The service as surveillance on the work of midwives. Some colleagues appeared to hold the view that their role was to act as 'whistleblowers' on those midwives

who had been prominent in stories, and would take those particular midwives aside to discuss issues of substandard care

(3) The service as a good public relations exercise – we are listening to you
(4) The service as a way of promoting midwifery care, in the face of obstetric intervention
(5) The service as a method of helping women come to terms with their childbirth experience
(6) The service as a way of auditing general midwifery care within the unit
(7) The service as a way of empowering women, to express distress and anger.

I was confused. I felt there was validity with each agenda, but that the first six were ultimately midwife-centred – they remained controlling to the extent that the end goal had to be a woman's silence, a signal that all was now well, and that there was no further threat to the provider of that service from its clients or customers. Silence in the context of service delivery feedback feels safe. I began to feel that I was very much a part of the buffer zone between what I was listening to, and my employer. This was not because I felt unable to tell senior managers about the issues arising from stories, but that 'the issues' somehow went deeper. When I went out to visit a woman, a different way of thinking and talking was deployed. To be woman-centred, required me absolutely to allow the free expression of anger and distress, to 'take her side' at least as far as curbing controlling responses. I could not remain impartial, objective or neutral *and* connect, offer comfort, and follow discussion honestly. Tensions were building up that I had little idea what to do with. These tensions find expression within the roles I was developing for myself, bounded by the listening visit (Fig. 10.4).

Summary: Anne, Alice and Lynda

There is a move away from the expert, reassuring, fixing midwife in these visits. I sense through the records that the listening role was dominant, along with a concern to offer ways of ensuring that future birth experiences are less traumatic. There is an assumption within those strategies, that the initial trauma stems from women lacking control and partnership within their care, and this issue is discussed 'openly' with Lynda.

I am also beginning to express an allegiance with the women I see, a connection that I wish to maintain through future caring. I am uneasy about entrusting their care to unknown people, finding the confidence to offer myself as a future contact, particularly in the case of Lynda about whom I am worried.

Ursula and Kate

Ursula

'Ursula's problems were multiple – social +++: violent husband (now separated), lack of support (two friends locally – no family support – did not feel confident in her health visitor). Past history of depression with suicidal ideation, wanted to know why previous c/sections had been necessary. First because of no progress in second stage – explained that although

Role expressions →	Midwife as carrier of expert knowledge Midwife as facilitator Midwife as resistance strategist with woman Midwife as advocate	Words and language ↓
The hospital records – the official truth of each event The experiences of others – attempts to normalise and offer reassurance Lynda's deep seated unhappiness	**Anne** **Alice** **Lynda**	Use of underscoring words to add emphasis Unsupported/poor care 'she felt...' Language focused on attempts to convey women's voices
↑ **The unsaid/ignored**	Greater openness to the voices of women – use of actual phrases and words in speech marks. Very little reliance on medical jargon and official records	← **Permeability**

Fig. 10.4 Anne, Alice and Lynda's cultural template.

vertex visible, head failed to deliver probably because shoulders had not descended into pelvis (11 lb + baby with wide shoulders) and that it is doubtful that greater mobility would have helped much (Ursula was in lithotomy in second stage of labour). Explained that in fact we sometimes used lithotomy position to aid delivery when other positions have failed. Second baby – c/section for previous c/section – emergency elective – SROM with contractions.

Ursula has consulted VBAC [vaginal birth after caesarian] and been told that her risk of scar rupture is minimal. Explained that no-one was going to force her to have a c/section electively. Explained however, that Mr C. (consultant) worried about scar rupture and that if it does happen it is a dire emergency, often without much warning. Ursula well aware of this but feels that she could deliver naturally. Explained that we will support her to have the delivery experience she wants: but that it may well be necessary for her to have a c/section. Ursula accepts this. We moved on to discussing childcare arrangements in the event of either SVD [spontaneous vaginal delivery] or c/section. I advised her that this was perhaps the salient issue and that with reliable childcare arrangements she may feel far less anxious. Her husband had refused to have them and she has no family or friends who can accommodate them. *Action:* contact social services re: possible fostering whilst she was in hospital. Ursula very happy for me to do this. Tina took referral and was very helpful – said she would contact Ursula and that something should be possible. Telephoned Ursula to let her know that I had spoken to childcare division and that they would be in touch. She was happy with this.

Postscript: Ursula delivered normally! She was booked for c/section but went into labour the evening of admission (and didn't tell anybody until delivery imminent). Childcare arrangements were made without social services having to provide for childcare, although they had followed the referral through. Ursula was discharged home the day after delivery.'

Initial reflection post postscript

I remember getting into trouble over this one – had my wrists slapped for becoming too involved – had community midwife, management and social services telling me I'd been duped by an overly needy woman: basically that I had been manipulated. When she had a normal delivery, I went to congratulate her on the labour ward and it really did feel like a triumph! However, I had overstepped the boundaries on this one.

Ursula was resisting from the start. The reason she had called me to see her had, I believe, less to do with an immediate need for 'debriefing' and more to do with finding an advocate, or at least an ally, in her difficult social situation. I was worried by her intentions to labour at home, and this visit really tested my resolve to act for the woman I was visiting. She was determined not to go into hospital; I remember her telling me how she would labour without telling anyone if need be. I could not accept the risks this put both herself and her baby in, given her obstetric history in particular. I explained that 'we will support her to have the delivery experience she wants: but that it may well be necessary for her to have a c/section'; there is a fundamental contradiction here. How could I both support her in her wishes, and believe that she will more than likely need an operative delivery, and tell her so? There was an urgent need to find a compromise, and I felt that the issue of childcare was the one that she was most worried about. Ursula seemed to be socially isolated, with only one close friend who herself was suffering from severe postnatal depression. She was very happy when I told her that we may be able to sort out short term fostering for her children while she was in hospital, even though in the end she had no need for it. (A family member turned up to look after them.)

Ursula resisted medical care in a number of ways here, and one of them was through me. She let it be known, on her own territory, that she was not prepared to accept that her labour and birth would be controlled by medical processes. Faced with that knowledge, I had no option but to act to find some sort of compromise, to recontextualise the medical process as a back-up, a safety net, to the normal processes of birth. Later in the pregnancy, Ursula was convinced to come into hospital for a caesarian section. On admission, she was in early labour, but told no-one of her discomfort or her suspicions that her baby was on its way. She still resisted those powerful discourses quite brilliantly, by simply not entering into dialogue. She kept the fact of her progressing labour a secret (by hiding in the bathroom on her own). Only when she felt delivery was imminent did she seek help, when it was obvious that she would deliver normally without medical assistance. She successfully mobilised help, found a place of safe compromise, and managed her own experience. The price she paid for this was to be alone in labour, lacking support and comfort and the fear this engendered in her (as she told me afterwards). Following the birth, she was triumphant – both she and her baby were well – but it might have been otherwise. What does it say about our 'caring' that a woman feels compelled to hide from it in order to feel respected, and in control of her own destiny?

Kate

'Kate very upset by birth experience. "No-one listens any more", "I felt like a slab of meat", "She didn't care for me, I was a nuisance, I was in the way". Kate felt totally abandoned by her midwife in labour – she felt out of control and that the midwife was too busy looking after another woman. She felt like a second class citizen. She tried to establish a relationship with the midwife to no avail. Then she gave up. She felt the midwife wasn't interested in her at all. Then she got frightened. It all kept coming back to the midwife *not listening*. Kate and her partner so wanted the birth to be a happy event, they had suffered a lot in the past 12 months. She feels robbed – betrayed. She *hates* the midwife involved. Also: on postnatal ward, midwives didn't talk to anyone – were *cold* – no-one asked how she was. Wants to relay that it's the "trivial" things that count – the human touch. Experiencing flashbacks and panic attacks. Having listening visits from health visitor. Explained that this not unknown – that they will subside with time. Kate cried quite a lot to start with – still *very* angry with midwife for deserting her. Says it's not about doing things to people but being there with them. Felt better having talked the experience through – I assured her that her feelings would be taken seriously and that a growing voice of dissent may well lead to changes in practice. Kate was relieved that I wasn't defensive of midwives – she said she needed acknowledgement – that her feelings mattered.'

I sense my own feelings of anger here; the sentences are staccato, the words and phraseology are powerful (slabs of meat; abandoned; second class citizen; robbed; betrayed; hates; cold; very angry for deserting her) and the italicising of certain words adds emphasis to the effect that Kate's story had on me. Permeability is high, and there is the suggestion of a rage shared. I remember that Kate opened the door with her initial line 'No-one listens any more', and I remember how long it took for her to relax with me, eying me cautiously for a while before talking freely. There is no reference to hospital records, and no attempt to detract from the uniqueness of her experience, although the reference to a 'growing voice of dissent' suggests that her feelings are shared by others.

How could I assure her that her feelings would be taken seriously? There was no recognised forum for allowing the 'dissenting voice' expression within the midwifery unit. This was part of the process that I never did attend to, and that was mostly due to an anxiety about feeling isolated in a potentially hostile culture. I was no longer the midwife I once was, and I no longer shared the 'midwifery culture' that I had become so critical of. I also knew that whilst individual midwives were occasionally responsible for abusive acts within 'caring' relationships, there was a greater social perspective underlying all of that, and requiring exploration. I felt a confusion of roles: as a facilitator of healing through storytelling; as the harbinger of evidence of poor care; as an advocate for women using the service; as a neophyte political activist in the realm of women's rights. I was beginning to feel less wedded to the label 'midwife' as I sought to understand the image of 'midwife' I heard in these women's stories. Crucially, perhaps due to this confusion, I had a sense of 'going underground', as doing so relieved me of the burden of responsibility and the strength required to confront poor care at its source. It was relatively easy to bring one women's story back for satisfaction, but to turn this into a real force for change required the support of like-minded and powerful colleagues. Interestingly, I do not remember looking too hard for them, and I wonder if the new power I found both in these women's stories and in their company was something I was jealous of.

Summary: Ursula and Kate

There is a fundamental shift within these last two entries (Ursula and Kate), and my analysis of them proceeds as in Fig. 10.5.

These visits are in chronological order – the fallout I experienced after involvement with Ursula's problems may have presaged my reactions with Kate. I felt almost 'beyond the pale' at this point, and took refuge with the women I was seeing. It is hard to resist the interpretation that I had somehow switched camps, and the implications of this are huge for both women and midwives meeting within the maternity services. If these 'camps' exist as social relationships, and are not just a product of my imagining, then what influences do they exert on women and midwives, and what do they tell us of the culture of midwifery and maternity in our society? Why did I feel a gulf between the camps? Why was mediation such a difficult role to maintain, in as much as I felt propelled (or pulled?) into a different role to that which I understood it to be at the start? What traditions of thought and practice inhabit each end of this continuum?

Role expressions →	Midwife as (worried) expert Midwife as advocate Midwife as interprofessional link Midwife as ally Midwife as neophyte political activist	Words and language ↓
Hospital records	**Ursula** **Kate**	Expressions of anger Expressions of solidarity
↑ Unsaid/ignored	Open to women's concerns and needs Midwifery knowledge and expertise overlaid Conduit for Kate's rage	← **Permeability**

Fig. 10.5   Ursula and Kate's cultural template.

The form of the intervention

Close examination of these entries, and my reflections on them, lead me to propose the following model of listening as I experienced it. This model (Fig. 10.6) attends to the political nature of this intervention, seeking the fundamental assumptions underlying each category. This is not presented as a watertight, all-encompassing explanatory model of 'what happens' – rather as an analytical guide of ideal types.

Reflection reveals to me four basic ways in which I, as a midwife, responded to these women. Each is based on a different set of assumptions about the power relationships between women and midwives, and the understanding of the role of the listener. I have labelled these according to the dominant role I assumed in the dia-

1. Normalising the story.	2. Mediating the story
3. Validating the story.	4. Activating the story.

Fig. 10.6 The form of the intervention.

logue; no one listening intervention will be a 'pure' form. I repeat, it would be impossible to fit any entry neatly into one box only. In practice, each is dominated by one or two. The interesting point is that there is a progressive journey from 1 to 4 represented in the journal. In other words, as my involvement grows, so the way I relate to women changes, and this is reflected both in the language I use to describe stories and visits, and my actions within the narratives. The following are what I see as the 'pure' forms of each box.

(1)   Normalising the story

This is essentially to do with fixing and appeasing an angry, hurt person who may be directing their anger at me. It contains within it the following assumptions:

- Women are ignorant of the 'real' nature of childbirth. They do not understand that a lot of people experience traumatic births. Helping them to understand this will heal the hurt and anger they feel, and remove their isolation.
- Women need to 'move on', and to do this they must be reassured that everything is all right, and that other people feel the same.
- Women simply do not understand that all childbirth has the potential to be traumatic, therefore:
- Information and explanation from the midwife will improve understanding, and alter the woman's perception of events.

The midwife who normalises a woman's story is simultaneously attempting to offer comfort through a sharing of experiences ('I know other women to whom this has happened, believe me you are not alone), and watering down the power of this narrative to shock and provoke beyond a local response. Normalising relies on the midwife maintaining the role of expert with regard to this woman's experience, maintaining a pedagogical relationship. It may also carry within its appeasement a self-defence mechanism for the listening midwife as she attempts to dissolve the burden of responsibility, perhaps for insensitive care delivery, amongst the various personnel involved. This one woman's story thus becomes diluted amongst many others, both in the mind of the midwife and potentially in the woman's understanding. It is effectively neutralised as a political force.

(2) *Mediating the story*

This has to do with negotiating one version of events with another (or more). This is the type of intervention that develops when the debriefing midwife refers to the hospital notes for the 'true' version of events, perhaps attempting to correct the woman's story. It belies a lack of faith in women to remember or construct for themselves their own history. Mediating is superficial listening in so far as it embodies the following assumptions:

- Your perceptions of events matter in so far as they have real consequences for your emotional state – they matter for you
- Your memories are, however, inevitably flawed as they are too subjective
- Your version can be corrected with reference to the objective, official version of events that is enshrined in the hospital records
- I hear what you say, and make note of it as I recognise it has validity for you. However, we will make sense of your perceptions via the real version.

Mediating is about comfort and healing, but may also have the effect of disempowering the story (and therefore the woman whose story it is) in its potential to alter the way midwives see their work, and may also disguise the part midwifery care played in the initiation of traumatic memories. It pays closer attention to the individual woman's distress, but in the final analysis has little faith in the truth of it. Again, this intervention is about altering the woman's perceptions of events.

(3) *Validating the story*

Validating involves the beginnings of real concern on the midwife's part. It involves the beginnings of resistance to uncaring attitudes and practices, and the facilitation of others' wishes. It says 'I am listening to your story and I am troubled and concerned by it'. It assumes the validity of women's stories *as they are told by the women themselves,* in other words they no longer require mediation with the 'proper' version. Objectivity is increasingly irrelevant in this context, as the uniqueness of each person's narrative becomes apparent as powerful in its own right. Validation therefore relies on the following assumptions:

- Your story matters for you, and is special and unique for you
- We can resist a repeat of this for you by using a variety of tools at our disposal. In a midwifery context this may be in the form of birth plans, arranging home births, etc.
- If we change the way you interact with the system, there may be improvements in your care
- I believe that what happened had traumatic consequences for you; it does not necessarily help to know that others feel the same.

The focus here is still on creating a better 'fit' between institutional and individual needs, rather than altering the shape of the institution. However, the narrative is allowed to exercise its power to provoke responses of resistance – the 'watering down' of one story among many is no longer used as a strategy to manage distress.

There is a gradual politicising of the role of the midwife as we move along this continuum from normalising through to activating. It is in the last quadrant that the relationship between midwife and woman has changed from a pedagogical to a facilitative, empowering one as the midwife turns advocate.

(4)   *Activating the story*

This involves emotional connection to the woman telling you her story. It resists 'professional distancing' and entails a response by the whole midwife to a woman's narrative. In eschewing objectivity as a superior response, this way of acting has the potential to be truly 'with woman'. The midwife uses her professional knowledge as well as her emotional imagination and intelligence to listen attentively, suspending as many preconceptions as she can about the 'case' in front of her. Stories are distressing in themselves, and sometimes tell us of our shortcomings as midwives. These may be about our failure to connect in a caring way. Activating these women's stories requires us to offer resistance to institutional, depersonalising and disempowering processes and individuals. Activating stories assumes we believe that:

- There is inequality of voice within caring institutions and processes. This inequality is greatest between midwife and client (in this context), but also exists *between* professions and *within* them.
- Women need advocates, because caring is essentially profession-centred in its delivery. It is organised more around the needs of the profession and the institution, than around women or clients generally.
- Listening to women's stories is the first stage of politicising them, and therefore opening a channel for dissenting voices. Dissenting voices may together be synthesised into a force for change, and the listening midwife is the channel for that synthesised voice.
- Mediation will not 'fix' this – because mediation waters down the immediacy and power of the personal narrative.

If these ways of relating are considered as discourses, then the question of their social and ideological origin must be addressed. The following discussion seeks to provide an initial insight into the range of issues emanating from this analysis.

Normalising – the medical model in midwifery practice

The notion that midwives have become 'medicalised' in their approach to pregnancy and childbirth is not a new one. Midwives and women have been battling with the pathological/physiological debate for decades (Donnison 1977). What is of interest here is the way in which our practice at an interpersonal level has been affected in subtle ways by the more powerful discourses of risk and pathology.

In his examination of the discourses of childbirth, Hewison (1993) argues that the language midwives use in interaction with women tends to be dominated by rational, medical terminology and is directly linked to the aims of the midwife within that moment. Aspects of women's experience are discounted, and emotive words avoided. He argues that resistance to this has been evident through the choice of imagery that critics of the maternity services employ, for example, 'slabs of meat', 'cattle herds', 'hacked' (into perineum), etc. It is disturbing to see so many references to butchery here as an illumination of the subjective experiences of childbirth for women, but unsurprising when one considers the consequences of a process that objectifies, fragments and depersonalises individual women. Fleming (1998) recommends that midwives remove themselves from the hegemonic structures that surround their work in order to meet in true and equal partnership with women. She argues that there are clear contradictions between midwives' personal and professional knowledge. The origins of midwifery knowledge and practice, based on an oral culture and expressed in emotive terms, are seen as illegitimate, and are undervalued by midwives as well as the medical profession. Hagell (1989) is concerned that by allying themselves ever closer to medicine, nursing and midwifery are losing their ability to acknowledge values and personal meanings. As they do so, they relinquish knowledge that is contextual and phenomena centred:

'In other words, as nurses become more and more scientific they will lose what is essential to nursing, i.e caring itself, because science cannot conceptualise caring nor can caring be measured, only experienced.' (p. 231)

Part of this undermining of midwifery knowledge is found in the striving for professional status that midwifery craves. Woodward (1997) argues that the discourse of professionalism actually places carers and clients in opposition, as instrumental activities take precedence over expressive ones. Porter (1992) explores this theme further in what he calls the 'poverty of professionalisation'. He argues that it is not possible to be a genuine patient advocate while we cling to dominant ideology; that this opens an 'inevitable chasm' between the nurse and her patient in terms of power and knowledge. Furthermore, the pursuit of professional status using the medical discourse ignores the fact that the power to grant occupations autonomy rests with those who already have it. Nursing and midwifery will always be subordinate to medicine while they seek to attain status through the same discourse. This drive undermines the potential for connectedness between midwives and women, as it renders midwives 'expert' and women 'ignorant', maintaining a pedagogical relationship in favour of the midwife's status but simultaneously stripping her of the real social power she wields in terms of her caring role. Midwifery is becoming subsumed into 'techno-rational' models of problem solving, and away from its roots 'with women' (Fahy 1998). In critical theory, this is what Connerton (1976) refers to as the triumph of instrumental reason thus:

'Practical reason is found in the liberation from externally imposed compulsions and it implies the good life, both private and collective, of individuals as well as citizens. Instrumental reason is found in the technical control of nature. This appears intellectually in the natural sciences and practically in modern technology. In the course of time the second type of reason has eclipsed the first . . . The success of instrumental reason blocks the possibility of achieving practical reason.' (p. 27)

Within midwifery this is, then, the familiar story of ongoing conflict between care and cure, pathology and physiology. In reality, both these perspectives are required to attend effectively and compassionately to the needs of women and their families within our care. Midwifery must reconcile two divergent demands – the positive, instrumental benefits of western medicine and sensitivity to the cultural and social meanings attached to traditional birthing practices (Parker & Gibbs 1998). The difficulty is that it is not only midwives and medical personnel who tend to view childbirth from the perspective of risk and control, but also women and their families. If we unwittingly offer this notion of pregnancy and childbirth, then women internalise it, resorting to the cultural props that we offer in what is seen as a time of crisis (Machin & Scammell 1997). I resisted women's interpretations of their experiences, because they did not fit with my received notion of 'what should normally happen'. This left me unable to 'fix' their problems, and disempowered me as a professional. The danger here is that if this mentality is maintained in the context of 'listening visits', then we are creating another powerful discourse that envelops the whole woman. Our 'gaze' wants to see all (tell me everything that happened to you), but admits no fundamental wrongdoing on our part. The relationship becomes one of a 'confessional' (May 1992).

If we accept that midwifery is more about 'being with' than 'doing to' (Haggart 1996), then we must value the restoration of 'care' over 'cure' as a primary concern. This emphasis attends both to the individual needs of women as whole human beings, and admits the social nature of midwifery practice. In the process, it resists the temptation to see midwives as all powerful, and instead places greater trust in women to find their own safe place, with support. Professional discourses atomise and fragment, they isolate and are essentially male in their emphasis on techno-rationality. Women's discourses, released from such constrictions, have been shown to offer more support and tolerance (Holmes 1997), but this runs counter to the stories of 'nasty midwives' and bullying both between midwives, and midwives and women (RCM 2000; Robinson 1998). Treichler (1990) argues that resistant discourses arise from within the dominant culture, that they inhabit them from the inside out and are therefore never 'pure' but grown in response to the discourse they wish to undermine. This view accords with the assumptions inherent here – that we are all essentially social actors in a particular historical context. Could our frustrations as women working within midwifery give rise to a form of horizontal violence that directs itself at those people we have most in common with? If this is so, then how can these responses be channelled into a more constructive resistance?

Footnote

The research is a story of self-development. It is a process of constant reflection on working practices, as I struggle to uncover what, for me, are the most pertinent issues around women's experiences of childbirth, and the midwifery care they receive. As I write, these issues are still being named, and the writing becomes not the culmination of a project but the creation of its own discourse – many parts adopted from others but reworked for my own use.

References

Alexander, J. (1998) Confusing debriefing and defusing postnatally: the need for clarity of terms, purpose and value. *Midwifery*, 14, 122–4.

Audit Commission (1997) *First Class Delivery: Improving Maternity Services in England and Wales*. Audit Commission Publications, Abingdon.

Axe, S. (2000) Labour debriefing is crucial for good psychological care. *British Journal of Midwifery*, 8(10) 626–31.

Ballard, C., Stanley, A. & Brockington, I. (1995) Post-traumatic stress disorder after childbirth. *British Journal of Psychiatry*, 166, 525–8.

Butler, M. & Jackson, L. (1998) The value of listening skills to midwifery practice. *British Journal of Midwifery*, 6(7) 454–7.

Connerton, P. (1976) *Critical Sociology*. Penguin, London.

Crowe, M. (1998) The power of the word: some post-structural considerations of qualitative approaches in nursing research. *Journal of Advanced Nursing*, 28(2) 339–44.

DoH (1993) *Changing Childbirth: Report of the Expert Maternity Group*. Department of Health, London.

DoH (1999) *Making a Difference. Strengthening the nursing, midwifery and health visiting contribution to health and health care*. Department of Health, London.

Donnison, J. (1977) *Midwives and Medical Men: A History of Inter-professional Rivalries and Women's Rights*. Schocken, New York.

Fahy, K. (1998) Being a midwife or doing midwifery? *Australian College of Midwives Journal*, 11(2) 11–16.

Fleming, V. (1998) Women and midwives in partnership: a problematic relationship? *Journal of Advanced Nursing*, 27, 8–14.

Hagell, S. (1989) Nursing knowledge: women's knowledge. A sociological perspective. *Journal of Advanced Nursing*, 14, 226–33.

Haggart, M. (1996) Nursing the soul. *Contemporary Therapies in Nursing and Midwifery*, 2, 17–20.

Hewison, A. (1993) The language of labor: an examination of the discourses of childbirth. *Midwifery*, 9, 225–34.

Holbrook, T. (1995) Finding subjugated knowledge: personal document research. *Social Work*, 40(6) 746–52.

Holmes, J. (1997) *Gender and Discourse*. Sage, California.

Johns, C. & Whitehead, J. (1999) *Reflective Practice*, 1(1) 105–12.

Lavendar, T. & Wilkinshaw, S. (1998) Can midwives reduce post-partum psychological morbidity? A randomised trial. *Birth*, 25(4) 215–19.

Machin, D. & Scamell, M. (1997) The experience of labour: using ethnography to explore the irresistible nature of the bio-medical metaphor during labour. *Midwifery*, 13, 78–84.

Marchant, S. & Garcia, J. (2000) The need to talk after birth: evaluating new services. In *Midwifery Practice. Core Topics 3* (eds J. Alexander, C. Roth & V. Levy). Macmillan Press, Basingstoke.

May, C. (1992) Individualised care? Power and subjectivity in therapeutic relationships. *Sociology*, 26(4) 589–902.

May, C. & Fleming, C. (1997) The professional imagination: narrative and symbolic boundaries between medicine and nursing. *Journal of Advanced Nursing*, 25, 1094–1100.

Menage, J. (1996) Post-traumatic stress disorder following obstetric/gynaecological procedures. *British Journal of Midwifery*, 4(10) 532–3.

Parker, J. & Gibbs, M. (1998) Truth, virtue and beauty: midwifery and philosophy. *Nursing Inquiry*, 5, 146–53.

Porter, S. (1992) The poverty of professionalisation: a critical analysis of strategies for the occupational advancement of nursing. *Journal of Advanced Nursing*, 17, 720–26.

Robinson, J. (1998) Consumer comments. Dangers of debriefing. *British Journal of Midwifery*, 6(4) 251.

Rolfe, G. (1997) Writing ourselves: creating knowledge in a post-modern world. *Nurse Education Today*, 17, 442–8.

Stewart, K. & La Nae, V. (1990) Recursiveness in qualitative research: The story about the story. *The Qualitative Report* 1(1). www.nova.edu/ssss/QR/QR1-1/stewart.html

Treichler, P. (1990) Feminism, medicine and the meaning of childbirth. In *Body/Politics: Women and the Discourses of Science* (eds M. Jacobus, E. Fox Keller & S. Shuttleworth). Routledge, New York.

UKCC (1998) *Midwives Rules and Code of Practice*. United Kingdom Central Council for Nursing Midwifery and Health Visiting, London.

UKCC (1999) *Practitioner Client Relationships and the Prevention of Abuse*. United Kingdom Central Council for Nursing Midwifery and Health Visiting, London.

Woodward, V. (1997) Professional caring: a contradiction in terms? *Journal of Advanced Nursing*, 26, 999–1004.

Part 3

Reflections

Chapter 11

Reflections

'Our lives have become narrow enough. Our dreams strain to widen them, to bring to our waking consciousness the awareness of greater discoveries that lie just beyond the limits of our sights. We must not force our poets to limit the world any further.'

(Okri 1997, p. 4/5)

In constructing narratives we become the poets of our own lives. We stir ourselves from our complacency to open the shutters of our lives to reveal the full landscape of our practice. This is the beauty and great gift of a carefully constructed narrative, to reveal the world, not as something to view but to experience. If you choose to research self through guided reflection, you become a poet and contribute to a new way of researching and writing grounded in the passion, beauty and terrors of everyday nursing practice. Theoretical texts that constrain our horizons or make us feel safe by prescribing how we should think, feel and act are no longer tenable. Nursing is a creative act that is interpreted within the unfolding moment. We need texts written by poets to inspire and challenge us, to take us on journeys where the mundane becomes profound simply because it makes a difference to people's lives, and where caring resides in its moment to moment unfolding. We need such texts as we need breath.

Each narrative is a snapshot of nursing practice that reveals the subtlety and complexity of caring, alongside the practitioner's effort to realise desirable practice, whatever that might be. Using Wilber's four quadrants model (see Fig. 1.2), the narrative sets the practitioner's reflections on self within the various contexts of interpersonal relationships and cultural background, behavioural, and social systems – layers of contexts unfolding that give shape and meaning to practice, and yet are shaped themselves in the process.

Value of narratives

What are the value of these narratives? We know that a narrative is an account of the practitioner's journey to realise desirable practice as reflexively unfolded through a series of experiences. We know that such accounts reveal the layers or contexts of practice within which the practitioner seeks to realise desirable practice. It is these contexts that set up the nature of contradiction and reveal the constraints that limit the practitioner's realisation of desirable practice. As such, the narratives have a profound intrinsic value to the practitioner irrespective of their value to the reader.

As I indicated in chapter 3, the validity or congruence of narrative can be established to ensure the sincerity or integrity of each narrative, or in other words, to answer the reader's question – can the narrative be trusted to be a true account? Perhaps this question is irrelevant because the reader will relate to the stories within the narratives in terms of their own experiences and interpretations. From this perspective it does not matter if the factual nature of the experience has become pure fantasy. Narratives are critical ethnographies in their exposition of the contextual nature of practice and the critique and effort to resolve contradiction. Many readers will have experienced similar situations and will be able to frame themselves within the stories. Readers will also be able to reflect on the way the practitioners have critiqued and assimilated extant theory within their personal knowing. We know that listening to another's story is a powerful trigger for personal reflection. Moreover the narratives portray complex and subtle aspects of practice that can never be adequately dealt with in more conventional abstract theoretical texts.

Reflective texts by their very nature do not set out to predict or generalise but always to inform others through rich description and reflection. This was how it was for me – make of it what you will. It is the context that makes it possible for the reader to relate to the experiences set out in the narratives. Any claims to generalisability to do with issues of human-human encounter are always illusory simply because all situations are inherently unique and ultimately unpredictable. Yet practitioners can be informed by the experiences of others. And as I have argued, this type of knowledge may be more useful than abstract theory.

The idea of theory as predictive is a relic of scientific thinking that has always been inadequate for human encounter even though such a *modern* world view continues to dominate what counts as the most valid knowledge.

From a post-modern perspective, all truths are at risk of being held up as relative, and that reality is always socially constructed rather than grounded in universal truths. As the narratives portray, there are always multiple voices clamouring their view, whereby a pluralistic minefield of competing perspectives awaits. Wilber (2000) emphasises that such a relative world cut free from some anchoring point is inevitably a descent into nihilism and narcissism where anything goes, where discipline breaks down. Self-inquiry might be open to a criticism of narcissism by researchers or readers locked into modernity, because it does focus on self – 'what makes you so special?'. The value of the four quadrant model is that it always places the self in context. Hence guided reflection is always grounded. The world is viewed as relational and dynamic, unfolding in non-linear patterns. It is not static or predictable, but does have patterns of universal truths within it. As Wilber (2000) sees it – a world of 'universal deep features and local surface features' (p. 288). The narratives weave the patterns of the universal and local within the uniqueness of the unfolding situation.

The significance of narrative can be summarised as follows:

- The narratives enable the development of the individual practitioner's personal knowing, a knowing that is subjective and contextual within the particular situation, and evolving in new patterns in response to new situations within the reflexive spiral of being and becoming. The value of this knowing is to inform other practitioners who may experience similar scenarios to those set out within the narratives. It is a form of self-disclosure that reveals ways of perceiving and responding that the reader can utilise. The reader can more easily relate to this knowing because such knowing is contextual rather than abstract.

- The narratives illuminate the context or the background of the practitioner's experience, highlighting the shifting gestalt relationship between foreground and background and the way the background forces enhance or constrain the realisation of desirable practice, enabling a deep understanding of these factors to emerge.
- The narratives integrate extant theory within personal knowing in ways that illuminate the relevance of theory to inform practice and in ways that test the value of theory to inform practice. In doing so extant theory is transcended.
- The narratives illuminate the development of insights and ideas as a product of co-creating meaning, the effort to make sense of unfolding situations. Such ideas and insights become available to readers to utilise in their own particular circumstances.
- The narratives illuminate the process of guided reflection and the reflexive development of guided reflection theory. For example, the analysis of guided reflection research has led to the development of specific frameworks that can be used and further developed in subsequent research.

Becoming an effective practitioner through guided reflection

The origins of this work were my guided reflection relationship with Gill as outlined in Chapter 1. This relationship became part of a research project working with practitioners within guided reflection relationships at Burford Community Hospital and subsequently in other clinical areas. The aim of the project was three-fold:

- To enable practitioners to become effective through guided reflection
- To understand and develop the process of guided reflection
- To understand the nature of effective practice and those factors that constrain it.

This project had two distinct phases. The first phase was working with six practitioners at Burford Hospital in relationships that spanned between 12 and 18 months. This enabled me to construct a series of sequential narratives over a four year span. These narratives were reflexive in the sense that insights gained from earlier narratives were applied to subsequent narratives, thus enabling the reflexive development of guided reflection and refining interpretative frameworks to frame the nature of desirable and effective practice.

In the second phase I guided six clinical leaders in guided reflection relationships whilst they simultaneously guided in guided reflection relationships ten practitioners who were accountable to them in line-management relationships (with the exception of one clinical leader who had a practice development role rather than line-management role). The comparison of the narratives from this study offered a vivid picture of clinical practice across seven units from multiple perspectives, as well as a vivid picture of guidance style and dynamics and its impact on enabling the practitioner to learn through experience and realise desirable and effective work.

Many of the insights that were developed within this study have been applied to subsequent narratives, including the narratives within this book. Examples include the being available template, the model for structured reflection, and the framing perspectives. Each time these frameworks are used, they are reflexively developed. Similarly, each subsequent narrative has nourished and enriched the philosophical understanding of guided reflection simply because nothing is ever taken for granted and must be critiqued for its relevance into practice. This is the key principle of reflexive growth. Everything develops from what is. It is an unfolding or emergence.

As with the narratives within this book, each guided reflection relationship was written as an individual narrative. They were written between 1990 and 1993, and pre-empted the emergence of clinical supervision. I actually called guided reflection 'professional supervision' (Johns 1993).

Individual narratives

I am going to reflect on each of the narratives (Chapters 4–10) to highlight some of the insights that have emerged through the guided reflection process.

Aileen's narrative

Aileen's narrative (Chapter 4) reflects the way reflection gives her permission to let go of containing a self that had become constrained, conformed, afraid, exhausted, frustrated and helpless. In this respect, reflection is reclaiming control of the self. The reader may ask 'what theory lies here?'. Perhaps theory is a misleading word. Perhaps insight of the relationship between things would be a better descriptor.

At the core of Aileen's narrative is the idea that reflection facilitates the expression of her voice as cathartic expression. Finding a voice that sheds light on the shadows within, a voice that is accepted and honoured, a voice nurtured and allowed to soar, a voice that reconnects the authentic self. Aileen notes, 'Zerwekh (1995) wrote that it is always a turning point when nurses can find and celebrate humanity and competence that at first may be hidden by suffering and degradation'. Zerwekh's insight is confirmed.

As Aileen noted, 'one positive aspect of listening to others reflecting is to realise my stresses are shared by others'. Aileen recognised herself in the words of others, both the spoken word of the group and the literary word of Zerweck, confirming Belenky *et al.*'s (1986) observation that women need to be reconnected to communities of caring, then recovery is possible and possibilities emerge.

Tessa's narrative

Tessa and Caitlin's narratives (Chapters 5 and 6) were part of a project – clinical supervision as a model for clinical leadership – that involved me working with 14 practitioners of varying grades in guided reflection relationships over periods ranging from seven months to two years. The aim of the project was to guide each practitioner to fulfil their clinical leadership role. Each relationship, for example Tessa's, was written as an individual narrative. I then did an analysis of all the narratives to draw out significant issues in being and becoming an effective clinical leader:

- Ward sisters embodied a hierarchical anxiety that was transmitted by their managers concerned with 'smooth running' of the organisation within a 'blame-shame' culture.
- As a consequence ward sisters were motivated to avoid issues of conflict and hence unable to resolve situations of conflict.
- Just as their managers endeavoured to manage anxiety by control so did the ward sisters.
- This control was manifest in parental-hierarchical behaviour that reinforced lack of responsibility that diminished the learning organisation.
- Parental-hierarchical behaviour manifested in two simultaneous roles: as the 'critical' mother – berating staff for their lack of responsibility; and as the 'protective' mother – comforting staff when hurt.
- As a consequence ward sisters were unable to fulfil leadership roles of enabling and supporting staff to fulfil role responsibility.
- There was a strongly perceived lack of nursing leadership at the organisational level for developing clinical practice that created an impoverished learning and change culture at ward level.
- Ward sisters had poorly developed visions of nursing and felt entrenched in the medical model and subordinate to doctors reinforced through nurse-doctor patterns of relating.
- As a consequence it was felt that nursing was not valued, which led to a strongly perceived lack of morale.
- As a consequence ward sisters were reactive to events rather than proactive, and hence unable to fulfil their roles for developing clinical practice.
- As a consequence ward sisters were unable to fulfil their clinical leadership roles.
- Clinical supervision (as per the research conditions) was of limited value in affecting the development of clinical leadership within the particular organisational context.

However, the project, as Tessa's narrative vividly portrays, illuminated the way the practitioners were constrained to realise their leadership potential. The project had a critical ethnography feel about the way the practitioner's experiences revealed embodied and embedded organisational and cultural norms within the workplace. Perhaps it is easy to dismiss or marginalise a single narrative as not being representational of the 'general' experience. Yet 14 narratives offer 14 perspectives of similar intention that become much harder to marginalise as insignificant.

The analysis also offered deep insights into the impact of clinical supervision on the practitioners, both in general and in terms of realising its intended outcomes. Given the current interest in clinical leadership, the narratives are useful references for other leadership studies and for focusing leadership development.

Caitlin's narrative

Caitlin illuminates the nature of resistance within the nurse-patient relationship and the way resistance was transformed, liberating Caitlin to be available to her patients and relatives. Caitlin's experiences also focus on the significance of her ability to create and sustain an environment that supports being available, not just for herself but for all ward staff. Caitlin's work supports a reflective theory that managing conflict within the nursing team is particularly difficult work. Caitlin's experience gives credence to the harmonious team as an insidious and resistance culture that is the antithesis of therapeutic work (Johns 1992, 2000).

Alexia's narrative

Alexia tests the being available template as a model for framing her development of effective practice (Chapter 7). Pivotal within the experiences is Alexia's ability to know the other in order to respond appropriately. This is true for both patients and staff. Alexia's experiences, like those of Jane and Caitlin (Chapters 9 and 6), illuminate her effort to read the pattern of her patients in her effort to tune in and get on her patient's wave-length and manage the resistance between herself and the patient. This gives the narrative great poignancy. In doing so she illuminates her embodied responses that have constrained her ability to achieve this work, and the resilience of learnt ways to be shifted. Alexia's narrative is a testament of the power of caring to make a significant difference to lives.

It is interesting to read Alexia's narrative as text from a hermeneutic perspective. So for example take session one in which we read, 'I unwittingly took it home with me and it impacted on my home life'. What sense shall we make of that? That Alexia draws a boundary between her home life and work life? That sometimes these boundaries are punctured? That working in more intimate ways with patients cannot be contained at work? That Alexia is stressed by this encounter? That her coping mechanisms are inadequate? From one line these ideas emerge. In one respect they are dormant cues that might have been picked up within the dialogue. Yet they remain cues for the discerning reader to pick up and consider.

The next sentence states, 'I also know it will happen again'. How does Alexia know this? Is it true that nurses (and here we move from Alexia into a challenging generalisation) know that certain events are inevitable? Of course knowing that it will happen again helps Alexia focus on how she might respond differently, and helps her focus her sense of self in response... 'Will I cope better with it next time? Will I not take it home with me next time?'

The next sentence states, 'It's about the amount of support patients need'. In this line Alexia generalises from the one patient to the patients in general. She is saying at least three very significant things about her practice. Firstly patients experience considerable anxiety and distress on her ward; secondly, nurses do not have adequate time to respond to these needs; thirdly, nurses absorb this anxiety and blame themselves for this failure to create enough time to adequately be with patients. Perhaps a fourth issue is – what is the nature of support and are nurses skilled to be supportive?

A few sentences later she says: 'Body image was a problem for him. I knew it would be'. In this line Alexia illustrates how she draws conclusions based on prior experience in the context of interpreting the present situation. In the next sentences she says, 'I didn't admit him... I wish I had done'. Alexia again blames herself with hindsight. It raises issues about how well prepared nurses are to assess patients within holistic frameworks and gives credence to Lydia Hall's claim that we can only nurse what the person enables us to see.

In the next line Alexia states, 'He was very British'. I love this line. Alexia reveals the way we (and again I move from Alexia to nurses in general) naturally categorise and stereotype people. Alexia does this as a way of making sense of the patient's behaviour. It also reveals the way people respond to bad news. Much research has been done on labelling theory and bad news, so it becomes possible to see the way Alexia's responses 'fit' within such research findings.

In the next sentence Alexia says, 'I challenged him then'. Alexia had to make a decision either to accept the man's position or challenge it. Was that the best ethical decision? I might have used the ethical mapping (see Fig. 1.5) to help her explore this decision. It reflects a wider issue that I find working in palliative care – should we confront the way people cope or their denial? If we do, for whose benefit do we do this? Do we imagine that it is in the patient's best interests to confront his reaction? As Alexia illustrates later in the text it did create a space for him to 'break down' (his defences).

In the next line Alexia states, 'I felt the family dynamics were odd'. This reflects the way Alexia is constantly reading the pattern of the patient and family, seeking for and interpreting cues. My challenge might have been – what is odd? And how did you respond to this oddness? What were the wife's concerns? Why did you not pursue this sense of oddness? So many questions tumble out from the text. Alexia partly answers the questions in her next line, 'This made it difficult for me to talk to them as a couple'. What was difficult about this? Does it reflect her own limitations? Is she being protective to the patient? The text suggests that Alexia senses a conflict within the family and positions herself with the patient. The text also challenges us to examine to what extent we know and respond to families and manage conflict within families at times of great distress. This is powerful stuff.

A few sentences later: 'Then on Sunday afternoon the ward was very quiet and I could chat to him without guilt'. This picks up the earlier text about guilt and confirms the impression that Alexia (and here we can say again all nurses) experience guilt. We might also reflect that guilt is related to sense of concern, that the more we care then the more likely we will experience guilt when we perceive we fail to care. The text suggests a hierarchy of work within the ward – the ward was quiet and I could chat with him – suggesting what? That chat work is less important than 'busy' work? This fits in with cultural norms of the nature of work and priorities that are fundamental to understand to successfully realise holistic practice. The existence of this norm is further captured a few paragraphs further on when Alexia says, 'It was really busy . . . I couldn't create the opportunity to be with him'.

And so on. Using dialogue as text creates this interpretative potential. I could also use this approach to reflect on my responses to Alexia, and in doing so, develop ideas about the style and techniques of guidance and dialogue.

My relationship with Alexia was established as a clinical supervision relationship as advocated by the NHSME (1993) Vision for the Future strategy. Much has been written about the nature of clinical supervision, and my work with Alexia, Tessa and Caitlin in particular offers vivid insights into the way supervision might work using guided reflection techniques.

Yvonne's narrative

Yvonne's narrative (Chapter 8) culminates in a grand claim for a new way of health visiting that finds balance in the apparently contradictory roles of protecting the child and working therapeutically with the mother/family. Yvonne illustrates that an emphasis on therapeutic work whilst managing risk is empowering for the mother. Yvonne suggests a reciprocal relationship between her own empowerment and the empowerment of her client. As Yvonne became empowered through guided reflection (as marked by the work of Kieffer (1984) and Belenky *et al.* (1986)) so did her client, as both emerged from an almost victimic sense of self to an agentic sense of self as they took control of their respective lives. The notion of mother agency as being most significant in preventing child abuse is worthy of focused research.

Jane's narrative

Jane strengthens the theory that a vision for practice is fundamental to her being available to the patient (Chapter 9). She confronts herself – 'what is my role in working with self harm patients in Accident & Emergency?' Indeed, what *is* the nurse's role in responding to these patients? Does the way the nurse respond have a significant therapeutic effect on these people's lives? Why are nurses prejudiced against this type of patient when they espouse holistic intent?

Jane's responses to these patients suggest a strong therapeutic benefit. Yet it is tentative. What is significant is Jane's own sense of integrity by responding with 'caring' responses, as if her previous responses (and those by the unit in general) had been less caring, or even uncaring, which is known to be life depleting (Halldórsdóttir 1991). Jane uses and tests the being available template to mark her sense of reflexive transformation. Her work gives new dimensions of knowing and managing her resistance in tuning into the patient's wave-length, of nurturing her concern for these people, and responding appropriately. Jane's emergence to find a way of being with self harm patients is immensely satisfying for her. Her work gives credence to the theory of energy dissipation within guided reflection – the way she was able to release her energy tied up in her anxiety into the guided reflection space and convert this energy into positive energy for taking action. It is pure transformation. She is happy, her self-esteem rises, her integrity is intact, she feels caring; and if she feels like that so her distressed and desperate patients will feel this transmission of energy and will experience deep caring.

Bella's narrative

Bella constructed a 'cultural template' as a way of making sense of the way she responded to and subsequently worked towards constructing genuine therapeutic relationships with women in home visits following traumatic childbirth. Reflection emerges as a powerful tool for revealing and questioning her responses to these women on home visits. Her cultural template is a penetrating self-analysis that helped her to penetrate and shift her embodied ways of responding to the women, which she came to realise were contradictory with her values. Guided reflection helped her to surface and question her values, not just her values in the context of these visits but more broadly her values as a woman working with women. Hence Bella immersed herself within a feminist perspective that shifted the topic of her narrative as she realigned her values in tune with these women. This was not initially comfortable because she had to fathom the purpose of these visits. The rhetoric was a listening service for complaining women, yet she felt her role was to dampen the conflict rather than really give these women a voice. She also sensed she had failed these women. Her narrative is resolving her discomfort by realigning the purpose of her visit in tune with her now articulated values. Inevitably Bella's work raises disturbing questions about the role of the service. Is it genuinely concerned for the women's experience? If so, can it respond genuinely or is it contaminated by inappropriate mental models?

Post-script

This book is a personal landmark to gather up the fragments of ideas that have influenced me in developing guided reflection as a collaborative research process, and at the same time to release the ideas so others can develop them if interested. I wonder what I would have done if I had had this book to guide me when tentatively stepping out to construct my first guided reflection narratives. I think that part of me would have held it tight for security, while another part would have pushed it aside as stifling my own imagination and creativity. So, as with all theory, treat the book with respect because it is deeply written, yet view it with curiosity. Now – how does this book inform my practice? Where do these ideas come from? I trust you to respond wisely.

> A good traveller has no fixed plans
> and is not intent upon arriving.
> A good artist lets his intuition
> lead him wherever it wants.
> A good scientist has freed himself of concepts
> and keeps his mind open to what is.
>
> Lao Tzu (1999)

References

Belenky, M., Clinchy, B., Goldberger, N. & Tarule, J. (1986) *Women's ways of knowing: the development of self, voice and mind.* Basic Books, New York.

Halldórsdóttir, S. (1991) Five basic modes of being with another. In *Caring: the compassionate healer* (eds J. Watson & D. Gaut), pp. 37–49. National League for Nursing, New York.

Johns, C. (1992) Ownership and the harmonious team: barriers to developing the therapeutic nursing team in primary nursing. *Journal of Clinical Nursing*, 1, 89–94.

Johns, C. (1993) Professional supervision. *Journal of Nursing Management*, 1, 9–18.

Johns, C. (2000) *Becoming a Reflective Practitioner.* Blackwell Science, Oxford.

Kieffer, C. (1984) Citizen empowerment: a developmental perspective. *Prevention in Human Services*, 84(3) 9–36.

NHSME (National Health Service Management Executive) (1993) *Vision for the Future.* Department of Health, The Stationery Office, London.

Okri, B. (1997) *A Way of Being Free*. Phoenix House, London.

Tzu, L. (1999) *Tao Te Ching* (trans. Stephen Mitchell). Frances Lincoln, London.

Wilber, K. (2000) *Sex, Ecology, Spirituality: the spirit of evolution*. Shambhala, Boston.

Zerwekh, J. (1995) Making the connection during home visits: narratives of expert nurses. *The Hospice Journal*, 10, 27–44.

Chapter 12

Guided Reflection in the Context of Post-Modern Practice

Dawn Freshwater

Introduction

It is crucial that authors working in similar areas of research and development stay in dialogue with one another. This is particularly the case when the work is aimed at surfacing the hegemony and hidden contradictions of practice discourses through the expansion of a critical mass – this with a view to bringing about a change in those practices (and indeed the practitioner's) through the development of a collective consciousness. Chris Johns strives to place his work within an ongoing dialogue with others (myself included) and I welcome this opportunity to engage in genuine conversation with practitioners, researchers and academics in the creation of what becomes a processual text (Ponge 1969). This is, of course, no more important than in a text that majors not only on dialogue and conversation, but also on relationship.

My aim for this chapter is to highlight the main concepts and processes as I see them, referring to the practitioner's narratives by way of amplifying the subtext and extending the margins of the dialogue. Having read this book there may be many themes that you identify as significant for you, some that inspire ideas and imagination, and others that evoke emotions. Many of these I will not address, some of them I may be aware of but have chosen to ignore, many others will be visible only to you because of the way you have engaged with the text, creating your own individual dialogue (and possibly reconstructing yourself) as you read.

This chapter, then, is based on some of the reflections that took place in the pauses between the lines of the text in the act of looking up from the reading. Although the pauses are ordered around some central discussion points, these are not as discrete as they might, at first glance, seem, that is to say that the divisions in the text are arbitrary; what I have chosen to bring to the foreground is related to and interdependent upon those issues that remain background. To use an earlier metaphor, I aim to bring light to bear upon certain elements of the text, whilst recognising that this casts a shadow on other aspects of the dialogue.

The self in guided reflection

Self-awareness is deemed to be central to the process of successful reflection, with the 'self' being the main instrument of both the practice and guidance of reflection.

Knowing self is not only a pivotal component of reflective practice but also a central tenet of the reflexive research process and to nursing and caring, here the emphasis being placed on the therapeutic use of self. Few theorists, however, consider the complex nature of the self and just what is involved in developing an awareness of the self through reflection, and indeed whether all practitioners can (and want to) achieve this. The notion of what constitutes the 'self' is a subject that has interested poets, artists and philosophers alike. Writers have described theories of self in philosophical terms (Sartre 1956), in psychological terms (Freud 1963; Lacan 1966), in spiritual and transpersonal terms (Wilber 1981) and in biological terms (Ginsburg 1984). The first section of this book (indeed the whole text could be said to be concerned with the self) makes several references to the pursuit of self-knowing. One could question if in the construction of their narratives the practitioners have moved any closer to their selves. Further, how would they know that this was the case, and if it were the true (authentic) self or false self they had encountered? Have they merely reflected using their persona in the service of public relations (Jung 1960; Winnicott 1965)?

The concept of the self is largely taken for granted in the discussions around guided reflection; the self that is often referred to in reflective circles is the ego, this being the dominant mode of communicating and connecting with others in the world. Whilst the social aspect of the self is an important part of daily lives and indeed crucial to our existence, there is more to the self than this, as is evident in the practitioner's reflective dialogues with themselves.

The concept of a self possessed by a person is a product of both personal reflection and social interaction. Dawson (1998) cites Priest's (1991) definition of the self as:

> 'an individual that is conscious of the individual that it is while at the same time being conscious that it is the individual it is conscious of.' (p. 163)

The experiencing self as described by Bohart (1993) and Maddi (1989) is essentially anti-reductionist in nature. Life is apprehended through experiencing, which involves an interplay of thought and feeling, without either of these concepts being conceived of as polar opposites (Bohart 1993). This is interesting when related to the discussions undertaken in the first section of this book. Chris is clearly arguing that emotions and feelings are not an inferior function, something to be feared and relegated to the shadow, rather they are the heart's way of sensing, a way of contacting and transforming powerful primitive energies originating in both love and hate. Perhaps it is the power behind the emotions as opposed to the emotions themselves that leads to them being feared and avoided. This issue of power and the reflective practitioner is something that has been raised throughout the narratives of the practitioners, and as such forms a meta-narrative of its own and will be debated later in this chapter. Meanwhile, the reduction of emotions to the Cinderella of the psyche continues to be a problem in society in general (Freshwater & Robertson 2001) and in caring communities (see for example the works of Isobel Menzies-Lyth 1970, 1988).

For Carl Jung the self was buried in the unconscious and full of creative potential. Jung believed that the aim of the psyche was towards individuation, that is the growth of an individual towards becoming aware of all aspects of their personality, which in turn leads to a better balance between their internal and external worlds and an integration of opposites. Through the process of socialisation, the self is repressed and thwarted; a *persona* is developed as the individual becomes absorbed in enacting roles. Thus the individual becomes alienated from who they are and who they might become. Dawson describes self-alienation as that in which the 'subject is no longer the author of the ongoing narrative of his self' (1998, p. 164), implying a loss of control over the self. This loss of control and the desperate need for control manifests itself in society's superficial illusion of coping, whilst the deeper level of angst associated with self-alientation is defended against. Guided reflection has the potential to open the door to self-alienation as the practitioner reconnects with their authentic self in the presence of another. But this process is fraught with difficulties and is never done in isolation, as Alexia's and Tessa's narratives demonstrate. Before moving on to discuss this in any depth, I would first like to expand the ideas around the self and authenticity.

Humanistic psychologists describe the self as conceived of separate entities. Rogers (1991), for example, speaks of the organismic self and the self-concept. The organismic self is that aspect of the self that is essentially the real inner life of the person and is present from birth. The organismic self consists of the basic force that regulates the individual's physiological and psychological growth; growth and maturity are seen then as the central aims of this aspect of the self (Hough 1994; Rogers 1991). The focus of the organismic self is therefore essentially internal. It is to the organismic self that the reflective practitioner turns when referring to their deep intuitive processes. This is an inward movement which requires not only a degree of awareness, listening and trust of one's inner voice but also an acceptance of one's own authority and responsibility as heard in that authentic voice. In relation to the self the process of guided reflection then might be seen as one of liberating the organismic self, challenging the self-concept and moving beyond the confines of personally and socially imposed prejudices.

The goal of any therapeutic alliance, including that of the supervisor and reflective practitioner and the nurse-patient relationship, is to facilitate the emergence of the authentic self (Freire 1972; Hall 1986). As already mentioned, from this vantage point the role of the nurse in caring can be seen to be to transcend the self-concept, the persona (or what Winnicott (1971) might term the false self) in order to give voice to the authentic self. How does reflection facilitate this process? Again one could argue that this is the implicit thread throughout this book, that is the process of facilitating the authentic voice of the practitioner (and indeed of the guide). But an even deeper question could be posed related to the purpose of reflective practice: 'Is the purpose of reflective practice one of adjustment or liberation?' Further is it always possible for practitioners (and do they always want) to be liberated from the constraints of the persona?

Chris begins Part 2 of the book with two courageous narratives that highlight the perils of not being able to move beyond the self-imposed constraints that can hinder liberation, but also the struggle that ensues when attempting to adjust to a context that feels alien. From a psychotherapeutic perspective this process belies the struggle both to belong to a community or group (the same) and to differentiate and be individual (special). This is a difficult balance to achieve without on the one hand marginalising oneself and on the other losing oneself. This is an interesting point to examine in the context of reflective practice; often those practitioners who opt for clinical supervision experience being marginalised by their colleagues not in supervision, yet find themselves belonging to a different order. The dangers are that this new order becomes yet another place in which the authentic self is usurped.

Alexia's narrative outlines a process of throwing off or challenging old habits and routines, in a bid to liberate the caring self that is gasping for air. This process of deconstruction, however, does not necessarily bring the practitioner closer to the self, but perhaps closer to a socially constructed view of what one's self should be doing, that is deconstructing. As Chris indicates very early in the text, this is one of the dangers not only of reflective practice but also of the research paradigm within which it is located (see for example Alvesson & Skoldberg 2000; Rolfe *et al.* 2001). That is, it becomes yet another technique which when normalised becomes oppressive; a literal should or ought, a schema, rather than one of many doors leading to the development of meaning and purpose in practice and therein for the self. The process of reflective practice and the development of the self becomes encultured and, as Chris argues, is in danger of being colonised in nursing in a mechanistic way. Chris is of course in danger of colluding with this colonisation and imposition of a schema himself, for looking at the practitioners and guiding them through the prejudice of the lens of reflection and of not knowing, is as much a schema as is trying not to be blocked by one's own filters. This trying involves the ego and reflects an act of attempting to gain control.

Guided reflection as research

No matter what one's theoretical standpoint on the concept of the self, from the viewpoint of reflexivity the person is always at the centre of the inquiry process and the inquiry is always part of the person, whether this is research, psychotherapy or assessment of the patient's needs in nursing. The living reality of the inquiry process, however, is not always presented in the research texts that report on this process. Research or any process of inquiry is intimately linked with one's awareness of oneself and oneself in the world (and I view reflective practice as a process of guided inquiry with reflexive inquiry being synonymous with research, again see Alvesson & Skoldberg 2000; Freshwater & Rolfe 2001; Rolfe *et al.* 2001 for further elaboration). As Bentz and Shapiro (1998) comment:

> 'Good research should contribute to your development as a mindful person, and your development as an aware and reflective individual should be embodied in your research.' (p. 5)

In this way the process of reflective inquiry might seem like a selfish endeavour. Once again this takes us back to the concept of the self, whether that is as a separate ego, a rather reductionist view, or as an entity that is connected to everything, part of what Jung might term the collective unconscious. The danger of any model or approach to research is that it becomes literalised and technicalised. This is also true of models of guided reflection which at times appear to be rather prescriptive, as do some of the interventions, something that Chris comments on in his reflective responses. Perhaps using Heron's (1989) six-category intervention model, the prescriptive interventions form part of a bigger containing process – that of providing a structure in order to create a container for less structured work. In the move towards independent practice and authenticity it is important to ensure that the (metaphorical) container is (metaphorically) smashed by the practitioner at an appropriate point in the work, and that the guide encourages this killing off of the leader rather than foster a move to their own guru status. The practitioner may initially locate their power and authority in the guide/researcher; the role of the researcher/guide is to allow themselves to be depotentiated (this is different to being rendered impotent).

The guide/researcher of reflective practice aims to demystify not only reflective practice but also the process of research, to uncover a ruse. The ruse though is not the treachery of the research or practices itself, but the fact that the myth of objective research, and of objective practice, has been literalised through explanation. Explanation, as opposed to narrative, relies on the notion of cause and effect and fails to plumb the depths of symbolic images and intuitive intelligence, although narratives can in themselves, and often do, contain explanations (Paris 1995).

Jung used amplification to describe a phenomenon, which involved setting the narrative in a larger archetypal and mythical context, that is, moving away from concretisation and literalisation of a narrative into the imaginal realms of the symbolic. In this sense the writing of the narrative is itself reductionist and literalised, something that is always a problem in any qualitative inquiry involving the experience of others. Chris reflects on the difficulty of winnowing the narratives for the purpose of the word limit; what Jung offers in his notion of amplification is both an expansion of the self and a distillation of the collective, reduction being different to the notion of distillation. This process necessitates a degree of reflexivity.

Reflexivity

Definitions of reflexivity differ, with the term now having a multiplicity of inter-pretations and usages. In Chapter 3 Chris describes reflexivity as the looking back and seeing self as a changed person through the series of unfolding experiences that have been reflected on and learnt through. Freshwater and Rolfe (2001) identify three different and distinct ways in which the term reflexivity can be related to practice; risking the label of reductionism they organise these into a typology, although this is not presented as a hierarchical model. More significantly Freshwater and Rolfe (2001) identify reflexivity as an ethical and political endeavour involving personal and social challenges, conflict and bids for power. This is associated with experiences of discomfort and disorder. Chris similarly refers to Prigonine and Stengers' (1984) theory of dissipative structures, whilst Joyce terms this discomfort the process of dynamic disequilibrium (1984).

Whatever your definition of reflexivity, one cannot avoid the fact that it essentially involves the subjective self, and the ability of the self to turn back on itself. This is important in the context of both reflective inquiry and reflexive research, for as Bentz and Shapiro (1998) comment:

'Research is always carried out by an individual with a life and a *lifeworld*, a personality, a social context, and various personal and practical challenges and conflicts, all of which affect the research, from the choice of a research question or topic, through the method used, to the reporting of the project's outcome'.

They go on to say that 'the very act of posing a research question will shape and influence the answer' (p. 2). Or as Paris (1995) prefers: 'Wherever there is a Narrator (and how could there not be?), there is no objective biography, no more than objective history...' (p. 50). The narrator (researcher/guide) is part of the process of transforming practice and is in the same instance transformed. It is therefore not possible for them to be available in a therapeutic manner whilst being concerned with the process of phenomenological 'bracketing'.

This leads me to reflect on Chris's model of the influences on guided reflection methodology. It appears to me that Chris is attempting to say that reflective practice includes and is part of the whole. From a transpersonal point of view it might be more apt to observe that the whole is in reflective practice and that reflective practice is in the whole; in other words, Chris does not only choose these collective influences, they choose him. In allowing the particular influence to present itself in any given forum as opposed to going into a session with a predetermined model or agenda, the guide is less likely to become rigidly attached to any particular theoretical influence. Bentz and Shapiro's (1998) model of mindful inquiry, which synthesises four traditions (phenomenology, critical social science, hermeneutics and Buddhism), is a good example of how the reflective practitioner can move between approaches using a mindful approach both to practice and to the practice of reflection. Mindfulness then *is* the process of inquiry rather than the progression through any predetermined set of established criteria. I am saying here that transformation occurs through mindfulness of the narrative.

Transforming professional practice through narrative

'Rarely do different forms of life intersect so intimately as in clinical settings' (Frank 2000, p. 362).

Both Chris and I have commented that reflection begins with a sense of discomfort and an awareness of contradictions, or as Frank points out:

'Transformations of professional practice start with confrontation of ambiguity that calls for reflection.' (p. 191)

We would do well to question how narrative serves this process of transformation. Frank (2000) in his exposition of storytelling goes on to say that:

'Stories are powerful tools in change, because they are one of the most fundamental ways to order experiences and events'.

Abma (1998) concurs with Frank, observing that the aim of stories is not primarily to describe a situation but to 'motivate people to act in a certain way so that a practice is continued or changed' (p. 170). But are stories the same as narratives? As Chris points out in the preface, we are in agreement that the term narrative is imbued with all manner of interpretations we may not, however, agree on our own interpretations. Before I move on to expand these ideas further, I would like to make an additional observation in relation to the connection between story and professional practice.

Abma (1998) argues:

> 'Every professional practice is guided by a set of stories that professionals have constructed for the constraints in their work.' (p. 171)

She defines a standard story as 'a story that is repeated over and over again and gives stability to a professional practice' (Abma 1998, p. 171). Stability is of course important to any profession, but it could be argued that it is not helpful if it rules the lives of those living within its walls. Standard stories are useful in that they sustain; however stories that transform are also needed. One standard story is that there should be a practical guide to professional practice, but practice like the process of guided reflection is not linear, tidy and ordered, but chaotic, spontaneous and creative and as such does not follow a prescribed practical guide. Space needs to be made within the standard stories for synchronicity and happenstance. As I have already mentioned, the problem with guides to professional practice and indeed to research and reflection is that they become literalised, squeezing out the juice; establishing a co-operative inquiry (and I include in this guided reflection) is as much about establishing a relationship as it is about following a prescribed set of rules, although Reason and Heron (1998) themselves provide practical guidelines to the process of co-operative inquiry. These I believe should come with a cautionary note. The authority then is not in the practical guidance, nor in the guide (who might tell a standard story), but in the discriminant application of the same.

Narrative, story and plot

Narrative is generating a great deal of interest in health related disciplines and appeals to the masses because it functions so readily as a focus for anti-positivist analyses of medical interventions. As such it is ripe for appropriation. Researchers and practitioners using the narrative approach need to ensure that if narrative and story are to become a 'genuine focus for nursing inquiry', then it is important that the meaning of these concepts is adequately defined and delimited (Wiltshire 1995). Currently there is little, if any, distinction between the term story and narrative in the context of healthcare, where it is used interchangeably.

According to Frank (2000) the difference between story and narrative is that story is a relational activity which takes place within a fluid social context and ethical matrix, whereas narrative is more sophisticated and structured than a story; stories and tales are causal, informal and contingent. Narratives, he argues, are premeditated, organised and have a structure which is their own. The distinction then is that narratives contain a reflective or theoretical component involving meditation and contemplation. Frank (2000) offers a clear insight into the subtle differences between narrative and story in saying that:

'The subtle semantics of narrative suggest a structure underpinning the story, and narrative analysis locates the structures that storytellers rely on but are not fully aware of.' (p. 354)

Wiltshire (1995) makes a clear distinction not only between story and narrative but also between these and the notions of explanation and account, the latter two being more closely aligned with power and authority. He discusses the concept of story and narrative and its relationship to other concepts such as explanation and account, arguing that story and narrative are different from account and explanation by the nature of the fact that they tend to imply a democracy of equals; explanation, he argues, usually suggests that one person has more knowledge than the other.

The narrator, in contrast to the storyteller, selects and arranges material, participating by means of implicit reflection on the information and events being described. Narrative is thus:

'a reflective practice, whereas story is not. And because it is a reflective practice, narrative is connected, as story is not, with authority.' (Wiltshire 1995, p. 77)

This link with authority is significant given my earlier reference to power and autonomy, and has implications for who is writing/reading the narrative. Narration then is part of a reflective self-conscious and an interventionary process which requires abstract thought. It is integrational, requiring energy and intellectual and physical commitment. Chris and I obviously use the concept of narrative and plot in line with our own interpretations and whilst this is not a matter of either/or but of both/and being appropriate, I am keen to highlight the issue of power and authority, linked to voice, that I believe is inherent in the notion of narrative and plot.

The plot is the basic means by which specific events are brought into one meaningful whole (Abma 1998, p. 171). That is to say that the plot is the structure underpinning the story, which as Frank suggests may or may not be conscious. Emplotment is the central process in narrative, providing order and meaning to the previous chaotic flow of events; from this a configuration of succession procession is derived (Ricoeur 1987). Enplotment is not a finished event but an ongoing process – as new information arises the plot is adjusted accordingly; thus it is a dynamic process which is always in the process of becoming (Parse 1987). The basic modernist narrative has a beginning, middle and end. The beginning introduces the participants, the middle describes the main action sequences and the end describes the consequences (Murray 1999). Frye (1957), who actually coined the term enplotment, identified four archetypal plot structures; comedy, romance, tragedy and satire. These plots have been discussed in the context of wider life. I wonder if the practitioners were able to locate any of the underpinning structures (plots) to their own stories and how guided reflection does this, if it does. Perhaps you, the reader, can see archetypal plots in your own lives or in the stories of the practitioners. I am also curious about Chris' own plot, both in the creation of this text and its role in the progression of reflective practice.

Brooks (1984) suggests we both create narratives and are created by them; they are part of our very being. They bring order to disorder, but I would argue that disorder itself is a narrative with its own plot, which in turn gives order to disorder. The reflective practitioner, like the researcher, in their desire to avoid too much uncertainty can move too quickly to order and premature closure or ending. Through the telling of stories we intensify and clarify the plot structure of events as lived, eliminating events that in retrospect are not important to the development of that plot, which do not as we say contribute to the ending. But as Murray (1999) has already pointed out, the notion of an ending is in itself a narrative by which to order our experience. Reflective narratives may be full of purpose without knowing what it is that the reflective practitioner is tending towards. That purpose is not manifest as a clearly framed goal, more likely a troubling, as in the discomfort that spurs the practitioner into a reflective process. The fate of the narrative though is not sealed (from the past) but signified in the emerging plot. A narrative then is created through a person's narration, as is the narrator.

In telling their stories, the narrators shape their narratives to the audience, in this case Chris to the readers, and in the case of the practitioners, to Chris and consequently to the readers. Storytellers always require a cast of listeners; for the client it is the nurses, for the practitioner it is the guide, etc. Narrators can exaggerate certain elements of the story or downplay other aspects. The character of the relationship between the two partners in guided reflection is of vital importance in this interplay of connecting conversations. Importantly then, storytelling is for another just as much as it is for oneself. Here one could easily substitute the words nursing for guided reflection. For narrative practitioners do not regard conversations as expressions of meaning, but rather as the sites where meaning is created in people's lives; conversations do not only describe experience, they generate experience and are both unique in the moment and limited by the cultural assumptions and possibilities of their contexts. Narratives then as acts of telling '*are* relationships' Frank (2000, p. 354). The risk of reducing the story to a narrative is that of 'losing the purpose for which people engage in storytelling', which Frank argues is relationship building. Chris comments frequently throughout the narratives about his relationship (and sometimes lack of it) with the practitioners. He is clearly struggling with the tension between the issue of choice, freedom and autonomy, which he hopes to inspire, and the need for a professional ethical and personal meaningful relationship. This perhaps fits with Ricoeur's sense of narrative and its relationship to life. Life, he says, can be seen as 'an activity and a passion in search of a narrative' (Ricoeur 1991, p. 29). This begs some interesting questions regarding the notion of research ethics in narrative inquiry, which are relational and relationship and come before method; one cannot ever analyse a relationship without entering into it more knowledge may be less important than a sense of clearer value and authentic truth. What is the relationship between narrative inquiry (and guided reflection) and authentic truth and value?

Narrative inquiry

According to Josselson and Lieblich (1999), narrative research is 'a process of inquiry that embraces paradox and cannot therefore be defined in linear terms' (p. xi). It is cyclical and always in the process of becoming. Narrative analysis is not designed to make a new plot or new meaning, although this will inevitably occur should the research be reflexive, but to expose the limitations and constraints of old meanings and old plots. Many writers who emphasise the modality of narrative argue that all truth is 'constructed' and therefore local and contingent. There is not one knowledge or truth, but a variety of competing 'knowledges' each of which is developed within a specific cultural, professional or institutional framework. Emphasising the 'fictive' provisional and discursive aspects of all 'knowledge production', they draw on such sources as Kuhn's work on scientific paradigms and Foucault to dispute the outright truth claims of science. Post-modern theorists argue that narrative is already woven into the fabric of science; for example science itself is a story (Lyotard 1984). The notion of truth therefore that goes along with narrative (and guided reflection) is that of it being local and contingent and constructed in relation (Wiltshire 1995). This notion of relational truth is linked to the practice of co-operative inquiry and has implications for the understanding and experiencing of power and authority.

Co-operative inquiry is a systematic approach to developing understanding, and action involves what Reason and Heron (1998) call an 'extended epistemology' (p. 3), that is it extends beyond the primarily theoretical knowledge of academia to include many different ways of knowing. The researcher claims, inevitably and often effectively, to be the master of the code that makes some underlying phenomenon intelligible, just as Chris attempts to do through his surfacing of the underlying phenomena in the guided reflection sessions. That code may be termed any number of things (in this case framing perspectives, transactional analysis, etc.), but analysts who identify the code underlying some social order unavoidably present themselves as the masters of that order. The auspices of this knowing as mastery is often called a methodology (Frank 2000). These methodological codes are useful in their own way and describe some aspects of social life. Indeed I have used them and continue to use them myself. Nevertheless, one needs to view this whole issue of methodology and mastery of the data with suspicion when referring to the concept of co-operative inquiry and in the development of narrative approaches. There are of course a number of issues regarding the rigour of such reflexive approaches. Suffice it to say that I agree with other authors and researchers who argue a position on goodness that holds that the product of inquiry should serve the community studied, rather than one's discipline. The question for the purpose of this book appears to be, how does one know if the product serves the community studied? Perhaps the community being studied here is the discipline? I choose to reflect on this in relation to one of the main purposes of Chris' theory of guided reflection as I see it, this being emancipation and empowerment.

Guided reflection as emancipation: agency v. victim

The notion of agency, one of the most highly valued terms in social sciences, is a term that is ambiguous and disputed. As a theoretical concept it is closely aligned to the experience of power, impotence and locus of control. The notion of agency is particularly interesting when viewed within the context of guided reflection. One of the aims of guided reflection, it would appear, is to enable the practitioner to challenge dominant discourses, especially those which serve to keep the practitioner in the position of victim (these includes the practitioner's own internalised discourses). It is obviously a contradiction in terms for the supervisor of reflective practice to facilitate this in an environment in which they cast themselves as the authority on how the individual practitioner 'should' or 'could' best afford this shift. Further, whilst one would hope that the practitioner volunteers themselves for clinical supervision, they may not always be aware of the implied agenda of the facilitator. A crucial factor in the development of authenticity is that the guide is aware of their own power and authority. Hiding it under a pretension of democracy is just as exploitative as using it for one's own furtherance. Chris touches on this in Tessa's narrative (Chapter 5), as he reflects on the need to rescue. Even this urge presupposes a level of power, authority and potency beyond that of the practitioner.

In this sense the guide makes a reflective choice to be openly and unashamedly directive and indeed prescriptive at times. For if the guide doesn't own their power and authority then how can the reflective practitioner come to see power as something to be celebrated and honoured? Chris comments on his own authority and power as a guide, saying that he needs to 'pay attention to using authoritative responses such as "I believe that..." "I think that...", "do you think...", "have you read...".' I don't view these questions as problematic in themselves, but agree that what is necessary is a degree of mindfulness regarding the origin of these interventions. Being directive and using one's self authoritatively is not a fault in guiding reflection, rather the lack of awareness of the directing and its inherent motivation is the problem. Even co-operative inquiry needs a leader. Reason and Heron (1998) discuss this when they describe the different roles people may have in co-operative inquiry:

> 'it may be that one person has more knowledge of the subject, another knows more about the inquiry method. But it does mean that specialist knowledge is used in the service of the work.' (p. 4)

I applaud the fact that Chris addresses these issues within the text, but wonder if he might also be attending to his interventions, asking the question 'Is this intervention in the service of the work?' 'How do these questions serve my authentic self?' – reflecting on his relationship to himself both as an agent and victim.

A further contradiction inherent in the narrative method and in editing text for a book, is the desire to be seen to be equal in a co-operative and collaborative inquiry, striking, as Yvonne's narrative illustrates, at the very core of oppression, and yet to be the person who writes other people's stories. Perhaps the main concern here is for the narrator, who aims to be the biographer, to do so in a non-oppressive way. The writing of other people's stories with regard to agency and victim is an ethical concern in narrative inquiry. The process of winnowing and separating out experiences is an authoritative one if done in isolation. Frank (2000) comments on this, saying:

> 'My methodological quandary has been and remains the limits of what can be said *about* anyone else's story.' (p. 360)

It seems that Frank is articulating the struggle that reflexive inquirers have about empowering others to have a critical voice in regard to the dominant discourse, without falling into the trap of speaking for those others whom they aim to liberate. Even as I write I am aware that this last sentence is full of ambiguous terminology surrounding power, empowerment and voice. Nevertheless, it is important to at least begin to articulate what might be termed a standpoint or voice.

Taking a standpoint then requires self-consciousness and is an attempt to 'transform oneself into the ethical subject of one's behaviour' (Foucault 1985, p. 27). To have a voice means recognising, owning and expressing a standpoint; it is a political and ethical act of self reflection, which shifts the locus of control to internal and locates the practitioner as an agent responsible for one's own behaviour and its effects and consequences for self and others, even if that behaviour means being submissive (as in some of the narratives presented here). Developing a standpoint is something that can be achieved in guided reflection, which as Aileen reports (Chapter 4) is about giving oneself permission to break from performing in order to break from performance. What I have been attempting to make foreground is the problem of guided reflection becoming yet another performance; what gets put into the shadow is the critical reflection of guided reflection and, indeed, of the notion of a guide. This is particularly important in regard to Aileen's comments about repeating patterns. A critical reflective cue here might relate to how she is repeating her pattern in guided reflection *with* her guide. This also links to Chris' discussion surrounding gender. Gender-related issues also occur in guided reflection; the danger in trying not to appear patronising is that we risk appearing patronising. As Chris explicates in his model of influences, some theorists believe that science, at best, 'has neglected the influence of gender in the process of inquiry and in the interpretation of results' Bentz & Shapiro 1998, p. 6). If guided reflection is a process of inquiry then gender issues also need to be addressed in the relationship between practitioner and supervisor, irrespective of whether these are same gender relationships.

Summary

I would like to close where I began, that is to say something about complementary discourses. Bella, in her narrative (Chapter 10), spoke of guided reflection as something similar to confession; this is something that patients often feel about psychotherapy. Chris has referred briefly within the text to the differences and similarities between therapy and guided reflection. I believe this needs to be explored further (see Heath & Freshwater 2000). When Chris, using transactional analysis in Caitlin's narrative (Chapter 6), refers to himself as being the critical parent, he could just as easily be using the psychodynamic concepts of transference and countertransference in an exploration of repeating patterns in his relationships to Caitlin. What is of significance here is the intention behind the therapeutic alliance. Whether it is for therapy (either liberating or adjusting) or for guided reflection, both emphasise the centrality of the self. The intended agenda is always mutual to all the 'selves' involved in the work. Hence when Chris says that his only agenda is to 'enable the practitioner to learn well through the reflection to realise desirable work' I have to disagree. From a transpersonal perspective Chris does not choose the agenda. It chooses him; his work is part of a bigger picture which is attempting to become foreground. There are many more agendas to both therapy and guided reflection; it is not an altruistic venture, the supervisor always has an agenda other than that of enabling the other;

the self has an agenda even in enabling and empowering others. True co-operative inquiry is of benefit to all participants and *all* are transformed in the process. As Nielsen suggests:

'The passion inherent in the creating of a text is not only to make sense of what goes on around the narrator but also to make sense of the unconscious passions and sufferings within the narrator.' (p. 50)

References

Abma, T.A. (1998) Powerful stories: The role of stories in sustaining and transforming professional practice within a mental hospital. In *Making Meaning of Narratives* (eds R. Josselson & A. Lieblich). Sage, California.

Alvesson, M. & Skoldberg, K. (2000) *Reflexive Methodology*. Sage, London.

Bentz, V.M. & Shapiro, J.J. (1998) *Mindful Inquiry in Research*. Sage, California.

Bohart, A.C. (1993) Experiencing the basis of psychotherapy. *Journal of Psychotherapy Integration*, **3**(1) 51–67.

Brooks, P. (1984) *Reading for the Plot, Design and Intention in Narrative*. Knopf, New York.

Dawson, P. (1998) The self. In *Philosophical Issues in Nursing* (S.D. Edwards). Macmillan, London.

Foucault, M. (1985) *The Use of Pleasure: The History of Sexuality*, vol. 2. Vintage, New York.

Frank, A. (2000) The standpoint of storyteller. *Qualitative Health Research*, **10**(3) 354–65.

Freshwater, D. & Robertson, C. (2001) *Needs and Emotions*. Open University Press, Buckinghamshire.

Freshwater, D. & Rolfe, G. (2001) Critical reflexivity: A political and ethically engaged research method for nursing. *NT Research*, **6**(1).

Freud, S. (1963) Standard edition of the complete psychological works 1953–1974. Hogarth Press, London.

Freire, P. (1972) *Pedagogy of the Oppressed*. Harmondsworth: Penguin.

Frye, N. (1957) *Anatomy of Criticism*. Princeton University Press, Princeton.

Ginsburg, C. (1984) Towards a somatic understanding of the self. *Journal of Humanistic Psychology*, **24**, 66–92.

Hall, J.A. (1986) *The Jungian Experience*. Inner City Books, Toronto.

Heath, H. & Freshwater, D. (2000) Clinical supervision as an emancipatory process: avoiding inappropriate intent. *Journal of Advanced Nursing*. **32**(5) 1298–1306.

Heron, J. (1989) *The Facilitator's Handbook*. Kogan Page, London.

Hough, M. (1994) *A Practical Approach to Counselling*. Pitman, London.

Josselson, R. & Lieblich, A. (eds) (1999) *Making Meaning of Narratives*. Sage, California.

Joyce, B.R. (1984) Dynamic disequilibrium: the intelligence of growth. *Theory into Practice*, **23**(1) 26–34.

Jung, C. (1960) *On the nature of the Psyche*. Princeton University Press, Princeton.

Lacan, J. (1966) *Ecrits: A selection*. Tavistock, London.

Lyotard, J.P. (1984) *The Postmodern Condition*. Manchester University Press, Manchester.

Maddi, S. (1989) *Personality Theories: a comparative analysis*. Wadsworth, Pacific Grove.

Menzies-Lyth, I.E.P. (1970) *The Functioning of Social Systems as a Defence against Anxiety*. Tavistock, London.

Menzies-Lyth, I.E.P. (1988) *Containing Anxiety in Institutions: selected essays*. Free Association Books, London.

Murray, M. (1999) The storied nature of health and illness. In *Qualitative Health Psychology* (eds M. Murray & K. Chamberlain). Sage, London.

Paris, G. (1995) *Pagan Grace*. Spring Publications, Woodstock.

Parse, R.R. (1987) *Nursing Science: major paradigms, theories and critiques*. Saunders, Philadelphia.

Ponge, F. (1969) *Soap*. Stanford University Press, California.

Priest, S. (1991) *Theories of the Mind*. Houghton and Mifflin, Boston.

Prigonine, I. & Stengers, I. (1984) *Order out of Chaos*. Bantam, New York.

Reason, P. & Heron, J. (1998) A layperson's guide to co-operative inquiry. http://www.bath.ac.uk/carpp/layguide.htm

Ricoeur, P. (1987) Life: A story in search of a narrator. In *Ricoeur Reader: Reflect and Imagination* (ed. M.J. Valdes). University of Toronto Press, Toronto.

Ricoeur, P. (1991) Life in quest of narrative. In *On Paul Ricoeur: Narrative in Interpretation* (ed. D. Wood). Routledge, London.

Rogers, C.R. (1991) *Client-Centred Therapy*. Constable, London.

Rolfe, G. Freshwater, D. & Jasper, M. (2001) *Critical Reflection for Nurses and the Caring Professions*. Palgrave, Basingstoke.

Sartre, J.P. (1956) *Being and Nothingness*. Philosophical Library, New York.

Wilber, K. (1981) *Up from Eden: A transpersonal view of human evolution*. Routledge, London.

Wiltshire, J. (1995) Telling a story, writing a narrative: terminology in health care. *Nursing Inquiry*, 2, 75–92.

Winnicott, D.W. (1965) *The Maturational Processes and the Facilitating Environment*. Hogarth, London.

Winnicott, D.W. (1971) *Therapeutic Consultations in Child Psychiatry*. Hogarth Press, London.

Index